Personalized Treatment Options
in Dermatology

Thomas Bieber • Frank Nestle

Editors

Personalized Treatment Options in Dermatology

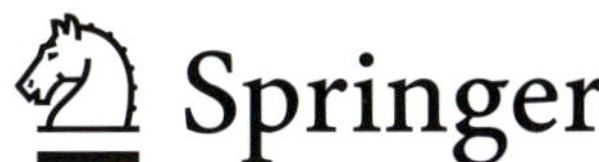 Springer

Editors
Thomas Bieber
Department of Dermatology and Allergy
Center of Translational Medicine
University of Bonn
Bonn
Germany

Frank Nestle
St. John's Institute of Dermatology
London
UK

ISBN 978-3-662-45839-6   ISBN 978-3-662-45840-2   (eBook)
DOI 10.1007/978-3-662-45840-2

Library of Congress Control Number: 2015932148

Springer Heidelberg New York Dordrecht London

Printed on acid-free paper

Springer is part of Springer Science+Business Media (www.springer.com)

Contents

Concept and Scientific Background of Personalized Medicine

Thomas Bieber

Contents

1.1 Introduction

In the history of medicine, it has always been the goal to understand the basic mechanisms leading to diseases and to develop appropriate therapeutic approaches based on this knowledge. Over the last several centuries, in the absence of appropriate pathophysiological knowledge, the development of medical care has been dominated by a rather empirical approach. In the end of the last century, the need for more scientific and economic evidences in the wide choice for appropriate treatment regimen became a primary goal. However, this approach was not able to take into account the wide heterogeneity of almost all diseases and the pharmacological development was driven by the idea of generating possibly one or a few medical products aimed to treat a large population of patients affected by one given disease. This kind of "one size fits for all" approach was of benefit for some selected situations such as pain or headache, while it became obvious that diseases such as various kinds of cancer were hardly responding to this classical approach [1].

The idea of personalized medicine can also be found in the literature under more or less synonymous terms [2] such as stratified medicine [3], precision medicine [4], molecular medicine [5], genomic medicine [6], or tailored medicine [7]. The ultimate goal of this approach is to reach an ideal stage of very early diagnosis, even before the first clinical symptoms, allowing the initiation of adapted prevention measures.

T. Bieber, MD, PhD, MDRA
Department of Dermatology and Allergy,
Center of Translational Medicine, University of Bonn, Sigmund Freud Str. 25, Bonn 53105, Germany
e-mail: Thomas.Bieber@ukb.uni-bonn.de

T. Bieber, F. Nestle (eds.), *Personalized Treatment Options in Dermatology*,
DOI 10.1007/978-3-662-45840-2_1, © Springer-Verlag Berlin Heidelberg 2015

Table 1.1 Key fields and potential of personalized medicine in dermatology

Key fields
Heterogeneity of a given target disease
Identification and validation of biomarkers and their development as companion diagnostic
Stratification of patient population with the biomarker/endophenotype
Improved genotype-phenotype relationship with information of improved computational medicine
Provide evidence for a better benefit-to-risk ratio and efficiency
Potential of personalized medicine in dermatology
Identification of still healthy individuals with high risk to develop a given disease and the opportunity to act preventively (e.g., atopic dermatitis)
Opportunity for early detection of a disease possibly even before the first symptoms appear (early intervention) and to control them effectively (e.g., psoriasis arthritis)
Better and more precise diagnostic of disease and stratification according to ways for a more adapted therapy (e.g., malignant melanoma)
Prognostic information (e.g., autoinflammatory skin diseases, skin cancers)
Development of more targeted therapies with more efficacies and less side effects (e.g., lupus, malignant melanoma)
Reduce the time, costs, and failure rate of clinical trials for new therapies
Stage adapted therapy decisions and improved treatment algorithms (e.g., skin cancers)
Better monitoring during therapy and more options for alternatives by nonresponders (e.g., skin cancers)
Opportunity for disease-modifying strategy (e.g., skin cancers, atopic dermatitis)

Once the disease becomes clinically visible and symptomatic, personalized medicine aims to identify and characterize an individual biomarker profile, the endophenotype [8], in order to propose a more precise and adapted, ideally curative treatment. Thereby, the prognosis of diseases such as cancer or other debilitating or life-threatening conditions can potentially be dramatically influenced or even reversed. This kind of disease-modifying strategy could be applied to many diseases including a number of dermatological conditions such as atopic dermatitis [9] and psoriasis [10]. Overall, there is substantial potential for personalized medicine in dermatology (Table 1.1).

1.2 The Concept and Goals of Personalized Medicine: The Right Patient with the Right Drug at the Right Dose at the Right Time

With the elucidation of the human genome at the beginning of this century [11] followed by the rapid development of bioanalytical high throughput technologies (the so-called omics) [12], a new area in our understanding of the genetic background of many monogenetic but also genetically complex diseases was introduced. Thus, the progress in understanding the genetic and epigenetic complexity for a number of clinical phenotypes has brought substantial information of putative predictive, diagnostic, and prognostic value [13]. The molecular pathways based on the genomic background are increasingly considered for the identification of putative therapeutic targets for some subgroups of patients within one seemingly single clinical phenotype or disease [14]. This kind of stratification of complex and heterogeneous groups of patients [15] ultimately leads to a better definition of disease subgroups where a substantial risk-to-benefit ratio can be afforded in responding patients. In selecting those patients who will respond to a given drug [16] and avoiding to expose unresponsive patients to the same drug with potential side effects will overall increase the effectiveness of a given medial product and decrease the risk for the generation of unnecessary side effects or drug interactions which may induce severe complications and costs.

1.3 The Tools of Personalized Medicine

The biomarkers are the most important tools on which personalized medicine strategies will be based on in the future [17]. The tremendous progress in the different "omics" areas has open an enormous field of investigation for a better understanding of the epi/genetics and the pathophysiological mechanisms leading to complex diseases with a wide clinical and heterogeneous phenotype. These technologies will allow to discover step by step new biomarkers enabling the endophenotype-based stratification of the patients according to elaborated criteria. Besides the aspects of discovery, many efforts will have to be invested in the validation of the biomarkers until they can be considered of clinical use [3]. The identification of relevant biomarkers and their validation can only be reached when they are originated from biobanks implemented by detailed clinical phenotypic information [18]. The huge amount of data which need to be handled in this context is strongly related to sophisticated algorithms integrated in bioinformatics-based system biology [19, 20]. More recently, it also became evident that the microbiome [21] (and the products of the metatranscriptome) must be considered as an important factor in the control of health and diseases. Thus, data from microbiome which is now considered as our second genome, particularly from the skin [22], will be of crucial importance to be included in the strategies mentioned herein. Therefore, establishing and combining (1) high-quality biobanks gathering representative biological samples, (2) high-quality phenotypic information, and (3) state of the art in systems biological tools are considered to be key for the discovery and validation of biomarkers.

1.4 Dissecting the Complex Clinical Phenotypes for Optimized Drug Development and Application

Each disease is characterized by a more or less wide spectrum of individual symptoms building up a complex clinical phenotype but under the heading of one diagnosis. This clinical heterogeneity often mirrors complex pathophysiological mechanisms which may have distinct epi/genetic origins. Similarly, the heterogeneity of the clinical response to the classical treatments includes the risk to apply potent drugs with serious side effects in patients who will not respond to that particular drug [23]. This is one particular and important aspect to which stratified medicine tries to find an answer. The progress in our knowledge on the

epi/genetic background and the diversity of the pathophysiological mechanisms leading to complex phenotypes will ultimately lead to a splitting of this heterogeneous phenotype in some more clearly and homogeneously defined subgroup potentially characterized by a given profile of biomarkers and endophenotype (Fig. 1.1). Therefore, it is expected that most diseases will be refined in subgroups according to a biomarker-based molecular taxonomy [24, 25]. Besides the genomic and epigenomic information as well as the biochemical and immunological pathways, a number of other information will be gathered and integrated such as the metatranscriptome [26], diet, lifestyle, exposure to environmental factors, and many others in order to better understand the individual profile of each patient in the hope to switch from the current attempt to cure diseases towards future prevention approaches. The current approach of personalized medicine is requesting the interaction of numerous stakeholders facing a number of challenges. The success is tightly dependent on the progress in the identification of relevant biomarkers [27] enabling us to stratify complex phenotypes and to identify those patients with the highest response to a given drug with the lowest possible side effects. Finally it should also be mentioned that personalized medicine generates substantial ethical [28] and socioeconomic issues [29, 30] which cannot be addressed in this short review but are of real concern at all levels.

1.5 Conclusion and Outlook

As a consequence of tremendous progress in biomedical research and diagnostic technologies, an endophenotype-based stratification of complex clinical phenotypes will allow to better address the patient population which will have the highest benefit of targeted therapy with a significantly improved safety profile. The combination of several biomarkers with different predictive and prognostic values [31] will enable to optimize the management of hitherto lethal or debilitating diseases. Thus, a kind of refinement with increasingly complex biomarker profiles will emerge, ultimately reaching the level of

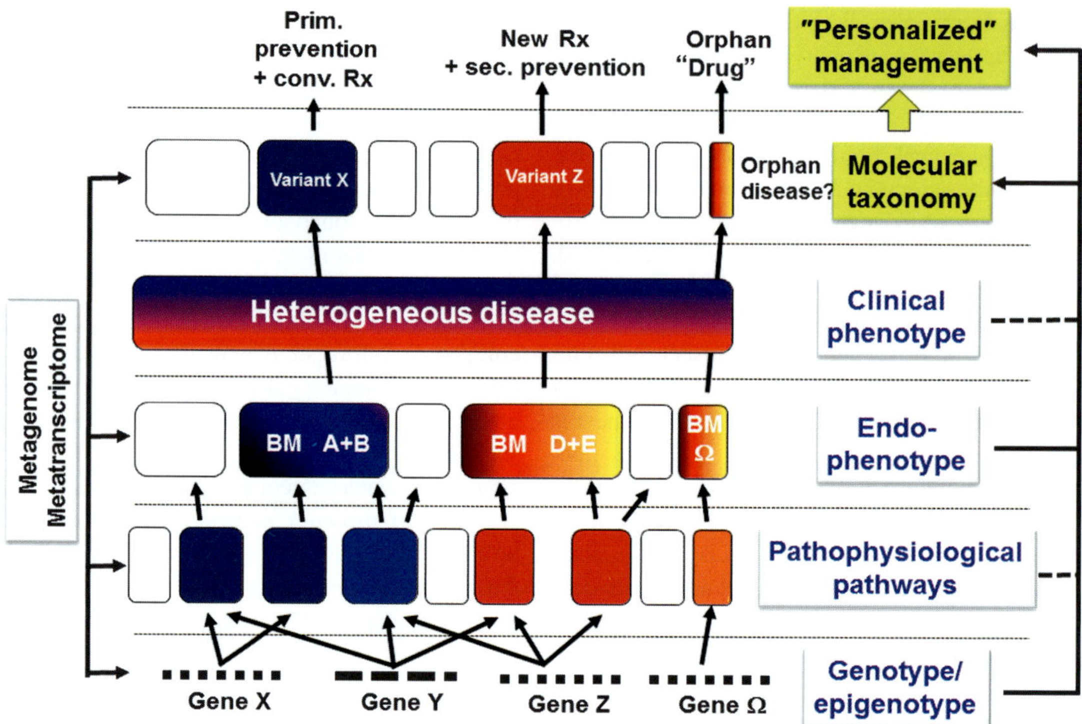

Fig. 1.1 Endophenotype-based stratification of heterogeneous clinical phenotypes into variants and the consequences for personalized management

truly individualized medicine. As an obvious consequence of a modern endophenotype-based strategy, it will be possible to intervene in a pathologic process before the symptoms become apparent or before it has caused irreversible damages, i.e., disease-modifying strategies will become a reality [9, 16].

While personalized medicine has experienced its innovative start in the field of life-threatening diseases with significant unmet medical needs, such as oncology and neurological diseases, it is expected that this trend will extend progressively to other fields such as autoinflammatory and autoimmune diseases. The further reduction of the costs for sequencing and overall genomics-based diagnostics will lead to its implementation to more and more fields less related to the unmet medical need but rather to, e.g., aging-related issue and ultimately to lifestyle aspects [3].

The wider acceptance and application of validated and qualified genomic markers may initiate a new medical evolutionary process, progressively shifting away from the traditional curative medicine. This putative future health system involves a transition to predictive, preventive, personalized, and participatory (P4) [32] medicine and will require a systems biologic approach including the collection of tremendous amounts of data from genomics, endophenotypic information, as well as those related to individual interactions with the environment. However, legal and ethical considerations in the context of an increasing risk of transparency should guarantee the privacy and autonomy of choice and decision of all individuals and patients. Otherwise, an uncontrolled overemphasizing of the significance of individual genomic information could lead the society into temptation to decide on an obligation of prevention for each individual.

References

1. Spear BB, Heath-Chiozzi M, Huff J. Clinical application of pharmacogenetics. Trends Mol Med. 2001;7(5):201–4.
2. Roden DM, Tyndale RF. Genomic medicine, precision medicine, personalized medicine: what's in a name? Clin Pharmacol Ther. 2013;94(2):169–72.
3. Bieber T. Stratified medicine: a new challenge for academia, industry, regulators and patients. London: Future Science; 2013.
4. Shen B, Hwang J. The clinical utility of precision medicine: properly assessing the value of emerging diagnostic tests. Clin Pharmacol Ther. 2010;88(6):754–6.
5. Ross JS, Linette GP, Stec J, Clark E, Ayers M, Leschly N, et al. Breast cancer biomarkers and molecular medicine. Expert Rev Mol Diagn. 2003;3(5):573–85.
6. Eng C. Molecular genetics to genomic medicine practice: at the heart of value-based delivery of healthcare. Mol Genet Genomic Med. 2013;1(1):4–6.
7. Smart A, Martin P, Parker M. Tailored medicine: whom will it fit? The ethics of patient and disease stratification. Bioethics. 2004;18(4):322–42.
8. Gottesman II, Gould TD. The endophenotype concept in psychiatry: etymology and strategic intentions. Am J Psychiatry. 2003;160(4):636–45.
9. Bieber T, Cork M, Reitamo S. Atopic dermatitis: a candidate for disease-modifying strategy. Allergy. 2012;67(8):969–75.
10. Suarez-Farinas M, Shah KR, Haider AS, Krueger JG, Lowes MA. Personalized medicine in psoriasis: developing a genomic classifier to predict histological response to Alefacept. BMC Dermatol. 2010;10:1.
11. Broder S, Venter JC. Whole genomes: the foundation of new biology and medicine. Curr Opin Biotechnol. 2000;11(6):581–5.
12. Ocana A, Pandiella A. Personalized therapies in the cancer "omics" era. Mol Cancer. 2010;9:202.
13. Chen R, Snyder M. Promise of personalized omics to precision medicine. Wiley Interdisc Rev Syst Biol Med. 2013;5(1):73–82.
14. Bieber T, Broich K. Personalised medicine. Aims and challenges. Bundesgesundheitsblatt Gesundheitsforschung Gesundheitsschutz. 2013;56(11):1468–72.
15. Dorfman R, Khayat Z, Sieminowski T, Golden B, Lyons R. Application of personalized medicine to chronic disease: a feasibility assessment. Clin Transl Med. 2013;2(1):16.
16. van den Broek M, Visser K, Allaart CF, Huizinga TW. Personalized medicine: predicting responses to therapy in patients with RA. Curr Opin Pharmacol. 2013;13(3):463–9.
17. Trusheim MR, Berndt ER, Douglas FL. Stratified medicine: strategic and economic implications of combining drugs and clinical biomarkers. Nat Rev Drug Discov. 2007;6(4):287–93.
18. Olson JE, Bielinski SJ, Ryu E, Winkler EM, Takahashi PY, Pathak J, et al. Biobanks and personalized medicine. Clin Genet. 2014;86:50–5.
19. Suh KS, Sarojini S, Youssif M, Nalley K, Milinovikj N, Elloumi F, et al. Tissue banking, bioinformatics, and electronic medical records: the front-end requirements for personalized medicine. J Oncol. 2013;2013:368751.
20. Fernald GH, Capriotti E, Daneshjou R, Karczewski KJ, Altman RB. Bioinformatics challenges for personalized medicine. Bioinformatics. 2011;27(13):1741–8.
21. Costello EK, Lauber CL, Hamady M, Fierer N, Gordon JI, Knight R. Bacterial community variation in human body habitats across space and time. Science. 2009;326(5960):1694–7.
22. Grice EA, Kong HH, Conlan S, Deming CB, Davis J, Young AC, et al. Topographical and temporal diversity of the human skin microbiome. Science. 2009;324(5931):1190–2.
23. Momper JD, Wagner JA. Therapeutic drug monitoring as a component of personalized medicine: applications in pediatric drug development. Clin Pharmacol Ther. 2014;95(2):138–40.
24. Robison JE, Perreard L, Bernard PS. State of the science: molecular classifications of breast cancer for clinical diagnostics. Clin Biochem. 2004;37(7):572–8.
25. Bieber T. Atopic dermatitis 2.0: from the clinical phenotype to the molecular taxonomy and stratified medicine. Allergy. 2012;67(12):1475–82.
26. Morgan XC, Huttenhower C. Chapter 12: Human microbiome analysis. PLoS Comput Biol. 2012;8(12):e1002808.
27. Kesselheim AS, Shiu N. The evolving role of biomarker patents in personalized medicine. Clin Pharmacol Ther. 2014;95(2):127–9.
28. Schleidgen S, Marckmann G. Re-focusing the ethical discourse on personalized medicine: a qualitative interview study with stakeholders in the German healthcare system. BMC Med Ethics. 2013;14:20.
29. Phillips KA, Ann Sakowski J, Trosman J, Douglas MP, Liang SY, Neumann P. The economic value of personalized medicine tests: what we know and what we need to know. Genet Med. 2014;16(3):251–7.
30. Koelsch C, Przewrocka J, Keeling P. Towards a balanced value business model for personalized medicine: an outlook. Pharmacogenomics. 2013;14(1):89–102.
31. Hayes DF, Markus HS, Leslie RD, Topol EJ. Personalized medicine: risk prediction, targeted therapies and mobile health technology. BMC Med. 2014;12:37.
32. Bousquet J, Anto JM, Sterk PJ, Adcock IM, Chung KF, Roca J, et al. Systems medicine and integrated care to combat chronic noncommunicable diseases. Genome Med. 2011;3(7):43.

Melanoma: From Tumor-Specific Mutations to a New Molecular Taxonomy and Innovative Therapeutics

Crystal A. Tonnessen and Nikolas K. Haass

Contents

C.A. Tonnessen, PhD • N.K. Haass, MD, PhD (✉)
Experimental Melanoma Therapy Laboratory,
The University of Queensland Diamantina Institute,
Translational Research Institute,
Woolloongabba, Brisbane, QLD 4102, Australia
e-mail: n.haass1@uq.edu.au

2.1 Introduction

Melanoma is an aggressive skin cancer that arises from melanocytes. Melanocytes produce the pigment melanin, which is pumped into the associated keratinocytes to act as a UV-protecting shield of the dividing cells in the basal layer of the epidermis and consequently results in darkened skin color and/or tanning. Benign lesions such as nevi result from an initial hyperproliferation of melanocytes, which then undergo senescence. However, due to certain mutations, proliferation of these melanocytic cells may become deregulated and result in the formation of a melanoma – usually a radial, then a vertical growth phase and eventually a metastatic melanoma. The challenge of diagnosing pigmented melanomas is mainly due to their similarity to dysplastic nevi [88] but also other pigmented lesions (e.g., pigmented basal cell carcinomas or pigmented seborrheic keratoses). There are also melanomas that display low pigment production and appear lighter in color (hypomelanotic) or pink or red (amelanotic). These melanomas are harder to diagnose as they are often either overlooked or mistaken for other types of skin disorders; however, they are relatively rare [88].

Melanocytes are found throughout the body, including the epidermis, mucosa (e.g., mouth, rectum, vagina), and uvea, but also in the inner ear, brain, and lymph nodes. Cutaneous melanoma, arising from melanocytes in the skin, is the most common form of melanoma, comprising

T. Bieber, F. Nestle (eds.), *Personalized Treatment Options in Dermatology*,
DOI 10.1007/978-3-662-45840-2_2, © Springer-Verlag Berlin Heidelberg 2015

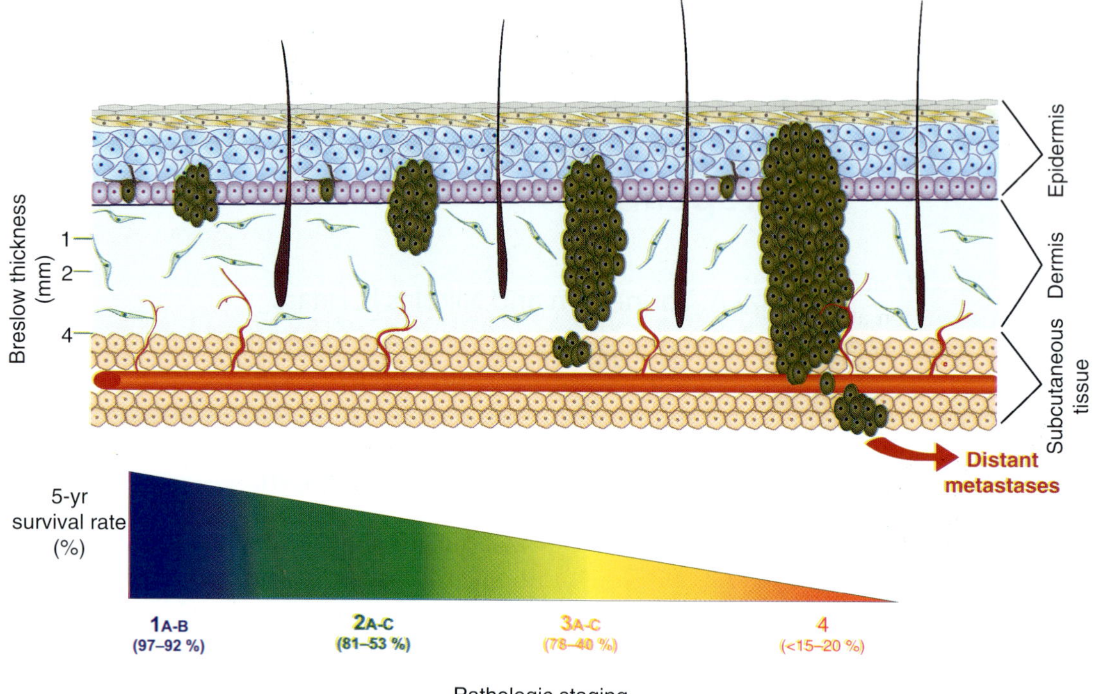

Fig. 2.1 Pathologic staging of melanoma progression and 5-year survival rates. The later stage of melanoma at the time of diagnosis is directly related to 5-year survival rates, as adapted from the AJCC melanoma staging database. Pathologic staging includes 1A–1B, 2A–2C, 3A–C, and stage 4. Breslow thickness, which is measured in millimeters from the *stratum granulosum* of the epidermis, also correlates with disease progression and survival

more than 90 % of all incidences [16], while noncutaneous melanomas, which arise in other locations than the skin, are much less common. When detected early, melanoma is highly curative by local surgical resection and retains a 98 % 5-year survival rate. However, the 5-year survival rate drops precipitously as staging progresses, resulting in 15 % 5-year survival rate if the patient presents with distant metastases upon initial diagnosis (Fig. 2.1) [101].

While less than 3 % of all skin cancers are melanomas, they are the cause of over 75 % of skin cancer-related deaths [1]. Overall incidence of melanoma varies by geographical location and race, with the highest incidence occurring in 40 of 100,000 males in Australia [35]. Melanoma is an extremely aggressive disease and has proven to be highly resistant to current therapies.

2.2 Early Therapies

Before 2011, there were few options for patients with advanced melanoma. Aside from surgical intervention, treatment was comprised of either dacarbazine, interleukin-2, or interferon [37].

Dacarbazine (DTIC, dimethyl triazeno imidazole carboxamide), an alkylating agent, was the only FDA-approved chemotherapy available for metastatic melanoma until recently. Even though dacarbazine was the standard treatment regimen, it has a low response rate of around 15–20 % and only an average 6–7-month overall survival time [29]. Temozolomide, an orally available derivative of dacarbazine, has also been tested for treatment of metastatic melanoma, but did not achieve a significant difference in overall survival compared to dacarbazine; however, progression-free survival was increased to 1.9 months compared to 1.5 months [82]. Additionally, multiple regimens combining chemotherapies have been attempted, such as the Dartmouth regimen. The Dartmouth regimen includes dacarbazine with cisplatin, carmustine, and tamoxifen. While response rate was slightly higher, overall survival was not significantly increased [17]. Other single-agent chemotherapies have also been attempted to treat malignant melanoma, such as gemcitabine and fotemustine, but none have received FDA approval. Gemcitabine has also been tested in the clinic for the treatment of advanced uveal melanoma. However, gemcitabine combined with treosulfan has shown promise in uveal melanoma in some trials, increasing median progression-free survival to 3 months when compared to 2 months of treosulfan alone [100].

In addition to chemotherapy, immune-based therapy is another tool used to combat melanoma. Approved by the FDA for melanoma treatment in 1998, high-dose interleukin-2 was shown in clinical trials conducted between 1985 and 1992 to result in partial regression in 10 % of patients and 7 % achieved complete regression [99]. Unfortunately, it has proven to have high toxicity, although readily reversible after treatment has ended, and for that reason only administered to healthier patients.

Another cytokine, interferon-α2b (IFN-α2b), is used as an adjuvant therapy for patients with a high risk of melanoma recurrence. Interferon-α2b was approved by the FDA after it was noted in 1996 to have a significant effect on disease recurrence after surgical intervention of late stage disease. Used as an adjuvant therapy after surgery, INF-α2b was shown to delay disease recurrence and to increase overall survival (1–1.7 years and 2.8–3.8 years, respectively) [66]. While these therapies did improve survival, it was only a modest increase and by no means a cure. Only in 2011 did the outlook of melanoma treatment change, bringing the hope of finding better treatments of melanoma through small molecule inhibitors and new immunotherapies, to name a few.

2.3 Staging and Genotype

Melanoma progression is well documented, beginning from a stage 1 localized lesion undergoing radial growth, then achieving vertical growth (stage 2) and lymph node metastases (stage 3), to finally populating distant metastases in stage 4 (Fig. 2.1). The stages of melanoma are further denominated by the TNM system, which is comprised of three different categories: tumor thickness and ulceration (T), number and size of metastatic positive lymph nodes (N), and presence and location of distant metastases (M) [5]. Depth of invasion into the dermis is also monitored by Breslow thickness (Fig. 2.1). The later stage at diagnosis, as outlined by these American Joint Committee on Cancer (AJCC) classifications, is generally associated with a more somber prognosis, as melanoma staging and survival are tightly intertwined (Fig. 2.1).

A number of molecular alterations have also been associated with the progression of melanoma. Early in the development of cancer, cells obtain the ability to undergo uncontrolled proliferation. Two pathways that are known to regulate cell proliferation are the mitogen-activated protein kinase (MAPK) and phosphatidylinositol-3-kinase (PI3K) pathways, and both have been found to be deregulated early in melanoma formation (Fig. 2.2). B-RAF, a serine-threonine kinase downstream of RAS in the MAPK pathway, is mutated in 80 % of nevi [91]. This mutation produces a constitutively active B-RAF, resulting in increased proliferation. Additionally, cell cycle arrest that may occur in response to oncogenic B-RAF activity is impaired by secondary inactivation of the *CDKN2A* locus, discussed in detail below. PI3K pathway activity is increased in melanoma progression by loss of its negative regulator, the tumor suppressor phosphatase and tensin homolog (PTEN). Cell proliferation is furthermore enhanced by increased expression and activity of cell cycle-regulated proteins, such as cyclin D. These highly proliferative cells then become malignant following enhanced cell motility and invasion through alteration of protein expression. These modifications include loss

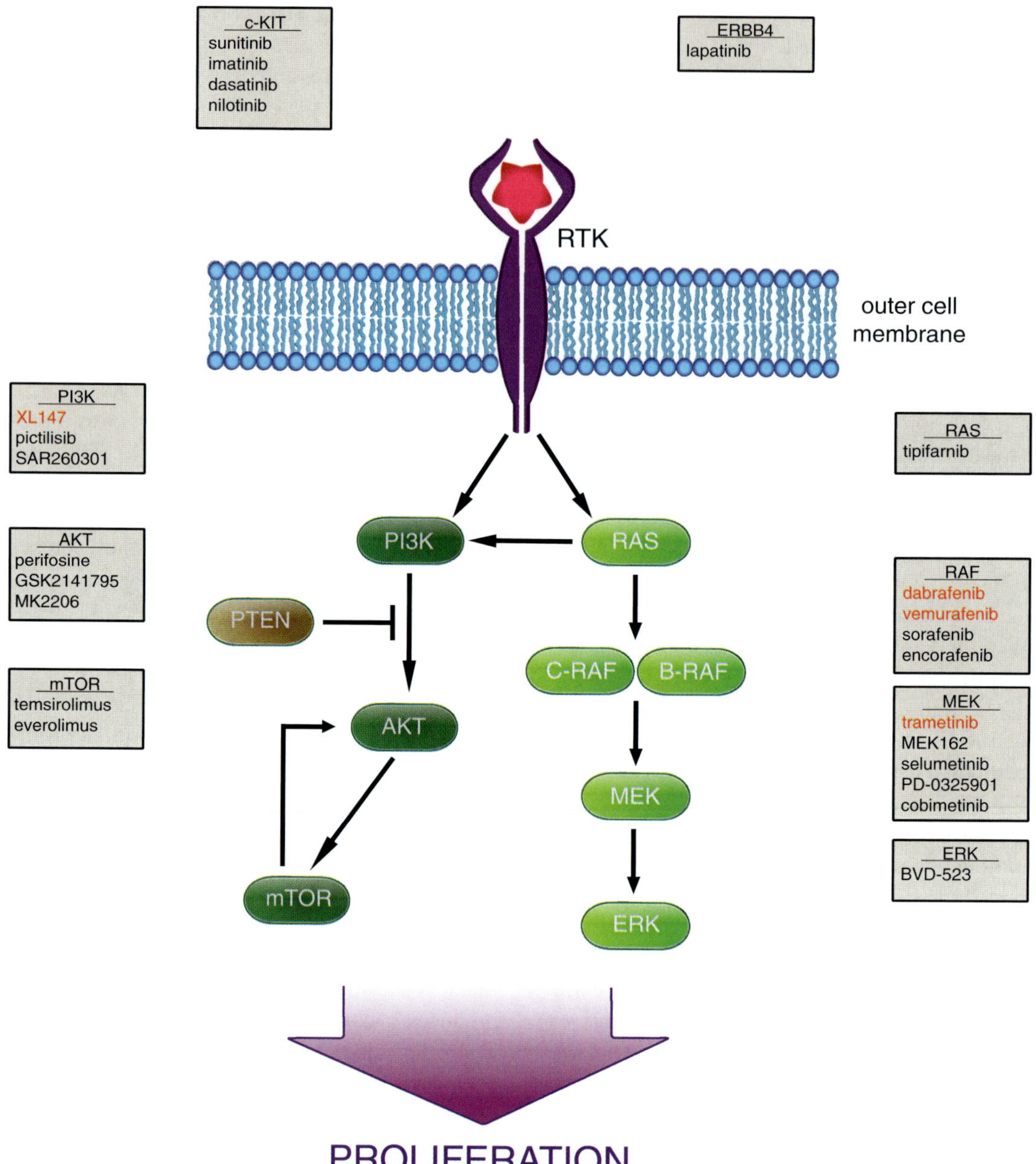

Fig. 2.2 MAPK and PI3K pathway targeting in melanoma. Upon ligand binding to transmembrane receptors, survival pathways such as PI3K (*left*) and MAPK (*right*) are stimulated, resulting in increased cell proliferation. Multiple members of these pathways are being explored as targets in therapy, and the protein targeted as well as the corresponding inhibitors are given in *gray boxes*. *Red writing* indicates FDA approval in melanoma

of E-cadherin, increased N-cadherin, as well as increased matrix metalloproteinase 2 (MMP-2) expression [83].

Not only are certain acquired mutations associated with the disease progression, but also inherited mutations can enhance the likelihood of developing melanoma. Ten percent of melanoma patients have a documented family history of melanoma [42]. The most common genetic alteration found in familial melanoma is that of *CDKN2A*. It is estimated that around 40 % of familial melanoma subjects carry a *CDKN2A*

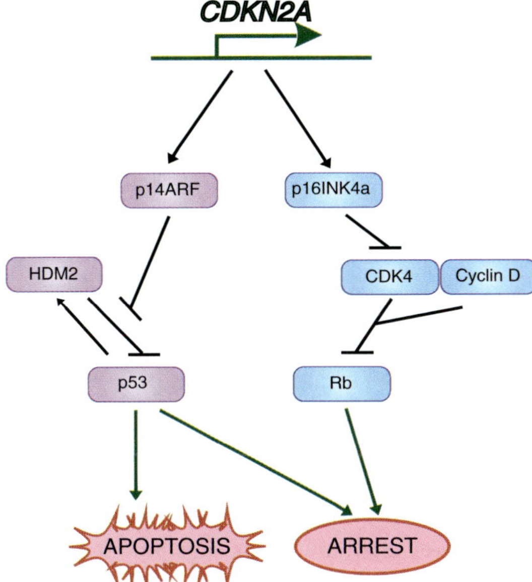

Fig. 2.3 Protein products and signaling pathways of the *CDKN2A* gene. The gene *CDKN2A* encodes p14ARF as well as p16INK4a, which are both involved in cell cycle control and can result in apoptosis or arrest

alteration [44, 81]. Thirty percent of *CDKN2A* mutation carriers develop melanoma by age 30 [11]. *CDKN2A* encodes two regulators of the cell cycle, p16INK4a and p14ARF. It is through inactivation of this locus that cancer cells are able to evade arrest and enhance proliferation by two mechanisms (Fig. 2.3) [123]. Normally p14ARF is able to inhibit the function of the ubiquitin ligase for p53, HDM2, resulting in increased p53 levels and cell cycle arrest. Without proper p14ARF function, HDM2 is free to target p53 for degradation, bypassing arrest mediated by p53. In addition to p14ARF, *CDKN2A* encodes p16INK4a. p16INK4a normally halts cell division at the G1-S checkpoint by inhibiting cyclin-dependent kinase 4 (CDK4), preventing Rb phosphorylation. Without this protein, Rb is phosphorylated and cancer cells are able to move into S phase, effectively evading another cell cycle checkpoint.

Germline mutation of the *CDK4* gene itself is also found in melanoma-prone families [103]. CDK4 binds cyclin D and promotes cell cycle progression. Mutation of *CDK4*, occurring at arginine 24, renders CDK4 unable to bind its inhibitor p16INK4a, resulting in increased

activity [125]. Both cyclin D overexpression and CDK4 mutation are found in melanoma, enhancing cell proliferation by the same network.

Microphthalmia-associated transcription factor (*MITF*) is another gene linked to familial melanomas and is amplified in 15 % of cases [124]. MITF is known as the master regulator of melanocyte differentiation, and mutation and loss of function of MITF in mice cause complete absence of the melanocyte lineage [70]. Increased in melanoma, MITF has been found to regulate multiple target genes important for cellular survival and proliferation [70]. Surprisingly, MITF expression has also been shown to inhibit melanoma cell proliferation [14, 71]. These conflicting results are reconciled by the rheostat model, where either extreme of expression (i.e., very high or very low) results in arrest or apoptosis, while intermediate levels enhance proliferation [46].

In addition to proteins that regulate the cell cycle, there are other altered cellular mechanisms known to enhance melanoma susceptibility. UV light, mainly UV-B, has specifically been linked to melanoma acquisition, as UV radiation is able to induce DNA damage. Melanocytes have developed a mechanism to produce the pigment melanin, which can shield DNA from incoming UV rays. The lack of skin pigment is one reason melanoma occurs far more frequently in those with lighter skin who sunburn easily [60]. Additionally, dysfunction in the regulation of the melanin production pathway is connected to familial melanoma. Melanocortin 1 receptor (MC1R) is important for UV-induced skin pigmentation in response to its ligand, α-melanocyte-stimulating hormone (α-MSH) [7]. Without proper MC1R function, the ability of melanocytes to produce melanin (specifically eumelanin) is impaired, leaving DNA exposed to incoming UV irradiation, therefore increasing susceptibility to melanoma [111]. It is important to note that non-UV-induced melanomas also occur. In mice that lack MC1R activity (and therefore eumelanin production) and harbor mutant B-RAF, invasive melanomas arose without any UV exposure. This was found to be due to increased pheomelanin synthesis and resulting oxidative DNA damage [86].

Surprisingly, the mutations common in cutaneous melanoma, such as *B-RAF* and *N-RAS*, are not found in uveal melanoma [20, 95]. Uveal melanoma, which arises from melanocytes in the choroidal plexus of the eye, comprises 5 % of diagnosed melanomas and portrays a distinct landscape of mutations. For example, BRCA1-associated protein 1 (BAP1) is mutated and activity lost in 84 % of metastatic uveal melanomas [53]. While germline mutation of BAP1 results in cancer predisposition, it also is found in spontaneous melanomas, with the highest prevalence in uveal melanoma (40 %) [117]. Another mutation also appears highly specific for uveal melanoma, GNAQ. GNAQ, a G-protein α-subunit, has an activating mutation in 46 % of uveal melanoma [112]. Even though all melanomas arise from melanocytes, not all present the same tendencies for mutations, highlighting the necessity for individualized molecular profiling before treatment.

One of the oddities of melanoma is the low prevalence of *TP53* mutations. p53, encoded by the gene *TP53*, is a tumor suppressor protein that in response to cell stress and DNA damage is increased and can result in cell cycle arrest or apoptosis [15]. While p53 is mutated in about half of cancers, mutation frequency in melanoma is very low, around 9 % [48]. Initial studies found high levels of p53 in many melanoma samples when staining by immunohistochemistry, which is normally indicative of accumulated mutant p53. However, these results turned out to be misleading. In fact, not only do melanomas rarely mutate *TP53*, but they are also found to express high levels of wild-type (wt) p53 [3]. It remains unclear what function high levels of wt p53 play in melanoma, although it is proposed that p53 activity is modified. Indeed, other members of the p53 pathway are found to be deregulated in melanoma. This includes loss of p14ARF and also amplification of HDM2, leading to increased inhibition and degradation of p53. Other proteins have also been found to alter the transcriptional ability of p53. Recent reports have attributed elevated levels of iASPP in modulating p53 transcriptional function [73]. While p53 is not commonly mutated in melanoma, its levels and activity are modulated, leading to a functional impairment.

Multiple acquired and inherited mutations are known to be prevalent in melanoma. These include proteins involved in different aspects of cancer progression, from growth and proliferation to loss of cell adhesion and increased invasion. Many of these proteins are being actively pursued for treatment therapies and will be discussed in detail below.

2.4 B-RAF Mutation and Targeted Therapy

B-RAF mutations are found in about 50 % of melanomas, and 90 % of these mutations occur at amino acid position 600. Furthermore, the vast majority of these mutations substitute the amino acid valine to glutamic acid (V600E) [24]. Not only is mutant B-RAF common in melanoma, it is also linked to more aggressive disease. While time of metastasis appearance from initial diagnosis was not affected by the presence of wt vs. mutant B-RAF, overall survival was shortened in patients that harbored mutant B-RAF from 8.5 to 5.7 months [72]. However, no prognostic impact of BRAFV600 mutations on overall survival was observed for patients with primary melanoma and also not for patients with distant metastasis treated with monochemotherapy [79, 80]. B-RAF is activated by RAS, as is its family member C-RAF, and both are able to activate MEK, the next kinase in the MAPK cascade (Fig. 2.2). Additionally, in N-RAS mutant melanoma C-RAF is preferentially activated over B-RAF [28]. Interestingly, unlike B-RAF, there are no known mutations of C-RAF in melanoma [32].

The first small molecule inhibitor to be tested in melanoma patients was sorafenib, a broad-spectrum tyrosine and serine-threonine kinase inhibitor. While sorafenib showed activity against B-RAF, it also inhibits C-RAF and other kinases such as PDGFR, VEGFR-2, and c-KIT [118]. Unfortunately, in clinical trials no benefit was found in those treated with sorafenib [30]. This may be due to the fact that even at the maximum tolerated dose, B-RAF was not inhibited sufficiently. This could be attributed to the inhibition of other kinases, resulting in counteractive effects and/or increased toxicity. In efforts to achieve more robust B-RAF inhibition, selective B-RAF inhibitors, such as PLX4720 and PLX4032 (vemurafenib), were generated [68, 110].

Vemurafenib and dabrafenib both selectively inhibit B-RAF, including the V600 mutant. In clinical trials, 85 % of patients saw some tumor regression, an unprecedented robust response. Unfortunately, it was shortly discovered that the median response for progression-free survival was only 5–7 months [107]. Interestingly, use of B-RAF inhibitors has shown to result in spontaneous growth of squamous cell carcinomas and keratoacanthomas in 20 % of patients. This is partly due to developed RAS mutation, which preferentially signals through C-RAF, not B-RAF. Fortunately, these lesions are easily removed by surgical resection [106]. Additionally, it has been discovered that B-RAF inhibition in B-RAF mutant melanoma cell lines results in loss of signaling through pERK, but in activation of the MAPK pathway in wt B-RAF lines. This is due to inhibitor binding to B-RAF increasing hetero- and homo-dimerization of B-RAF and C-RAF, leading to activation of C-RAF and increased downstream signaling [54]. These data highlight the necessity of knowing the molecular profile of tumors before therapy is designed. Not only do these small molecules have a low toxicity, they also had a high response rate. Unfortunately, relapse was common as the disease was able to compensate for B-RAF inhibition. These results, however, were very promising for future development of small molecule inhibitors.

In an effort to treat patients who have relapsed after B-RAF inhibition, multiple studies were undertaken to determine the mechanism of compensation within tumor cells. B-RAF itself was probed for second mutations that would hinder small molecule inhibitor binding, but none were found [113]. However, alternative splicing of B-RAF has been seen, resulting in a protein that can still bind the inhibitor but no longer binds RAS due to a deletion in that region, resulting in increased dimer formation and activity [92].

In addition to B-RAF splicing, it was more commonly observed that the MAPK pathway was reactivated by other means. This either occurred upstream by mutation of RAS or upregulation of tyrosine kinase receptors such as PDGFR and ERBB2, as well as upregulation of C-RAF [34]. Downstream members of the pathway were also affected, as activating mutations of MEK, or amplification of the gene encoding COT, were observed [61, 115]. Outside of the MAPK pathway, resistance also occurred through increased activity of a parallel pro-proliferative pathway, PI3K. All of these mediators of resistance exhibited by melanoma are now possible therapeutic targets.

2.5 The Role of N-RAS in Melanoma

N-RAS is found to be mutated in 15–30 % of melanomas. Interestingly, N-RAS mutations rarely overlap with B-RAF mutation, likely due to the redundancy of pathway activation this could create [24, 43]. The common mutations of N-RAS are substitutions at position Q61 (around 86 %) and result in an inability of N-RAS to hydrolyze GTP to GDP, resulting in a constitutively active kinase [36]. N-RAS activity can also be upregulated in melanoma by increased levels of its upstream RTKs, such as c-KIT, c-MET, and EGFR [6, 40].

Tipifarnib (R115777) is a farnesyltransferase inhibitor (FTI) currently being tested in melanoma to inhibit RAS activity. Farnesylation is an important posttranslational modification of RAS that promotes its localization to the cell membrane, which is necessary for activation. Treatment with tipifarnib did result in decreased RAS activity, as indicated by the loss of AKT and ERK phosphorylation, in tumor samples taken from patients. Unfortunately, there was no clinical response observed [41]. These results show that farnesyltransferase inhibition alone does not cause tumor regression in advanced melanoma, and a more specific RAS drug may be more efficacious. Additionally, downstream components of pathways mediated by RAS (MAPK and PI3K) are also attractive targets for melanoma, and many have multiple small molecule inhibitors already being explored.

2.6 MAPK Pathway Inhibition

Downstream of RAF in the MAPK pathway are MEK and ERK, both of which are under investigation as targets in melanoma therapy. Currently, there is one inhibitor specific for MEK1 and MEK2 which is FDA approved, trametinib. In a phase 3 clinical trial, trametinib was compared to standard dacarbazine treatment in patients with metastatic melanoma harboring mutant B-RAF. Those given trametinib had better progression-free survival and increased overall survival when compared to the chemotherapy group, with 81 % survival at 6 months compared to 67 %, respectively [39].

In addition to trametinib, multiple other MEK inhibitors are being explored in melanoma. These include MEK162, which has been tested in both B-RAF mutant and N-RAS mutant (B-RAF wild-type) patients, and both sets achieved 20 % partial response at 3.3 months [4]. However, there is dose-limiting toxicity because the MAPK pathway is blocked in all cells, not just those that are cancerous.

Selumetinib (AZD6244), a MEK1/2 inhibitor, was shown to suppress melanoma tumor growth in mice, and tumor regression was enhanced with combination with docetaxel, compared to either treatment alone [50]. This combination therapy is now currently undergoing clinical trial (NCT01256359). Other trials have also tested selumetinib for efficacy in patients with unresectable advanced melanoma. When compared to temozolomide treatment, selumetinib did not have a significant effect on progression-free survival [2]. However, of the partial responders to selumetinib, 83 % were B-RAF mutant [65]. These data led to the possibility that this MEK inhibitor would be most effective in patients with mutant B-RAF. Later, a clinical trial compared selumetinib in combination with dacarbazine vs. placebo with dacarbazine in mutant B-RAF patients with advanced melanoma. Progression-free survival was slightly improved with those treated with selumetinib in combination with dacarbazine, but unfortunately no significant difference in overall survival was observed [96].

As MEK inhibition proved to be effectual in mutant B-RAF patients, combination of MEK inhibition and B-RAF inhibition is being explored. In patients with mutant B-RAF, dabrafenib and trametinib were combined and compared to single dabrafenib treatment. Not only was progression-free survival increased to 9.4 compared to 5.8 months, less secondary squamous cell carcinoma was observed (7–19 %) [38]. Another MEK inhibitor, cobimetinib, is also in clinical trial in combination with vemurafenib, in hopes to improve upon mutant B-RAF and MEK inhibition therapy (NCT01689519). In addition to MEK inhibition, ERK is also a potential target, as it lies downstream of the MAPK pathway. Small molecule inhibitors of ERK are in use, such as SCH772984, and another molecule BVD-523 is currently in clinical trial [89] (NCT01781429).

2.7 PI3K Pathway Members in Therapy

The phosphatidylinositol 3-kinase (PI3K) pathway is activated by multiple growth factors and results in increased cell survival and proliferation (Fig. 2.2). After binding of growth factor to a receptor tyrosine kinase, PI3K is activated and in turn activates AKT, which regulates multiple downstream components to promote cell growth [75]. Multiple components of the PI3K pathway are found to be dysfunctional in melanoma. Loss of PTEN, a phosphatase and negative regulator of the PI3K pathway, has been found to be able to induce melanoma formation in concert with B-RAF mutation [23]. This pathway is also activated in cancer by mutations in AKT as well as amplifications of receptor tyrosine kinases such EGFR and c-KIT. There are multiple small molecule inhibitors currently being tested that target the PI3K pathway.

PI3K itself has several drugs in clinical trials for advanced metastatic disease, including SAR260301, XL147 (SAR245408), and pictilisib (GDC-0941). SAR260301 selectively inhibits the PI3Kβ isoform. Both XL147 and pictilisib directly bind isoforms of PI3K, effectively competing for ATP binding. However, the clinical efficacy for use of these drugs in melanoma has yet to be concluded.

AKT, a serine-threonine kinase downstream of PI3K, has been shown to be important for transformation to melanoma [45], and increased expression of phosphorylated AKT mirrors disease progression [22]. Increased AKT activity or by activating mutation (specifically AKT3) in melanoma can be due to either dysregulation of the PI3K pathway or by activating mutation and is observed in about half of nonfamilial melanomas [25, 104]. Thus, AKT is an attractive target for therapy. Initially, perifosine, an AKT inhibitor, was not found to exhibit a clinical response [33]. However, AKT targeting is still being explored, and MK2206 is currently in trial for advanced melanoma.

In addition to single-agent targeting of the PI3K pathway, it has been shown in melanoma cells that combination inhibition of the PI3K and MAPK pathways is a more efficient therapeutic [102]. GSK2141795, which is able to specifically bind and inhibit AKT, is being explored in combination with trametinib in uveal melanoma (NCT01979523). Additionally, a clinical trial combining the MEK inhibitor AZD6244 with the AKT inhibitor MK2206 is also proceeding (NCT01021748).

Mammalian target of rapamycin (mTOR) regulates cell proliferation and angiogenesis and is an upstream activator as well as a downstream target of AKT (Fig. 2.2). Temsirolimus is an inhibitor of mTOR and has been evaluated in phase 2 clinical trials in combination with other therapies. When temsirolimus is given to patients in combination with sorafenib compared to sorafenib with tipifarnib, no substantial difference was observed with either progression-free survival or overall survival [76]. While the downstream targets of the PI3K pathway have yet to be fully examined, upstream RTKs are also being studied.

2.8 Decreasing Melanoma Growth Through RTKs

c-KIT, encoded by the *KIT* gene, is found to be mutated in at least 2 % of melanomas [120]. Mutation or amplification of the *KIT* gene was found to be present in 28 % of melanomas with high sun exposure, as well as 36 % of acral and 39 % mucosal melanomas [21]. Stem cell factor (SCF) is the ligand for the RTK c-KIT and upon ligand binding c-KIT is able to activate both the

MAPK and PI3K pathways. As c-KIT mutations are found in other cancer types, small molecule inhibitors have already been created and are being tested in melanoma.

Nilotinib (Tasigna, AMN107) is a small molecule c-KIT inhibitor that is FDA approved for use in chronic myeloid leukemia and currently undergoing trials for use in melanoma (Fig. 2.2). A small phase 2 clinical trial of nilotinib in patients with c-KIT alterations showed low toxicity and promising inhibition of tumor progression, with a decrease in tumor size in 44 % of patients. Interestingly, greater progression-free survival was observed in treated patients harboring c-KIT mutation (8.4 months) than those with amplifications (1.7 months) [18]. This trend was also observed with imatinib mesylate (Gleevec®, Glivec®) which showed a higher response rate for those harboring *KIT* mutations rather than amplification [49, 56]. A study with sunitinib, a general tyrosine kinase inhibitor, also showed a higher percentage of response in those with *KIT* mutations vs. amplifications [85]. All of these drugs are tyrosine kinase inhibitors with activity not only against c-KIT but also other tyrosine kinases as well, such as PDGFR, and more specific drugs may have different outcomes. Dasatinib, another tyrosine kinase inhibitor that also shows high selectivity for SRC in addition to c-KIT, was examined in patients with advanced melanomas. No substantial effect was seen in melanoma and was found to be relatively toxic [67] (Fig. 2.2).

In addition to c-KIT, the RTK ERBB4 is also being targeted in melanoma. The *ERBB4* gene is found to be mutated in 19 % of patients with melanoma, which results in increased activity [93]. Lapatinib is a tyrosine kinase inhibitor that is already approved for use by the FDA in breast cancer. It is currently undergoing phase 2 trial in patients with advanced melanoma that are positive for *ERBB4* mutations (NCT01264081).

2.9 Inhibition of Angiogenesis

In order for a tumor to grow over a few hundred micrometers in diameter, new blood vessels must be formed to supply the new tissue mass with oxygen and nutrients, a process termed angiogenesis [84]. Development of new vasculature from existing vessels is orchestrated through expression of multiple proteins including cell surface receptors as well as secretion of growth factors. All of these aspects are found deregulated in cancers, including melanoma [31]. Destroying the ability of a tumor to create new vessels to support itself is an attractive therapy that could halt tumor growth. Additionally, the leaky, unorganized vessels found in tumors also make drug delivery much less efficient. Antiangiogenic therapies have been proposed to cause tumor vasculature normalization, instead of complete collapse, which may enhance drug delivery and therefore would be more successful as a combination therapy [58].

Vascular endothelial growth factor (VEGF) binding to its receptor VEGFR results in enhanced angiogenesis through endothelial cell proliferation as well as increased vessel permeability. VEGF and its receptor are overexpressed in melanoma, and inhibitors of this ligation are being explored in therapy. Bevacizumab is a humanized antibody that binds VEGF-A and inhibits receptor association and is currently FDA approved for use in colorectal cancer. Trials with bevacizumab in advanced melanoma include combination with other therapeutics. In a phase 2 trial, bevacizumab was combined with the mTOR inhibitor everolimus, and an average 4-month progression-free survival time and 8.6-month overall survival time were observed [51]. These results show that MAPK pathway inhibition combined with bevacizumab could be a promising therapeutic. Combination of bevacizumab with temozolomide resulted in an overall survival rate of 9.6 months, which was enhanced to 12 months if only considering B-RAF wt patients [114]. However, combination of bevacizumab with fotemustine showed an overall survival time of 20.5 months [26]. A large clinical trial including 214 patients compared treatment of paclitaxel and carboplatin with or without bevacizumab addition. Bevacizumab increased overall survival time to 12.3 months as compared to 9.2 months, and while the trend appeared to favor bevacizumab addition, it was not statistically significant [64]. While angiogenesis is an important part of tumor growth, the lack of compelling responses may be due to the fact that all these trials were given to late stage patients, at a point when new vessel formation is not as critical.

2.10 Immunotherapy

Normally the immune system works to clear pathogens and damaged cells; however, cancer cells have found a way to evade destruction and thrive. Many therapies being developed against cancers have been aimed to initiate clearance by the immune system. This is particularly true in melanoma, which is considered a highly immunologic tumor. High levels of tumor-infiltrating lymphocytes observed within tumor sites, as well as documented cases of spontaneous regression, have contributed to this label [19, 62]. Many mechanisms by which tumor cells evade immune system recognition are being targeted in melanoma and will be discussed below.

For T-cell activation during the immune response, a receptor presented on the surface of T cells, CD28, will bind a co-stimulatory molecule, B7, on the antigen-presenting cell (APC), in addition to a T-cell receptor binding antigen presented by the major histocompatibility complex (MHC) (Fig. 2.4). However, if cytotoxic T-lymphocyte-associated protein 4 (CTLA-4) is also presented on the T cell, it will compete with CD28 for B7 binding and inhibit T-cell activation, resulting in inhibition of cytokine production and T-cell proliferation [13]. Therefore, inhibition of CTLA-4 promotes T-cell response and enhances immune system response. Ipilimumab is a fully human IgG1 monoclonal antibody that targets and blocks CTLA-4 and is FDA approved for use in melanoma. In clinical trials, ipilimumab administered with gp100 peptide vaccine vs. vaccine alone produced an overall survival of 10 months compared to 6 months, respectively [57]. Furthermore, these results were supported by another clinical trial that compared ipilimumab in combination with dacarbazine to dacarbazine alone. Overall survival rates were increased to 11.2 months when ipilimumab was added, from 9.1 months of dacarbazine alone.

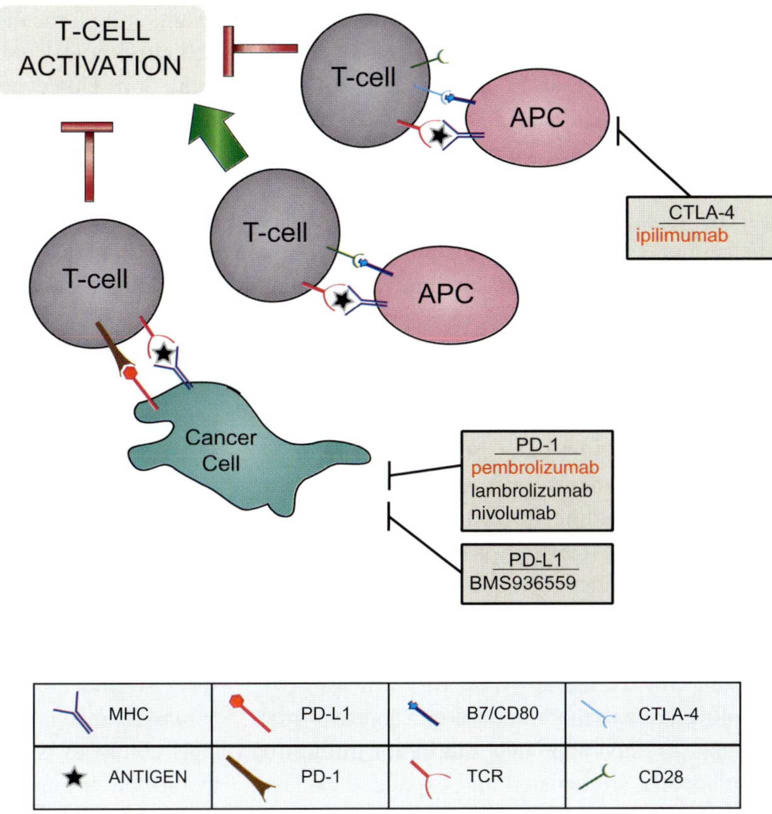

Fig. 2.4 Immune signaling being exploited in melanoma therapy. In hopes to increase immune response to melanoma, receptors and ligands that are deregulated in melanoma are being targeted to increase T-cell activation. *Red* writing indicates FDA approval in melanoma. *APC* antigen-presenting cell, *MHC* major histocompatibility complex, *TCR* T-cell receptor

Additionally, 20.8 % of patients treated with the combination were alive after 3 years, compared to 12.2 % of chemotherapy alone [97]. While response rates are low, the lasting results achieved by ipilimumab show promise for future immunotherapy, and it would be important to characterize the propensity for response.

In addition to CTLA-4, another inhibitory receptor expressed on activated T cells is programmed death-1 (PD-1), although it is mostly active during chronic inflammation (Fig. 2.4). Upon binding of PD-1 to its ligands (PD-L1 or PD-L2), T-cell response is reduced and apoptosis of the T cell can be induced. Notably, many cancers, including melanoma, have been found to overexpress PD-L1, which lends to tumor evasion [27]. Given the promise of ipilimumab, antibodies blocking PD-1 and PD-L1 are also being tested in melanoma. Blocking PD-L1 accessibility by treatment with a PD-L1 targeting antibody (BMS-936559) was explored in a 52 patient cohort. Of these patients, nine exhibited an objective response, and three achieved complete response [12]. Lambrolizumab (MK-3475) is an anti-PD-1 antibody that has shown effectiveness in patients with advanced melanoma, with a response rate of 25–52 %, depending on dosage [52]. Nivolumab (MDX-1106) is a genetically engineered fully human IgG4 monoclonal antibody specific for human PD-1. Phase 1 clinical trials have used nivolumab in combination with ipilimumab to block both CTLA-4 and PD-1 in advanced melanoma. High occurrence (at least 88 % of patients) of adverse events, including rash, fatigue, and diarrhea, was observed. However, these were generally reversible with treatment of immunosuppressants. In their treatment group that consisted of both nivolumab and ipilimumab for 3 weeks followed by nivolumab alone for 3 weeks, a clinical response was observed in 65 % of patients. Not only was their response rate higher than that observed previously for either treatment alone, but 31 % of patients had at least an 80 % reduction in tumor size at 12 weeks [121]. Overall, targeting CTLA-4 and PD-1 shows not only a high response rate but also a relatively high durable response.

The most recently FDA approved drug for melanoma is a PD-1 antagonist, pembrolizumab. In a phase 1 trial, patients with advanced melanoma who had already undergone treatment with ipilimumab achieved an overall response rate of 26 % at 8 months [126, 127]. These promising results, along with low toxicity, resulted in approval of the first PD-1 inhibitor by the FDA, to be used in patients with advanced disease that are not responding to other therapies. This approval emphasizes the promise immunotherapies hold, and identifying molecular markers of responding patients will provide more effectual results.

Adaptive cell therapy is another strategy being employed due to the immunologic nature of melanoma. In this approach antitumor-infiltrating lymphocytes are isolated and expanded ex vivo, then infused back into lymphocyte-depleted patient along with interleukin-2. Lymphocyte depletion by chemotherapy before injection of the expanded antitumor lymphocytes increased response rates from 49 to 72 %, with about half of patients still alive at 30 months [98]. Future trials aim to select tumor-infiltrating lymphocytes that are more effective. Results have shown that patients who achieve a complete response from adoptive cell transfer have a higher proportion of T cells that are CD8 positive and that also express the co-stimulatory molecule BTLA (B and T lymphocyte attenuator) [94].

2.11 Targeting ER Stress and Apoptosis

While multiple oncogenic pathways are disrupted in melanoma that result in increased proliferation, such as the PI3K and MAPK pathways, melanoma cells have also found a way to enhance their survival by resisting apoptosis. As already mentioned, the loss of *CDKN2A* locus expression results in two means the cell is able to overcome cell checkpoint control, thus thwarting apoptosis induction. However, that is not the only means melanomas escape death.

After protein translation, amino acid chains are brought into the endoplasmic reticulum (ER) for proper folding. However, under certain cellular insults that disrupt ER homeostasis, too much unfolded protein can accumulate in the ER, a condition known as ER stress. These protein aggregates can be very toxic to the cell, and ER stress can result in apoptosis [108]. ER stress can be compensated for by activation of the unfolded protein response, which can either halt protein synthesis or increase chaperone protein expression to help fold nascent proteins. During cancer progression and tumor growth, cancer cells experience hypoxic and nutrient deprived conditions, and this can trigger ER stress. In order to circumvent ER stress-induced apoptosis and survive, cancerous cells have found ways to either augment protein folding or sabotage apoptosis mechanisms. Impairment of a cancer cells ability to prevent apoptosis is a compelling therapeutic avenue, which could result in completion of apoptosis as well as render cancer cells more sensitive to cytotoxic drugs.

During the unfolded protein response, expression of chaperone proteins that help correctly fold proteins, such as heat shock protein 90(HSP90), is increased. It is also found that HSP90 expression is increased along with melanoma progression [8]. Additionally, oncogenic proteins are highly dependent on HSP90 for correct folding; this includes mutant B-RAF, making it an even more attractive therapeutic target [47]. Two inhibitors of HSP90 are currently undergoing clinical trials in advanced melanoma, XL888 and ganetespib (NCT01657591, NCT01551693) (Fig. 2.5).

Another way to induce apoptosis through ER stress has been explored through the use of bortezomib, a proteasome inhibitor [55] (Fig. 2.5). Inhibition of the proteasome causes accumulation of proteins, including NOXA, and results in apoptosis. Bortezomib is currently FDA approved for treatment of mantle cell lymphoma and multiple myeloma and is being explored for efficacy in melanoma. However, bortezomib alone did not have a significant clinical effect in melanoma [77].

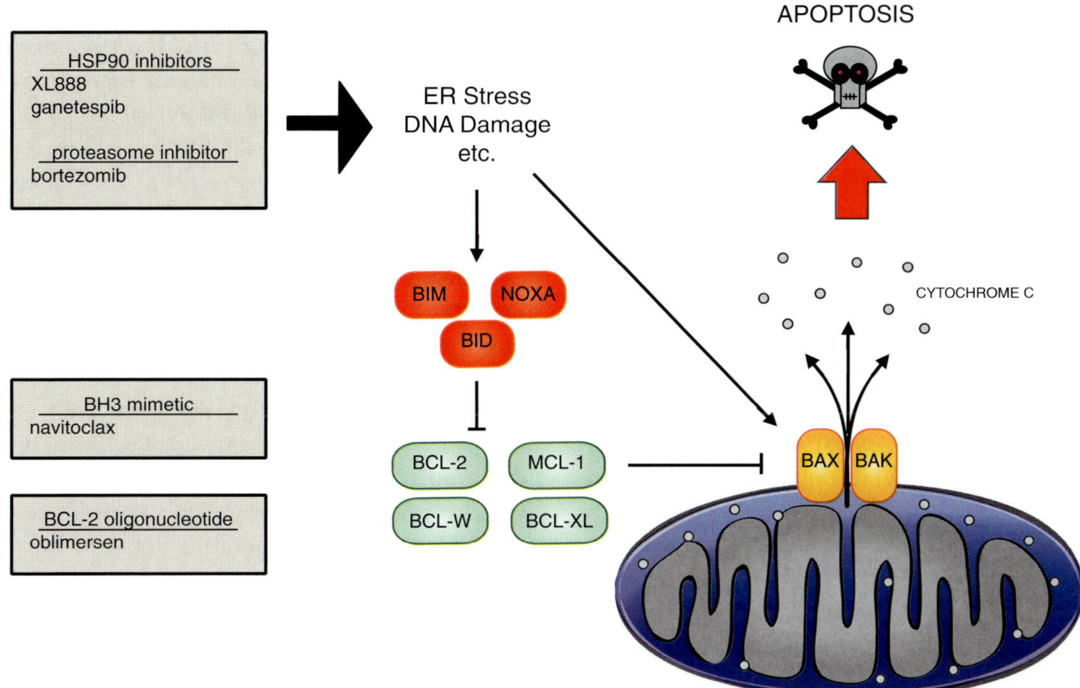

Fig. 2.5 Apoptosis signaling and experimental therapeutics. In response to multiple stimuli, including ER stress and DNA damage, apoptosis can be induced. Apoptosis is regulated by multiple BH3 domain containing proteins, which are divided into three classes. The *green*, antiapoptotic proteins, contains four BH3 domains. The other classes are both proapoptotic. The BH3 only proteins are indicated in *red*, and the proteins containing three BH3 domains are in *orange*. HSP90 inhibitors and proteasome inhibitors can induce ER stress and apoptosis. The BH3 mimetic navitoclax inhibits BCL-2, BCL-W, and BCL-XL. Oblimersen targets BCL-2

The intrinsic apoptosis pathway is triggered through formation of pores on the mitochondrial membrane, resulting in release of cytochrome c into the cytosol, generating a cascade of proteolysis (Fig. 2.5). These pores are either created or disrupted by BCL-2 protein family members, which are able to oligomerize with each other. There are three classes of proteins within the BCL-2 family, depending on their function (pro- or antiapoptotic) and basic homology (BH) domains [87].

1. One class of proteins contains four BH domains (BH1-4) and is anti- apoptotic; examples include BCL-2, BCL-XL, BCL-w, BFL-1/A1, and MCL-1 (Fig. 2.5, green).
2. The second class of proteins expresses three BH domains (BH1-3), is pro- apoptotic, and includes BAX and BAK (Fig. 2.5, orange).
3. A third class is the BH3 only proteins, which have only one BH domain and work to inhibit antiapoptotic BCL-2 proteins, therefore making themselves proapoptotic. These include, but are not limited to, NOXA, PUMA, BID, and BIM (Fig. 2.5, red).

For example, when activated, BAX will form pores with BAK in the mitochondrial membrane in order to release cytochrome c and cause apoptosis. However, the antiapoptotic BH1-4 proteins can bind BAX and BAK and inhibit pore formation. In addition, this process can be further regulated by BH3 proteins, such as PUMA, BIM, and BID, which bind antiapoptotic BCL-2 proteins, resulting in inhibition of apoptosis disruption [119]. Many of these proteins are deregulated in melanoma, resulting in enhanced resistance to apoptosis, and are currently being explored as drug targets [69].

BCL-2 is a target gene of MITF, both of which have been found overexpressed in melanoma cells [69, 78]. Additionally, other antiapoptotic BCL-2 proteins have been found in melanoma, such as BCL-XL and MCL-1 [109]. The overexpression of these proteins contributes to the cells ability to resist apoptosis and is therefore appealing for therapeutic targeting.

Oblimersen (a.k.a. G3139) is an antisense oligonucleotide that targets BCL-2 and has shown increased apoptosis and chemosensitivity when combined with dacarbazine in melanoma xenografts [59]. When taken into clinical trial, the use of oblimersen in addition to dacarbazine showed enhanced efficacy compared to dacarbazine alone, but the difference was moderate (progression-free survival was 2.6–1.6 months, respectively) [9]. While oblimersen showed poor clinical efficacy, other means by which to target BCL-2 proteins have been explored.

BH3 mimetics are small molecules that contain a BH3 domain and therefore can bind and inhibit antiapoptotic proteins. ABT-737 is a BH3 mimetic that targets multiple antiapoptotic proteins, such as BCL-2, BCL-W, and BCL-XL. While effective against melanoma cell lines, which is improved with combination of MCL-1 inhibition or NOXA induction, ABT-737 has yet to be brought into the clinic for melanoma [63, 74]. MAPK pathway inhibition upregulates BIM and downregulates the antiapoptotic protein MCL-1 and thus promotes apoptosis in melanoma [10]. Combination of the B-RAF inhibitor PLX4720 and ABT-737 killed melanoma cells synergistically in vitro, dependent on induction of BIM and downregulation of MCL-1 [122]. Consequently, the orally available derivative of ABT-737, navitoclax (ABT-263), that also preferentially inhibits BCL-2, BCL-XL, and BCL-W is currently recruiting for a clinical trial treating advanced metastatic disease, including melanoma, in combination with dabrafenib and trametinib (NCT01989585).

2.12 Therapies on the Horizon

In addition to optimizing the therapies mentioned above, other new strategies are also being explored but remain in early stages. The cyto-

skeleton is another potential target, and use of a tropomyosin inhibitor (TR100) to disrupt the actin cytoskeleton of tumor cells shows promise in melanoma lines [105]. Glutamine transport is also being investigated, as inhibition of glutamine transport results in diminished growth of some melanoma cell lines [116]. Decreased MITF expression could be achieved by histone deacetylase (HDAC) inhibitors. Additionally, the downstream target of MITF, cyclin-dependent kinase 2 (CDK2), is also being evaluated in melanoma. Targeting players in cell checkpoint control mechanisms, such as CHK1, also show promise in treatment of melanoma as well as increasing sensitivity to other therapies [90]. The use of small molecule inhibitors opens many doors for cancer treatment in addition to immunotherapies and chemotherapies, and these only represent a small amount of new approaches currently being explored in cancer.

Conclusion

As the molecular biology of melanoma becomes increasingly more clear, multiple proteins and pathways that are deregulated come to light. With this knowledge comes the ability to specifically target cancerous cells that are relatively indistinguishable from other normal tissue, as that is their origin. Early therapy banked on the fact that cancerous cells accumulated more DNA damage, due to inhibition of repair mechanisms, and used chemotherapy to damage all cells throughout the body. While all cells would be affected, normal cells would be able to recuperate, while cancerous cells would accumulate so much damage that they would no longer be functional and die. This strategy, while effectual in some cases, is highly toxic and the success rate in melanoma is strikingly low.

Using the knowledge gained by scientists in the laboratory, more specific strategies can be created to target specific mutated proteins. With the use of small molecule inhibitors, which are generally well tolerated, cancer therapy is evolving to more advanced treatments. The use of selective B-RAF inhibitors was remarkably effectual in melanoma treatment; unfortunately, the disease had a high rate of relapse. This, however, gives hope to a new approach to cancer treatment. Multiple targets can be exploited by this approach, as discussed above. In addition, mapping the molecular signature of a specific tumor can also uncover the probability of a patient's response to other therapies, such as immune-based or antiangiogenic therapies.

In the general populace there is a tendency to lump cancers by location, such as breast cancer or melanoma, for example. However, it is becoming increasingly clear that not all tumor types are equal, and subsets of each cancer types are apparent, each with their own molecular signature and each with varying responses to different therapies with unique results. The future of cancer therapy, especially melanoma therapy, lies in the molecular landscape of each patient's tumor and will require personalized strategies.

Acknowledgments N.K.H. is a Cameron Fellow of the Melanoma and Skin Cancer Research Institute, Australia, and a Sydney Medical School Foundation Fellow. N.K.H. also acknowledges contributing grant support from the Cancer Council NSW (RG 09-08, RG 13-06), Cancer Australia/Cure Cancer Australia Foundation (570778), Cancer Institute New South Wales (08/RFG/1-27), and the National Health and Medical Research Council Australia (1003637). We would also like to thank Dr. Lucas B. Murray, The University of Queensland Medical School, and Ms. Sheena Daignault, The University of Queensland Diamantina Institute, for carefully proofreading the manuscript.

References

1. Australian Institute of Health and Welfare & Australasian Association of Cancer Registries. Cancer in Australia: an overview, 2012. Cancer series no. 74. Cat. no. CAN 70. Canberra: AIHW; 2012.
2. Adjei AA, Cohen RB, Franklin W, Morris C, Wilson D, Molina JR, Hanson LJ, Gore L, Chow L, Leong S, Maloney L, Gordon G, Simmons H, Marlow A, Litwiler K, Brown S, Poch G, Kane K, Haney J, Eckhardt SG. Phase I pharmacokinetic and pharmacodynamic study of the oral, small-molecule mitogen-activated protein kinase kinase 1/2 inhibitor AZD6244 (ARRY-142886) in patients with advanced cancers. J Clin Oncol. 2008;26:2139–46.
3. Albino AP, Vidal MJ, McNutt NS, Shea CR, Prieto VG, Nanus DM, Palmer JM, Hayward NK. Mutation and expression of the p53 gene in human malignant melanoma. Melanoma Res. 1994;4:35–45.
4. Ascierto PA, Schadendorf D, Berking C, Agarwala SS, van Herpen CM, Queirolo P, Blank CU, Hauschild A, Beck JT, St-Pierre A, Niazi F, Wandel S, Peters M, Zubel A, Dummer R. MEK162 for patients with advanced melanoma harbouring NRAS or Val600 BRAF mutations: a non-randomised, open-label phase 2 study. Lancet Oncol. 2013; 14:249–56.
5. Balch CM, Gershenwald JE, Soong SJ, Thompson JF, Atkins MB, Byrd DR, Buzaid AC, Cochran AJ, Coit DG, Ding S, Eggermont AM, Flaherty KT, Gimotty PA, Kirkwood JM, McMasters KM, Mihm Jr MC, Morton DL, Ross MI, Sober AJ, Sondak VK. Final version of 2009 AJCC melanoma staging and classification. J Clin Oncol. 2009;27:6199–206.
6. Bardeesy N, Kim M, Xu J, Kim RS, Shen Q, Bosenberg MW, Wong WH, Chin L. Role of epidermal growth factor receptor signaling in RAS-driven melanoma. Mol Cell Biol. 2005;25:4176–88.
7. Beaumont KA, Liu YY, Sturm RA. The melanocortin-1 receptor gene polymorphism and association with human skin cancer. Prog Mol Biol Transl Sci. 2009;88:85–153.
8. Becker B, Multhoff G, Farkas B, Wild PJ, Landthaler M, Stolz W, Vogt T. Induction of Hsp90 protein expression in malignant melanomas and melanoma metastases. Exp Dermatol. 2004;13:27–32.
9. Bedikian AY, Millward M, Pehamberger H, Conry R, Gore M, Trefzer U, Pavlick AC, DeConti R, Hersh EM, Hersey P, Kirkwood JM, Haluska FG. Bcl-2 antisense (oblimersen sodium) plus dacarbazine in patients with advanced melanoma: the Oblimersen Melanoma Study Group. J Clin Oncol. 2006;24: 4738–45.
10. Berger A, Quast SA, Plotz M, Kuhn NF, Trefzer U, Eberle J. RAF inhibition overcomes resistance to TRAIL-induced apoptosis in melanoma cells. J Invest Dermatol. 2014;134:430–40.
11. Bishop DT, Demenais F, Goldstein AM, Bergman W, Bishop JN, Bressac-de Paillerets B, Chompret A, Ghiorzo P, Gruis N, Hansson J, Harland M, Hayward N, Holland EA, Mann GJ, Mantelli M, Nancarrow D, Platz A, Tucker MA. Geographical variation in the penetrance of CDKN2A mutations for melanoma. J Natl Cancer Inst. 2002;94:894–903.
12. Brahmer JR, Tykodi SS, Chow LQ, Hwu WJ, Topalian SL, Hwu P, Drake CG, Camacho LH, Kauh J, Odunsi K, Pitot HC, Hamid O, Bhatia S, Martins R, Eaton K, Chen S, Salay TM, Alaparthy S, Grosso JF, Korman AJ, Parker SM, Agrawal S, Goldberg SM, Pardoll DM, Gupta A, Wigginton JM. Safety and activity of anti-PD-L1 antibody in patients with advanced cancer. N Engl J Med. 2012;366:2455–65.
13. Callahan MK, Postow MA, Wolchok JD. Immunomodulatory therapy for melanoma: ipilimumab and beyond. Clin Dermatol. 2013;31:191–9.

14. Carreira S, Goodall J, Aksan I, La Rocca SA, Galibert MD, Denat L, Larue L, Goding CR. Mitf cooperates with Rb1 and activates p21Cip1 expression to regulate cell cycle progression. Nature. 2005;433:764–9.
15. Carvajal LA, Manfredi JJ. Another fork in the road–life or death decisions by the tumour suppressor p53. EMBO Rep. 2013;14:414–21.
16. Chang AE, Karnell LH, Menck HR. The National Cancer Data Base report on cutaneous and noncutaneous melanoma: a summary of 84,836 cases from the past decade. The American College of Surgeons Commission on Cancer and the American Cancer Society. Cancer. 1998;83:1664–78.
17. Chapman PB, Einhorn LH, Meyers ML, Saxman S, Destro AN, Panageas KS, Begg CB, Agarwala SS, Schuchter LM, Ernstoff MS, Houghton AN, Kirkwood JM. Phase III multicenter randomized trial of the Dartmouth regimen versus dacarbazine in patients with metastatic melanoma. J Clin Oncol. 1999;17:2745–51.
18. Cho JH, Kim KM, Kwon M, Kim JH, Lee J. Nilotinib in patients with metastatic melanoma harboring KIT gene aberration. Invest New Drugs. 2012;30:2008–14.
19. Cipponi A, Wieers G, van Baren N, Coulie PG. Tumor-infiltrating lymphocytes: apparently good for melanoma patients. But why? Cancer Immunol Immunother. 2011;60:1153–60.
20. Cruz 3rd F, Rubin BP, Wilson D, Town A, Schroeder A, Haley A, Bainbridge T, Heinrich MC, Corless CL. Absence of BRAF and NRAS mutations in uveal melanoma. Cancer Res. 2003;63:5761–6.
21. Curtin JA, Busam K, Pinkel D, Bastian BC. Somatic activation of KIT in distinct subtypes of melanoma. J Clin Oncol. 2006;24:4340–6.
22. Dai DL, Martinka M, Li G. Prognostic significance of activated Akt expression in melanoma: a clinicopathologic study of 292 cases. J Clin Oncol. 2005;23:1473–82.
23. Dankort D, Curley DP, Cartlidge RA, Nelson B, Karnezis AN, Damsky Jr WE, You MJ, DePinho RA, McMahon M, Bosenberg M. Braf(V600E) cooperates with Pten loss to induce metastatic melanoma. Nat Genet. 2009;41:544–52.
24. Davies H, Bignell GR, Cox C, Stephens P, Edkins S, Clegg S, Teague J, Woffendin H, Garnett MJ, Bottomley W, Davis N, Dicks E, Ewing R, Floyd Y, Gray K, Hall S, Hawes R, Hughes J, Kosmidou V, Menzies A, Mould C, Parker A, Stevens C, Watt S, Hooper S, Wilson R, Jayatilake H, Gusterson BA, Cooper C, Shipley J, Hargrave D, Pritchard-Jones K, Maitland N, Chenevix-Trench G, Riggins GJ, Bigner DD, Palmieri G, Cossu A, Flanagan A, Nicholson A, Ho JW, Leung SY, Yuen ST, Weber BL, Seigler HF, Darrow TL, Paterson H, Marais R, Marshall CJ, Wooster R, Stratton MR, Futreal PA. Mutations of the BRAF gene in human cancer. Nature. 2002;417:949–54.
25. Davies MA, Stemke-Hale K, Tellez C, Calderone TL, Deng W, Prieto VG, Lazar AJ, Gershenwald JE, Mills GB. A novel AKT3 mutation in melanoma tumours and cell lines. Br J Cancer. 2008;99:1265–8.
26. Del Vecchio M, Mortarini R, Canova S, Di Guardo L, Pimpinelli N, Sertoli MR, Bedognetti D, Queirolo P, Morosini P, Perrone T, Bajetta E, Anichini A. Bevacizumab plus fotemustine as first-line treatment in metastatic melanoma patients: clinical activity and modulation of angiogenesis and lymphangiogenesis factors. Clin Cancer Res. 2010;16:5862–72.
27. Dong H, Strome SE, Salomao DR, Tamura H, Hirano F, Flies DB, Roche PC, Lu J, Zhu G, Tamada K, Lennon VA, Celis E, Chen L. Tumor-associated B7-H1 promotes T-cell apoptosis: a potential mechanism of immune evasion. Nat Med. 2002;8:793–800.
28. Dumaz N, Hayward R, Martin J, Ogilvie L, Hedley D, Curtin JA, Bastian BC, Springer C, Marais R. In melanoma, RAS mutations are accompanied by switching signaling from BRAF to CRAF and disrupted cyclic AMP signaling. Cancer Res. 2006;66:9483–91.
29. Eggermont AM, Kirkwood JM. Re-evaluating the role of dacarbazine in metastatic melanoma: what have we learned in 30 years? Eur J Cancer. 2004;40:1825–36.
30. Eisen T, Ahmad T, Flaherty KT, Gore M, Kaye S, Marais R, Gibbens I, Hackett S, James M, Schuchter LM, Nathanson KL, Xia C, Simantov R, Schwartz B, Poulin-Costello M, O'Dwyer PJ, Ratain MJ. Sorafenib in advanced melanoma: a Phase II randomised discontinuation trial analysis. Br J Cancer. 2006;95:581–6.
31. Emmett MS, Dewing D, Pritchard-Jones RO. Angiogenesis and melanoma – from basic science to clinical trials. Am J Cancer Res. 2011;1:852–68.
32. Emuss V, Garnett M, Mason C, Marais R. Mutations of C-RAF are rare in human cancer because C-RAF has a low basal kinase activity compared with B-RAF. Cancer Res. 2005;65:9719–26.
33. Ernst DS, Eisenhauer E, Wainman N, Davis M, Lohmann R, Baetz T, Belanger K, Smylie M. Phase II study of perifosine in previously untreated patients with metastatic melanoma. Invest New Drugs. 2005;23:569–75.
34. Fedorenko IV, Paraiso KH, Smalley KS. Acquired and intrinsic BRAF inhibitor resistance in BRAF V600E mutant melanoma. Biochem Pharmacol. 2011;82:201–9.
35. Ferlay J, SI, Ervik M, Dikshit R, Eser S, Mathers C, Rebelo M, Parkin DM, Forman D, Bray F. GLOBOCAN 2012 v1.0, Cancer Incidence and Mortality Worldwide: IARC CancerBase No. 11 [Internet]. Lyon: International Agency for Research on Cancer; 2013. Available from: http://globocan.iarc.fr. Accessed on 13 Jan 2014.
36. Fernandez-Medarde A, Santos E. Ras in cancer and developmental diseases. Genes Cancer. 2011;2:344–58.
37. Finn L, Markovic SN, Joseph RW. Therapy for metastatic melanoma: the past, present, and future. BMC Med. 2012;10:23.
38. Flaherty KT, Infante JR, Daud A, Gonzalez R, Kefford RF, Sosman J, Hamid O, Schuchter L, Cebon J,

Ibrahim N, Kudchadkar R, Burris 3rd HA, Falchook G, Algazi A, Lewis K, Long GV, Puzanov I, Lebowitz P, Singh A, Little S, Sun P, Allred A, Ouellet D, Kim KB, Patel K, Weber J. Combined BRAF and MEK inhibition in melanoma with BRAF V600 mutations. N Engl J Med. 2012;367:1694–703.

39. Flaherty KT, Robert C, Hersey P, Nathan P, Garbe C, Milhem M, Demidov LV, Hassel JC, Rutkowski P, Mohr P, Dummer R, Trefzer U, Larkin JMG, Utikal J, Dreno B, Nyakas M, Middleton MR, Becker JC, Casey M, Sherman LJ, Wu FS, Ouellet D, Martin AM, Patel K, Schadendorf D, Grp MS. Improved survival with MEK inhibition in BRAF-mutated melanoma. N Engl J Med. 2012;367:107–14.

40. Furge KA, Kiewlich D, Le P, Vo MN, Faure M, Howlett AR, Lipson KE, Vande Woude GF, Webb CP. Suppression of Ras-mediated tumorigenicity and metastasis through inhibition of the Met receptor tyrosine kinase. Proc Natl Acad Sci U S A. 2001; 98:10722–7.

41. Gajewski TF, Salama AK, Niedzwiecki D, Johnson J, Linette G, Bucher C, Blaskovich MA, Sebti SM, Haluska F. Phase II study of the farnesyltransferase inhibitor R115777 in advanced melanoma (CALGB 500104). J Transl Med. 2012;10:246.

42. Gandini S, Sera F, Cattaruzza MS, Pasquini P, Zanetti R, Masini C, Boyle P, Melchi CF. Meta-analysis of risk factors for cutaneous melanoma: III. Family history, actinic damage and phenotypic factors. Eur J Cancer. 2005;41:2040–59.

43. Goel VK, Lazar AJ, Warneke CL, Redston MS, Haluska FG. Examination of mutations in BRAF, NRAS, and PTEN in primary cutaneous melanoma. J Invest Dermatol. 2006;126:154–60.

44. Goldstein AM, Chan M, Harland M, Gillanders EM, Hayward NK, Avril MF, Azizi E, Bianchi-Scarra G, Bishop DT, Bressac-de Paillerets B, Bruno W, Calista D, Cannon Albright LA, Demenais F, Elder DE, Ghiorzo P, Gruis NA, Hansson J, Hogg D, Holland EA, Kanetsky PA, Kefford RF, Landi MT, Lang J, Leachman SA, Mackie RM, Magnusson V, Mann GJ, Niendorf K, Newton Bishop J, Palmer JM, Puig S, Puig-Butille JA, de Snoo FA, Stark M, Tsao H, Tucker MA, Whitaker L, Yakobson E. High-risk melanoma susceptibility genes and pancreatic cancer, neural system tumors, and uveal melanoma across GenoMEL. Cancer Res. 2006;66:9818–28.

45. Govindarajan B, Sligh JE, Vincent BJ, Li M, Canter JA, Nickoloff BJ, Rodenburg RJ, Smeitink JA, Oberley L, Zhang Y, Slingerland J, Arnold RS, Lambeth JD, Cohen C, Hilenski L, Griendling K, Martinez-Diez M, Cuezva JM, Arbiser JL. Overexpression of Akt converts radial growth melanoma to vertical growth melanoma. J Clin Invest. 2007;117:719–29.

46. Gray-Schopfer V, Wellbrock C, Marais R. Melanoma biology and new targeted therapy. Nature. 2007;445:851–7.

47. Grbovic OM, Basso AD, Sawai A, Ye Q, Friedlander P, Solit D, Rosen N. V600E B-Raf requires the Hsp90 chaperone for stability and is degraded in response to Hsp90 inhibitors. Proc Natl Acad Sci U S A. 2006;103:57–62.

48. Greenblatt MS, Bennett WP, Hollstein M, Harris CC. Mutations in the p53 tumor suppressor gene: clues to cancer etiology and molecular pathogenesis. Cancer Res. 1994;54:4855–78.

49. Guo J, Si L, Kong Y, Flaherty KT, Xu X, Zhu Y, Corless CL, Li L, Li H, Sheng X, Cui C, Chi Z, Li S, Han M, Mao L, Lin X, Du N, Zhang X, Li J, Wang B, Qin S. Phase II, open-label, single-arm trial of imatinib mesylate in patients with metastatic melanoma harboring c-Kit mutation or amplification. J Clin Oncol. 2011;29:2904–9.

50. Haass NK, Sproesser K, Nguyen TK, Contractor R, Medina CA, Nathanson KL, Herlyn M, Smalley KS. The mitogen-activated protein/extracellular signal-regulated kinase kinase inhibitor AZD6244 (ARRY-142886) induces growth arrest in melanoma cells and tumor regression when combined with docetaxel. Clin Cancer Res. 2008;14:230–9.

51. Hainsworth JD, Infante JR, Spigel DR, Peyton JD, Thompson DS, Lane CM, Clark BL, Rubin MS, Trent DF, Burris 3rd HA. Bevacizumab and everolimus in the treatment of patients with metastatic melanoma: a phase 2 trial of the Sarah Cannon Oncology Research Consortium. Cancer. 2010;116:4122–9.

52. Hamid O, Robert C, Daud A, Hodi FS, Hwu WJ, Kefford R, Wolchok JD, Hersey P, Joseph RW, Weber JS, Dronca R, Gangadhar TC, Patnaik A, Zarour H, Joshua AM, Gergich K, Elassaiss-Schaap J, Algazi A, Mateus C, Boasberg P, Tumeh PC, Chmielowski B, Ebbinghaus SW, Li XN, Kang SP, Ribas A. Safety and tumor responses with lambrolizumab (anti-PD-1) in melanoma. N Engl J Med. 2013;369:134–44.

53. Harbour JW, Onken MD, Roberson ED, Duan S, Cao L, Worley LA, Council ML, Matatall KA, Helms C, Bowcock AM. Frequent mutation of BAP1 in metastasizing uveal melanomas. Science. 2010;330:1410–3.

54. Hatzivassiliou G, Song K, Yen I, Brandhuber BJ, Anderson DJ, Alvarado R, Ludlam MJ, Stokoe D, Gloor SL, Vigers G, Morales T, Aliagas I, Liu B, Sideris S, Hoeflich KP, Jaiswal BS, Seshagiri S, Koeppen H, Belvin M, Friedman LS, Malek S. RAF inhibitors prime wild-type RAF to activate the MAPK pathway and enhance growth. Nature. 2010;464:431–5.

55. Hill DS, Martin S, Armstrong JL, Flockhart R, Tonison JJ, Simpson DG, Birch-Machin MA, Redfern CP, Lovat PE. Combining the endoplasmic reticulum stress-inducing agents bortezomib and fenretinide as a novel therapeutic strategy for metastatic melanoma. Clin Cancer Res. 2009;15:1192–8.

56. Hodi FS, Corless CL, Giobbie-Harder A, Fletcher JA, Zhu M, Marino-Enriquez A, Friedlander P, Gonzalez R, Weber JS, Gajewski TF, O'Day SJ, Kim KB, Lawrence D, Flaherty KT, Luke JJ, Collichio FA, Ernstoff MS, Heinrich MC, Beadling C, Zukotynski KA, Yap JT, Van den Abbeele AD, Demetri GD, Fisher DE. Imatinib for melanomas harboring

mutationally activated or amplified KIT arising on mucosal, acral, and chronically sun-damaged skin. J Clin Oncol. 2013;31:3182–90.

57. Hodi FS, O'Day SJ, McDermott DF, Weber RW, Sosman JA, Haanen JB, Gonzalez R, Robert C, Schadendorf D, Hassel JC, Akerley W, van den Eertwegh AJ, Lutzky J, Lorigan P, Vaubel JM, Linette GP, Hogg D, Ottensmeier CH, Lebbe C, Peschel C, Quirt I, Clark JI, Wolchok JD, Weber JS, Tian J, Yellin MJ, Nichol GM, Hoos A, Urba WJ. Improved survival with ipilimumab in patients with metastatic melanoma. N Engl J Med. 2010;363:711–23.

58. Jain RK. Normalization of tumor vasculature: an emerging concept in antiangiogenic therapy. Science. 2005;307:58–62.

59. Jansen B, Schlagbauer-Wadl H, Brown BD, Bryan RN, van Elsas A, Muller M, Wolff K, Eichler HG, Pehamberger H. bcl-2 antisense therapy chemosensitizes human melanoma in SCID mice. Nat Med. 1998;4:232–4.

60. Jhappan C, Noonan FP, Merlino G. Ultraviolet radiation and cutaneous malignant melanoma. Oncogene. 2003;22:3099–112.

61. Johannessen CM, Boehm JS, Kim SY, Thomas SR, Wardwell L, Johnson LA, Emery CM, Stransky N, Cogdill AP, Barretina J, Caponigro G, Hieronymus H, Murray RR, Salehi-Ashtiani K, Hill DE, Vidal M, Zhao JJ, Yang X, Alkan O, Kim S, Harris JL, Wilson CJ, Myer VE, Finan PM, Root DE, Roberts TM, Golub T, Flaherty KT, Dummer R, Weber BL, Sellers WR, Schlegel R, Wargo JA, Hahn WC, Garraway LA. COT drives resistance to RAF inhibition through MAP kinase pathway reactivation. Nature. 2010;468:968–72.

62. Kalialis LV, Drzewiecki KT, Klyver H. Spontaneous regression of metastases from melanoma: review of the literature. Melanoma Res. 2009;19:275–82.

63. Keuling AM, Felton KE, Parker AA, Akbari M, Andrew SE, Tron VA. RNA silencing of Mcl-1 enhances ABT-737-mediated apoptosis in melanoma: role for a caspase-8-dependent pathway. PLoS One. 2009;4:e6651.

64. Kim KB, Sosman JA, Fruehauf JP, Linette GP, Markovic SN, McDermott DF, Weber JS, Nguyen H, Cheverton P, Chen D, Peterson AC, Carson 3rd WE, O'Day SJ. BEAM: a randomized phase II study evaluating the activity of bevacizumab in combination with carboplatin plus paclitaxel in patients with previously untreated advanced melanoma. J Clin Oncol. 2012;30:34–41.

65. Kirkwood JM, Bastholt L, Robert C, Sosman J, Larkin J, Hersey P, Middleton M, Cantarini M, Zazulina V, Kemsley K, Dummer R. Phase II, open-label, randomized trial of the MEK1/2 inhibitor selumetinib as monotherapy versus temozolomide in patients with advanced melanoma. Clin Cancer Res. 2012;18:555–67.

66. Kirkwood JM, Strawderman MH, Ernstoff MS, Smith TJ, Borden EC, Blum RH. Interferon alfa-2b adjuvant therapy of high-risk resected cutaneous melanoma: the Eastern Cooperative Oncology Group Trial EST 1684. J Clin Oncol. 1996;14:7–17.

67. Kluger HM, Dudek AZ, McCann C, Ritacco J, Southard N, Jilaveanu LB, Molinaro A, Sznol M. A phase 2 trial of dasatinib in advanced melanoma. Cancer. 2011;117:2202–8.

68. Lee JT, Li L, Brafford PA, van den Eijnden M, Halloran MB, Sproesser K, Haass NK, Smalley KS, Tsai J, Bollag G, Herlyn M. PLX4032, a potent inhibitor of the B-Raf V600E oncogene, selectively inhibits V600E-positive melanomas. Pigment Cell Melanoma Res. 2010;23:820–7.

69. Leiter U, Schmid RM, Kaskel P, Peter RU, Krahn G. Antiapoptotic bcl-2 and bcl-xL in advanced malignant melanoma. Arch Dermatol Res. 2000;292:225–32.

70. Levy C, Khaled M, Fisher DE. MITF: master regulator of melanocyte development and melanoma oncogene. Trends Mol Med. 2006;12:406–14.

71. Loercher AE, Tank EM, Delston RB, Harbour JW. MITF links differentiation with cell cycle arrest in melanocytes by transcriptional activation of INK4A. J Cell Biol. 2005;168:35–40.

72. Long GV, Menzies AM, Nagrial AM, Haydu LE, Hamilton AL, Mann GJ, Hughes TM, Thompson JF, Scolyer RA, Kefford RF. Prognostic and clinicopathologic associations of oncogenic BRAF in metastatic melanoma. J Clin Oncol. 2011;29:1239–46.

73. Lu M, Breyssens H, Salter V, Zhong S, Hu Y, Baer C, Ratnayaka I, Sullivan A, Brown NR, Endicott J, Knapp S, Kessler BM, Middleton MR, Siebold C, Jones EY, Sviderskaya EV, Cebon J, John T, Caballero OL, Goding CR, Lu X. Restoring p53 function in human melanoma cells by inhibiting MDM2 and cyclin B1/CDK1-phosphorylated nuclear iASPP. Cancer Cell. 2013;23:618–33.

74. Lucas KM, Mohana-Kumaran N, Lau D, Zhang XD, Hersey P, Huang DC, Weninger W, Haass NK, Allen JD. Modulation of NOXA and MCL-1 as a strategy for sensitizing melanoma cells to the BH3-mimetic ABT-737. Clin Cancer Res. 2012;18:783–95.

75. Luo J, Manning BD, Cantley LC. Targeting the PI3K-Akt pathway in human cancer: rationale and promise. Cancer Cell. 2003;4:257–62.

76. Margolin KA, Moon J, Flaherty LE, Lao CD, Akerley 3rd WL, Othus M, Sosman JA, Kirkwood JM, Sondak VK. Randomized phase II trial of sorafenib with temsirolimus or tipifarnib in untreated metastatic melanoma (S0438). Clin Cancer Res. 2012;18:1129–37.

77. Markovic SN, Geyer SM, Dawkins F, Sharfman W, Albertini M, Maples W, Fracasso PM, Fitch T, Lorusso P, Adjei AA, Erlichman C. A phase II study of bortezomib in the treatment of metastatic malignant melanoma. Cancer. 2005;103:2584–9.

78. McGill GG, Horstmann M, Widlund HR, Du J, Motyckova G, Nishimura EK, Lin YL, Ramaswamy S, Avery W, Ding HF, Jordan SA, Jackson IJ, Korsmeyer SJ, Golub TR, Fisher DE. Bcl2 regulation by the melanocyte master regulator Mitf modulates

lineage survival and melanoma cell viability. Cell. 2002;109:707–18.

79. Meckbach D, Bauer J, Pflugfelder A, Meier F, Busch C, Eigentler TK, Capper D, von Deimling A, Mittelbronn M, Perner S, Ikenberg K, Hantschke M, Buttner P, Garbe C, Weide B. Survival according to BRAF-V600 tumor mutations – an analysis of 437 patients with primary melanoma. PLoS One. 2014;9.

80. Meckbach D, Keim U, Richter S, Leiter U, Eigentler TK, Bauer J, Pflugfelder A, Buttner P, Garbe C, Weide B. BRAF-V600 mutations have no prognostic impact in stage IV melanoma patients treated with monochemotherapy. PLoS One. 2014;9:e89218.

81. Meyle KD, Guldberg P. Genetic risk factors for melanoma. Hum Genet. 2009;126:499–510.

82. Middleton MR, Grob JJ, Aaronson N, Fierlbeck G, Tilgen W, Seiter S, Gore M, Aamdal S, Cebon J, Coates A, Dreno B, Henz M, Schadendorf D, Kapp A, Weiss J, Fraass U, Statkevich P, Muller M, Thatcher N. Randomized phase III study of temozolomide versus dacarbazine in the treatment of patients with advanced metastatic malignant melanoma. J Clin Oncol. 2000;18:158–66.

83. Miller AJ, Mihm Jr MC. Melanoma. N Engl J Med. 2006;355:51–65.

84. Minchinton AI, Tannock IF. Drug penetration in solid tumours. Nat Rev Cancer. 2006;6:583–92.

85. Minor DR, Kashani-Sabet M, Garrido M, O'Day SJ, Hamid O, Bastian BC. Sunitinib therapy for melanoma patients with KIT mutations. Clin Cancer Res. 2012;18:1457–63.

86. Mitra D, Luo X, Morgan A, Wang J, Hoang MP, Lo J, Guerrero CR, Lennerz JK, Mihm MC, Wargo JA, Robinson KC, Devi SP, Vanover JC, D'Orazio JA, McMahon M, Bosenberg MW, Haigis KM, Haber DA, Wang Y, Fisher DE. An ultraviolet-radiation-independent pathway to melanoma carcinogenesis in the red hair/fair skin background. Nature. 2012;491:449–53.

87. Mohana-Kumaran N, Hill DS, Allen JD, Haass NK. Targeting the intrinsic apoptosis pathway as a strategy for melanoma therapy. Pigment Cell Melanoma Res. 2014;27:525–39.

88. Moloney FJ, Guitera P, Coates E, Haass NK, Ho K, Khoury R, O'Connell R, Raudonikis L, Schmid H, Mann GJ, Menzies SW. Detection of primary melanoma in individuals at extreme high risk: a prospective five-year follow up study. JAMA Dermatol. 2014;150:819–27.

89. Morris EJ, Jha S, Restaino CR, Dayananth P, Zhu H, Cooper A, Carr D, Deng Y, Jin W, Black S, Long B, Liu J, Dinunzio E, Windsor W, Zhang R, Zhao S, Angagaw MH, Pinheiro EM, Desai J, Xiao L, Shipps G, Hruza A, Wang J, Kelly J, Paliwal S, Gao X, Babu BS, Zhu L, Daublain P, Zhang L, Lutterbach BA, Pelletier MR, Philippar U, Siliphaivanh P, Witter D, Kirschmeier P, Bishop WR, Hicklin D, Gilliland DG, Jayaraman L, Zawel L, Fawell S, Samatar AA. Discovery of a novel ERK inhibitor with activity in models of acquired resistance to BRAF and MEK inhibitors. Cancer Discov. 2013;3:742–50.

90. Pavey S, Spoerri L, Haass NK, Gabrielli B. DNA repair and cell cycle checkpoint defects as drivers and therapeutic targets in melanoma. Pigment Cell Melanoma Res. 2013;26:805–16.

91. Pollock PM, Harper UL, Hansen KS, Yudt LM, Stark M, Robbins CM, Moses TY, Hostetter G, Wagner U, Kakareka J, Salem G, Pohida T, Heenan P, Duray P, Kallioniemi O, Hayward NK, Trent JM, Meltzer PS. High frequency of BRAF mutations in nevi. Nat Genet. 2003;33:19–20.

92. Poulikakos PI, Persaud Y, Janakiraman M, Kong X, Ng C, Moriceau G, Shi H, Atefi M, Titz B, Gabay MT, Salton M, Dahlman KB, Tadi M, Wargo JA, Flaherty KT, Kelley MC, Misteli T, Chapman PB, Sosman JA, Graeber TG, Ribas A, Lo RS, Rosen N, Solit DB. RAF inhibitor resistance is mediated by dimerization of aberrantly spliced BRAF(V600E). Nature. 2011;480:387–90.

93. Prickett TD, Agrawal NS, Wei X, Yates KE, Lin JC, Wunderlich JR, Cronin JC, Cruz P, Rosenberg SA, Samuels Y. Analysis of the tyrosine kinome in melanoma reveals recurrent mutations in ERBB4. Nat Genet. 2009;41:1127–32.

94. Radvanyi LG, Bernatchez C, Zhang M, Fox PS, Miller P, Chacon J, Wu R, Lizee G, Mahoney S, Alvarado G, Glass M, Johnson VE, McMannis JD, Shpall E, Prieto V, Papadopoulos N, Kim K, Homsi J, Bedikian A, Hwu WJ, Patel S, Ross MI, Lee JE, Gershenwald JE, Lucci A, Royal R, Cormier JN, Davies MA, Mansaray R, Fulbright OJ, Toth C, Ramachandran R, Wardell S, Gonzalez A, Hwu P. Specific lymphocyte subsets predict response to adoptive cell therapy using expanded autologous tumor-infiltrating lymphocytes in metastatic melanoma patients. Clin Cancer Res. 2012;18:6758–70.

95. Rimoldi D, Salvi S, Lienard D, Lejeune FJ, Speiser D, Zografos L, Cerottini JC. Lack of BRAF mutations in uveal melanoma. Cancer Res. 2003;63:5712–5.

96. Robert C, Dummer R, Gutzmer R, Lorigan P, Kim KB, Nyakas M, Arance A, Liszkay G, Schadendorf D, Cantarini M, Spencer S, Middleton MR. Selumetinib plus dacarbazine versus placebo plus dacarbazine as first-line treatment for BRAF-mutant metastatic melanoma: a phase 2 double-blind randomised study. Lancet Oncol. 2013;14:733–40.

97. Robert C, Thomas L, Bondarenko I, O'Day S, Garbe C, Lebbe C, Baurain JF, Testori A, Grob JJ, Davidson N, Richards J, Maio M, Hauschild A, Miller Jr WH, Gascon P, Lotem M, Harmankaya K, Ibrahim R, Francis S, Chen TT, Humphrey R, Hoos A, Wolchok JD. Ipilimumab plus dacarbazine for previously untreated metastatic melanoma. N Engl J Med. 2011;364:2517–26.

98. Rosenberg SA, Dudley ME. Adoptive cell therapy for the treatment of patients with metastatic melanoma. Curr Opin Immunol. 2009;21:233–40.

99. Rosenberg SA, Yang JC, Topalian SL, Schwartzentruber DJ, Weber JS, Parkinson DR, Seipp CA, Einhorn JH, White DE. Treatment of 283 consecutive patients with metastatic melanoma or renal

cell cancer using high-dose bolus interleukin 2. JAMA. 1994;271:907–13.

100. Schmittel A, Schmidt-Hieber M, Martus P, Bechrakis NE, Schuster R, Siehl JM, Foerster MH, Thiel E, Keilholz U. A randomized phase II trial of gemcitabine plus treosulfan versus treosulfan alone in patients with metastatic uveal melanoma. Ann Oncol. 2006;17:1826–9.

101. Siegel R, Naishadham D, Jemal A. Cancer statistics, 2013. CA Cancer J Clin. 2013;63:11–30.

102. Smalley KS, Haass NK, Brafford PA, Lioni M, Flaherty KT, Herlyn M. Multiple signaling pathways must be targeted to overcome drug resistance in cell lines derived from melanoma metastases. Mol Cancer Ther. 2006;5:1136–44.

103. Soufir N, Avril MF, Chompret A, Demenais F, Bombled J, Spatz A, Stoppa-Lyonnet D, Benard J, Bressac-de Paillerets B. Prevalence of p16 and CDK4 germline mutations in 48 melanoma-prone families in France. The French Familial Melanoma Study Group. Hum Mol Genet. 1998;7:209–16.

104. Stahl JM, Sharma A, Cheung M, Zimmerman M, Cheng JQ, Bosenberg MW, Kester M, Sandirasegarane L, Robertson GP. Deregulated Akt3 activity promotes development of malignant melanoma. Cancer Res. 2004;64:7002–10.

105. Stehn JR, Haass NK, Bonello T, Desouza M, Kottyan G, Treutlein H, Zeng J, Nascimento PR, Sequeira VB, Butler TL, Allanson M, Fath T, Hill TA, McCluskey A, Schevzov G, Palmer SJ, Hardeman EC, Winlaw D, Reeve VE, Dixon I, Weninger W, Cripe TP, Gunning PW. A novel class of anticancer compounds targets the actin cytoskeleton in tumor cells. Cancer Res. 2013;73:5169–82.

106. Su F, Viros A, Milagre C, Trunzer K, Bollag G, Spleiss O, Reis-Filho JS, Kong X, Koya RC, Flaherty KT, Chapman PB, Kim MJ, Hayward R, Martin M, Yang H, Wang Q, Hilton H, Hang JS, Noe J, Lambros M, Geyer F, Dhomen N, Niculescu-Duvaz I, Zambon A, Niculescu-Duvaz D, Preece N, Robert L, Otte NJ, Mok S, Kee D, Ma Y, Zhang C, Habets G, Burton EA, Wong B, Nguyen H, Kockx M, Andries L, Lestini B, Nolop KB, Lee RJ, Joe AK, Troy JL, Gonzalez R, Hutson TE, Puzanov I, Chmielowski B, Springer CJ, McArthur GA, Sosman JA, Lo RS, Ribas A, Marais R. RAS mutations in cutaneous squamous-cell carcinomas in patients treated with BRAF inhibitors. N Engl J Med. 2012;366:207–15.

107. Sullivan RJ, Flaherty K. MAP kinase signaling and inhibition in melanoma. Oncogene. 2013;32:2373–9.

108. Tabas I, Ron D. Integrating the mechanisms of apoptosis induced by endoplasmic reticulum stress. Nat Cell Biol. 2011;13:184–90.

109. Tang L, Tron VA, Reed JC, Mah KJ, Krajewska M, Li G, Zhou X, Ho VC, Trotter MJ. Expression of apoptosis regulators in cutaneous malignant melanoma. Clin Cancer Res. 1998;4:1865–71.

110. Tsai J, Lee JT, Wang W, Zhang J, Cho H, Mamo S, Bremer R, Gillette S, Kong J, Haass NK, Sproesser K, Li L, Smalley KS, Fong D, Zhu YL, Marimuthu A, Nguyen H, Lam B, Liu J, Cheung I, Rice J, Suzuki Y, Luu C, Settachatgul C, Shellooe R, Cantwell J, Kim SH, Schlessinger J, Zhang KY, West BL, Powell B, Habets G, Zhang C, Ibrahim PN, Hirth P, Artis DR, Herlyn M, Bollag G. Discovery of a selective inhibitor of oncogenic B-Raf kinase with potent antimelanoma activity. Proc Natl Acad Sci U S A. 2008;105:3041–6.

111. Valverde P, Healy E, Sikkink S, Haldane F, Thody AJ, Carothers A, Jackson IJ, Rees JL. The Asp84Glu variant of the melanocortin 1 receptor (MC1R) is associated with melanoma. Hum Mol Genet. 1996;5:1663–6.

112. Van Raamsdonk CD, Bezrookove V, Green G, Bauer J, Gaugler L, O'Brien JM, Simpson EM, Barsh GS, Bastian BC. Frequent somatic mutations of GNAQ in uveal melanoma and blue naevi. Nature. 2009;457:599–602.

113. Villanueva J, Vultur A, Herlyn M. Resistance to BRAF inhibitors: unraveling mechanisms and future treatment options. Cancer Res. 2011;71:7137–40.

114. von Moos R, Seifert B, Simcock M, Goldinger SM, Gillessen S, Ochsenbein A, Michielin O, Cathomas R, Schlappi M, Moch H, Schraml PH, Mjhic-Probst D, Mamot C, Schonewolf N, Dummer R. First-line temozolomide combined with bevacizumab in metastatic melanoma: a multicentre phase II trial (SAKK 50/07). Ann Oncol. 2012;23:531–6.

115. Wagle N, Emery C, Berger MF, Davis MJ, Sawyer A, Pochanard P, Kehoe SM, Johannessen CM, MacConaill LE, Hahn WC, Meyerson M, Garraway LA. Dissecting therapeutic resistance to RAF inhibition in melanoma by tumor genomic profiling. J Clin Oncol. 2011;29:3085–96.

116. Wang Q, Beaumont KA, Otte NJ, Font J, Bailey CG, van Geldermalsen M, Sharp DM, Tiffen JC, Ryan RM, Jormakka M, Haass NK, Rasko JE, Holst J. Targeting glutamine transport to suppress melanoma cell growth. Int J Cancer. 2014;135:1060–71.

117. Wiesner T, Obenauf AC, Murali R, Fried I, Griewank KG, Ulz P, Windpassinger C, Wackernagel W, Loy S, Wolf I, Viale A, Lash AE, Pirun M, Socci ND, Rutten A, Palmedo G, Abramson D, Offit K, Ott A, Becker JC, Cerroni L, Kutzner H, Bastian BC, Speicher MR. Germline mutations in BAP1 predispose to melanocytic tumors. Nat Genet. 2011;43:1018–21.

118. Wilhelm SM, Carter C, Tang LY, Wilkie D, McNabola A, Rong H, Chen C, Zhang XM, Vincent P, McHugh M, Cao YC, Shujath J, Gawlak S, Eveleigh D, Rowley B, Liu L, Adnane L, Lynch M, Auclair D, Taylor I, Gedrich R, Voznesensky A, Riedl B, Post LE, Bollag G, Trail PA. BAY 43-9006 exhibits broad spectrum oral antitumor activity and targets the RAF/MEK/ERK pathway and receptor tyrosine kinases involved in tumor progression and angiogenesis. Cancer Res. 2004;64:7099–109.

119. Willis SN, Adams JM. Life in the balance: how BH3-only proteins induce apoptosis. Curr Opin Cell Biol. 2005;17:617–25.

120. Willmore-Payne C, Holden JA, Tripp S, Layfield LJ. Human malignant melanoma: detection of BRAF- and c-kit-activating mutations by high-resolution amplicon melting analysis. Hum Pathol. 2005;36:486–93.
121. Wolchok JD, Kluger H, Callahan MK, Postow MA, Rizvi NA, Lesokhin AM, Segal NH, Ariyan CE, Gordon RA, Reed K, Burke MM, Caldwell A, Kronenberg SA, Agunwamba BU, Zhang X, Lowy I, Inzunza HD, Feely W, Horak CE, Hong Q, Korman AJ, Wigginton JM, Gupta A, Sznol M. Nivolumab plus ipilimumab in advanced melanoma. N Engl J Med. 2013;369:122–33.
122. Wroblewski D, Mijatov B, Mohana-Kumaran N, Lai F, Gallagher SJ, Haass NK, Zhang XD, Hersey P. The BH3-mimetic ABT-737 sensitizes human melanoma cells to apoptosis induced by selective BRAF inhibitors but does not reverse acquired resistance. Carcinogenesis. 2013;34:237–247.
123. Yang G, Rajadurai A, Tsao H. Recurrent patterns of dual RB and p53 pathway inactivation in melanoma. J Invest Dermatol. 2005;125:1242–51.
124. Yokoyama S, Woods SL, Boyle GM, Aoude LG, MacGregor S, Zismann V, Gartside M, Cust AE, Haq R, Harland M, Taylor JC, Duffy DL, Holohan K, Dutton-Regester K, Palmer JM, Bonazzi V, Stark MS, Symmons J, Law MH, Schmidt C, Lanagan C, O'Connor L, Holland EA, Schmid H, Maskiell JA, Jetann J, Ferguson M, Jenkins MA, Kefford RF, Giles GG, Armstrong BK, Aitken JF, Hopper JL, Whiteman DC, Pharoah PD, Easton DF, Dunning AM, Newton-Bishop JA, Montgomery GW, Martin NG, Mann GJ, Bishop DT, Tsao H, Trent JM, Fisher DE, Hayward NK, Brown KM. A novel recurrent mutation in MITF predisposes to familial and sporadic melanoma. Nature. 2011;480:99–103.
125. Zuo L, Weger J, Yang Q, Goldstein AM, Tucker MA, Walker GJ, Hayward N, Dracopoli NC. Germline mutations in the p16INK4a binding domain of CDK4 in familial melanoma. Nat Genet. 1996;12:97–9.
126. Robert L, Tumeh PC, Harview CL, Yearley JH, Shintaku IP, Taylor EJ, Chmielowski B, Spasic M, Henry G, Ciobanu V, West AN, Carmona M, Kivork C, Seja E, Cherry G, Gutierrez AJ, Grogan TR, Mateus C, Tomasic G, Glaspy JA, Emerson RO, Robins H, Pierce RH, Elashoff DA, Robert C, Ribas A. Anti-programmed-death-receptor-1 treatment with pembrolizumab in ipilimumab-refractory advanced melanoma: a randomised dose-comparison cohort of a phase 1 trial. Lancet. 2014;384(9948):1109–17.
127. Tumeh PC, Harview CL, Yearley JH, Shintaku IP, Taylor EJ, Robert L, Chmielowski B, Spasic M, Henry G, Ciobanu V, West AN, Carmona M, Kivork C, Seja E, Cherry G, Gutierrez AJ, Grogan TR, Mateus C, Tomasic G, Glaspy JA, Emerson RO, Robins H, Pierce RH, Elashoff DA, Robert C, Ribas A. PD-1 blockade induces responses by inhibiting adaptive immune resistance. Nature. 2014;515(7528):568–71.

Targeted and Personalized Therapy for Nonmelanoma Skin Cancers

3

Chantal C. Bachmann and Günther F.L. Hofbauer

Contents

Abbreviations

5-FU	5-Fluorouracil
AK	Actinic keratosis
ALA	5-Aminolevulinic acid
AZA	Azathioprine
BCC	Basal cell carcinoma
CLL	Chronic lymphocytic leukemia
CNI	Calcineurin inhibitors such as cyclosporin A, tacrolimus
COX-2	Cyclooxygenase-2
CsA	Cyclosporin A
LSRs	Local skin reactions
MAL	Methyl aminolevulinate
MMF	Mycophenolate mofetil
NHL	Non-Hodgkin lymphoma
NMSC	Nonmelanoma skin cancer
OTR	Organ transplant recipients
PDT	Photodynamic therapy
RCT	Randomized controlled trial
REAKT	Swiss Registry of Actinic Keratosis Treatment
SA	Salicylic acid
SCC	Squamous cell carcinoma
UV	Ultraviolet
UVA	Ultraviolet-A

C.C. Bachmann, MD • G.F.L. Hofbauer, MD (✉)
Department of Dermatology, UniversitätsSpital
Zürich, Zürich 8091, Switzerland
e-mail: hofbauer@usz.ch

T. Bieber, F. Nestle (eds.), *Personalized Treatment Options in Dermatology*,
DOI 10.1007/978-3-662-45840-2_3, © Springer-Verlag Berlin Heidelberg 2015

3.1 Introduction

Chronic ultraviolet (UV) radiation is the main risk factor for actinic keratoses (AKs). Patients with field cancerization (defined as two or more AKs on photodamaged skin) are at an increased risk for invasive nonmelanoma skin cancer (NMSC).

Further field cancerization is also associated with other forms of NMSC – including Bowen's disease, squamous cell carcinoma (SCC), and basal cell carcinoma (BCC).

3.2 Actinic Keratosis and Field Cancerization Background

AKs are intraepidermal lesions typically presenting as rough, scaly, keratotic macules, papules, or plaques. The lesions typically appear on the skin that has been subject to chronic exposure – the so-called sun terraces of the skin, including the face, chest, ear lobes, balding scalp, and backs of arms and hands – and are an indicator of cumulative UV exposure. Some patients may present with a single lesion, but the typical clinical presentation is multiple lesions across an area of sun-damaged skin. 7.7 AKs per person have been found in a seminal Australian study of more than 1,000 people over the age of 40 [1].

Before invasive SCC develops, intraepithelial changes occur in the clinical forms of AK and Bowen's disease. While only the latter is traditionally called carcinoma in situ due to its total loss of regular architecture of the epidermis, we believe that AK is part of the continuum of SCC development based on histological and molecular changes common to AK, Bowen's disease, and invasive SCC [2].

Histologically, AK is characterized by atypia or dysplasia of the keratinocytes in the basal layer of the epidermis and with progression in epidermal layers above. Disordered maturation of the superficial layers results in alternating areas of parakeratosis and hyperkeratosis [3].

A significant advance leading to more effective treatment of AK is acceptance of field cancerization as an underlying condition driving disease pathology and progression. UV exposure is believed to generate field cancerization. It is widely accepted that visible AK lesions (whether few or many) are a manifestation of pervasive damage and that the surrounding area ("field") of sun-damaged skin contains subclinical lesions and cellular changes. Bowen's disease, SCC, and BCC are also visible indicators of this damage. The presence of any of these NMSC lesions (to include AK) represents evidence of field cancerization.

The current focus of AK treatment is to target field cancerization, rather than limiting treatment to clinically apparent individual lesions.

3.3 Epidemiology and Risk Factors

AKs occur more frequently in regions with higher UV exposure and in fair-skinned populations. A 2006 report from the World Health Organization noted a clear relationship between latitude and AK prevalence as well as the likelihood of multiple AKs at lower latitudes [4]. Prevalence rates of 40–60 % in adults in Australia and 11–25 % in various Northern Hemisphere populations have been reported [5]. Prevalence rates are greater in males than in females and increase with age [5].

The most notable risk factor for development of AK is accumulated chronic UV radiation exposure, and the person with AK typically presents with characteristic signs of photodamage, including freckles and solar lentigines. Recently published results from a multicenter study across eight European countries provide additional information about a number of risk factors [6]. Differences in risk were noted among hair and eye coloration: red hair conferred a seven times higher risk than black hair, and brown eyes about a 40 % reduced risk when compared to blue. The presence of even a few freckles on the face was found to confer greater risk. Outdoor occupation, history of sunburns as a child, and residency in a tropical country were all associated with increased risk, whereas higher education levels were associated with a significantly reduced risk. This study also noted potentially significant increased risks in patients taking photosensitizing thiazide diuretics and cardiac drugs and a possible protective effect from nonsteroidal anti-inflammatory drugs (NSAIDs).

Patients who are immunocompromised are at significant increased risk for development of NMSC, as are patients with genetic disorders such as xeroderma pigmentosum.

3.4 AK Progression to SCC

Although not all AKs will progress to SCC – and, indeed, some AKs will regress – there is a clear relationship between AK and SCC. A review of the evidence supporting this relationship found that approximately 90 % of SCCs may have contiguous AKs, consistent with the concept that AKs are preinvasive forms of SCC [3]. One study found that up to 60 % of SCCs arise directly from an AK [7]. Another study found that 136 of 165 cutaneous SCCs examined were closely associated with AKs; of these, 26.7 % of the SCCs were found to have arisen directly from an existing AK lesion, and another 55.7 % were in close proximity to an AK lesion [8].

A large majority of lesions remain stable and others will regress. The review found that annual rates of regression for single lesions ranged between 15 and 63 %, with recurrence rates of 15–53 % [9].

The uncertainty of the timing and likelihood of AK progression has stimulated much discussion regarding the best treatment approach to AK, with some advocating watchful waiting and others a more aggressive approach. It is the perspective of the REAKT Working Group that we must consider AK a serious precursor to more invasive disease and treat promptly. The treatment algorithm will present appropriate treatment path based on patient presentation and risk factors, balancing health, fiscal, and quality-of-life concerns (Fig. 3.1).

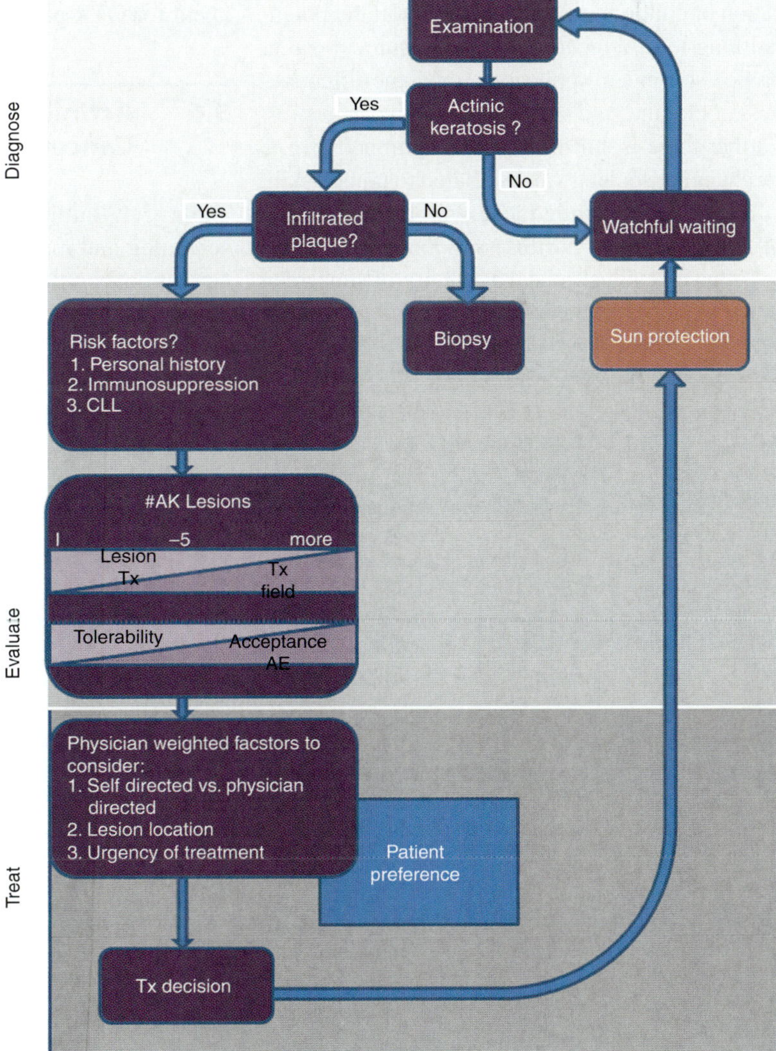

Fig. 3.1 Actinic keratosis and field cancerization treatment algorithm. The algorithm is intended to aid in the treatment decision process for actinic keratosis and field cancerization and is not intended to replace a physician's best judgment on the most appropriate treatment path for each individual patient

3.5 Prevention

As stated, chronic UV radiation exposure is understood to play an essential role in the development of AK and other forms of NMSC. Childhood and adolescence are pivotal periods for primary prevention efforts, which should focus on reducing overall exposure (minimizing the incidence of childhood sunburn) and helping to establish lifelong self-care habits. There is a need for primary prevention measures starting in childhood to reduce overall population-based risk for AK and NMSC.

Prevention measures focus on limiting UVA (ultraviolet-A) photodamage through avoidance of unnecessary exposure to UV light (including sunbeds) and the use of sunscreen when exposure is unavoidable. Despite wide-ranging skin cancer education, there remain needs for continued education of children and adolescent about the potential long-term effects of excessive sun exposure, proper sunscreen application, and the effectiveness of clothing and shade as protective measures. Further there is still a need for continued efforts on changing societal values related to tanned skin.

In adults, including those who have a history of AKs or other NMSC, randomized clinical trials have demonstrated that the use of sunscreen reduces the incidence of AKs and SCC. A randomized, controlled trial demonstrated reduction in SCC (but not BCC) through the regular use of sunscreen within 4.5 years [10]. In particular high-risk populations may also benefit from sunscreen use. Ulrich and colleagues studied the protective effects of regular sunscreen use on the development of NMSC in organ transplant recipients (OTR) and showed a reduction in lesion count from baseline and fewer lesions overall than the control group [11].

In very high-risk patients, the use of systemic chemoprevention like acitretin may also have some benefit [12]. In addition, two small, open-label studies demonstrated some protective benefits of oral capecitabine in OTR [13, 14]. The efficacy of afamelanotide, a first-in-class photoprotective drug, for use as a photoprotective agent for OTR patients is currently discussed.

3.6 Actinic Keratosis and Field Cancerization Management

Table 3.1 outlines the recommendations for screening and management of AK and field cancerization based on patient and disease factors.

Table 3.1 Management recommendations for actinic keratosis and field cancerization

Patient presentation	Recommended management	Suggested timing	Additional information
Photodamage; no other risk factors	Clinical skin examination	If new lesions occur	
	Patient-directed self-examination	Every 3 months	
Fewer than 5 lesions; no other risk factors	Clinical skin examination	Every 12 months	
	Patient-directed self-examination	Every 3 months	
Recurrent lesions and recalcitrant lesions	Clinical skin examination	Every 3, 6, and 12 months following treatment	Recalcitrant lesion requires biopsy by dermatologist
		At least every 6 months thereafter	
	Patient-directed self-examination	Every 3 months	
History of skin cancer	Clinical skin examination	Every 3, 6, and 12 months following treatment	Lymph node exam by dermatology specialist in high-risk patients
		At least every 12 months thereafter	
	Patient-directed self-examination	Every 3 months	
CLL/OTR	Clinical skin examination by dermatology specialist	For CLL:	Invasiveness of skin lesions can be clinically underestimated in CLL/OTR
		Every 12 months	
		For OTR:	
		One screening exam pretransplantation	
		Clinical exam at least every 12 months following transplantation	
	Patient-directed self-examination	Every month	

Absent specific risk factors, we recommend encouraging patients to perform skin self-examination every 3 months, with clinical examination if new lesions are noted. Certain risk factors require more frequent self- and clinical exams, as noted in the table. In any patient type, suspicious lesions necessitate timely professional inspection.

Professional screening for AK and field cancerization offers several important benefits. It enables the patient and physician to establish a baseline (at first screening) or note changes to the patient's skin since the last visit, thereby potentially promoting earlier identification of new or changing lesions. It also offers the opportunity to evaluate for other skin cancers, such as melanoma. Skin examinations should be comprehensive, including areas such as the scalp, palms, oral cavity, and genitalia. For patients at high risk for invasive skin cancer (e.g., those with history of melanoma or who have large lesions), it is recommended that the examination include palpation of the lymph nodes.

Clinician visits also offer the opportunity to introduce or reinforce prevention and self-care habits, as patients are typically noncompliant with regular self-examination as well as clinical examination of new lesions. Patients should be trained on how to effectively perform at-home skin self-examination.

Of course high-risk patients for NMSC like OTR, as well as patients with chronic lymphocytic leukemia (CLL) and other patients on long-term immunosuppression, require special consideration for screening. Annual clinical exams by a dermatology specialist and monthly skin self-examinations are encouraged for these patients; OTR should be screened by a dermatologist for NMSC prior to transplantation [15].

3.7 Clinical Assessment/ Diagnosis

AK lesions can often be diagnosed clinically. They broadly presents visually as a scaly, ill-defined macule, papule, or plaque, commonly flesh colored, pink, or reddish brown. A classic feature of many AKs is a rough "sandpaper" feel.

Firm, raised, and tender lesions are at greater risk for invasive carcinoma and should be biopsied. AK lesions may be solitary but more commonly present as multiple lesions in a photodamaged field.

Dermoscopy is very helpful for accurate diagnosis of AK. A red pseudonetwork is a widely cited characteristic dermatoscopic finding of AK and is significantly associated with AK [16, 17]. Other features include a pattern of linear wavy vessels in facial nonpigmented lesions and multiple gray or brown dots and globules around the follicular ostia in pigmented lesions [16].

If in a single patient two or more lesions of AK, Bowen's disease, invasive SCC, or BCC with accompanying photodamaged skin (with clinical signs such as skin atrophy, inhomogeneous pigmentation, dermatochalasis, purpura senilis of Bateman, or pseudocicatrices stellaires) have been diagnosed, the diagnosis of field cancerization should be considered.

3.8 Treatment Considerations

Although at this time it is not possible to predict which AKs will progress to invasive SCC, early diagnosis and treatment is believed to be key for minimizing disease progression and severity [18, 19].

Based on the patient's presentation and risk characteristics, the treatment strategy may differ (Table 3.2) [20].

Table 3.2 Factors that influence treatment decisions for actinic keratosis and field cancerization

Disease-specific factors
Progression/development of disease
Number of lesions
Localization and severity of disease
Location of lesions
Recurrence
Patient-specific factors
Age
Mental condition
Ability and willingness to adhere to therapy
History of skin cancer
Risk factors, especially immunosuppression

Treatment decisions must also be weighed against tolerability data and the burden presented by the treatment regimen in the context of the patient's disease considerations. For example, in a patient with no known risk factors and a single clinical lesion, the treatment path may appropriately be quite different from that of the patient with many visible lesions in a damaged field and a history of prior NMSC. Lesion location is an important factor, as lesions located in difficult-to-treat areas (e.g., the back) may prove too burdensome for patient-directed home-based treatment. There are different general paths dependent on the patient's disease severity and unique risk profile.

Specific considerations related to the patient's lifestyle, competence, and attitude toward treatment should significantly influence the treatment decision, as they are all important contributors to the patient's adherence behaviors [21]. Because treatment adherence is the foundation of good outcomes, it is essential to anticipate common factors associated with poor adherence and effectively work to overcome patient barriers.

3.9 Treatment Options

Treatment approaches to AK can be broadly divided into lesion directed or field directed. Lesion-directed therapies work by physically destroying individual clinically apparent lesions and are best reserved for use in patients who have only a few isolated lesions and no elevated risk for development of invasive NMSC. Field-directed therapies target both clinically visible lesions and preclinical lesions and other changes in keratinocytes in the skin surrounding the visible lesion. Because AK is a visible marker of more extensive damage caused by chronic UV radiation exposure, it is recommended field-directed therapy as the optimal treatment approach for most patients.

Figure 3.1 presents a visual guide designed to assist physicians with the important decision points inherent to determining the best treatment approach for each individual patient.

3.9.1 Sunscreen

Several studies have demonstrated benefit with regular sunscreen use for prevention of new AK lesions and mitigation of field cancerization progression to SCC and other invasive skin cancers [10, 11, 22, 23]. One Australian study [23] noted a clear dose-response relationship after the use of daily sunscreen that applied to both the formation of new lesions and remission of existing lesions. We recommend that all patients presenting with field cancerization be encouraged to use sunscreen frequently (daily is recommended). Education is recommended to ensure that patients use an appropriate dose; underdosing is a common mistake.

3.9.2 Curettage

Curettage is not a first-line therapy for treatment of AKs. The treatment is best reserved for treating a small number of AKs and/or thick, hyperkeratotic lesions. Any potential benefits of curettage must be balanced against common adverse outcomes, including infection, scarring, and pigmentary changes. Curettage has no benefit in treating subclinical lesions or the broader damaged field.

3.9.3 Cryotherapy

Cryotherapy is the most widely used nonsurgical technique for treatment of a broad range of skin cancers and remains the most common treatment for AKs [24]. Its procedure is simple, widely available, quick, and effective. So far there is no standardized approach to frequency, duration, intensity, or temperature of cryotherapy. This leads to a variety of physician-specific approaches with resulting differences in outcomes.

Study results [25] show in general that higher efficacy rates are linked to longer freeze times; longer freeze times, in turn, are associated with higher incidence of undesirable adverse effects. Cosmetic response was rated "good" or "excellent" in 94 % of the patients who had a 100 % response rate at 3 months following treatment.

Pain, redness, edema, and blistering are common side effects of treatment with cryotherapy. In addition, significant local adverse events, such as hyper- or hypopigmentation (up to 29 %), scarring, and hair loss, have been observed [25, 26]. Cryopeeling (diffuse cryotherapy) has been suggested as a possible approach for treating individual AKs as well as the broader damaged field [27]. Evidence for this treatment is limited, and no standardization in approach or methods exists.

3.9.4 5-Fluorouracil

Topical 5-FU interferes with deoxyribonucleic (DNA) and ribonucleic (RNA) synthesis in rapidly dividing cells, preventing cell proliferation and resulting in cell death. Clinical study of 5-FU has reported field clearance rates of 42–96 %, with recurrence rates up to 55 % [28–30]. 5-FU is associated with an almost 100 % incidence of local skin reactions. A 5 % formulation of fluorouracil is available for treatment of senile and actinic keratosis, requiring application once or twice daily for 3–4 weeks or longer in some cases. A 0.5 % fluorouracil formulation has demonstrated similar efficacy rates as the 5 % formulation but appears to cause less severe adverse events and is associated with improved patient satisfaction [30–32].

A combination product of 5-FU 0.5 % plus salicylic acid (SA) 10 % solution is approved in Switzerland for once-daily application over 12 weeks. In one trial [33], patients were treated with the combination 5-FU + SA and demonstrated significantly greater histological clearance (72 %) and complete clearance (55.4 %) rates at 20 weeks than either the vehicle or diclofenac 3 %. Application-site reactions were more common with the 5-FU + SA product but were mostly mild to moderate.

3.9.5 Diclofenac

Diclofenac sodium 3 % gel in a hyaluronic acid vehicle is approved for treatment of AK with a twice-daily administration for 60–90 days. Diclofenac is a nonsteroidal anti-inflammatory cyclooxygenase-2 (COX-2) inhibitor. Activation of COX-2 has been implicated in UV-induced skin cancers; inhibition of the COX-2 pathway has been shown to significantly reduce UV-induced tumorigenesis [34]. Diclofenac sodium 3 % gel in hyaluronic acid also induces apoptosis, which is believed to play an important role in its effectiveness as an AK treatment [35]. Forty percent complete clearance rate has been demonstrated in a meta-analysis of three trials [36].

Studies [37, 38] are suggesting that diclofenac sodium 3 % gel is also effective and well tolerated as a treatment of AKs in OTR. The complete clearance rate in a randomized controlled trial was 41 % and overall lesion counts decreased; importantly in this high-risk patient group, there were no cases of invasive SCC or aggressive AK in the 24-month follow-up period [38]. Diclofenac is typically associated with mild-to-moderate application-site reactions.

3.9.6 Imiquimod

Imiquimod is an immune-response modifier that is well studied for treatment of AK. The approved course of therapy for treatment of non-hyperkeratotic, non-hypertrophic AKs on the face or scalp is three times per week for 16 weeks. Complete clearance rates from clinical trials of this protocol range from 48.3 to 57.1 % [39, 40].

Long-term follow-up data revealed that 24.7 % of patients who applied imiquimod three times weekly had a recurrence of AK in the original treatment area after a median follow-up period of 16 months [41]. An overall complete clearance rate was shown ranging between 53.7 and 55 % in two studies [42, 43]. Topical imiquimod causes local skin reactions (LSRs), including severe erythema, scabbing, and ulceration. In addition, it has been associated with fairly significant but rare adverse events, including flares of previously controlled autoimmune diseases [44–47]. Despite these potential side effects, imiquimod is typically well tolerated.

In 2012, a 3.75 % imiquimod formulation was approved in Europe. Clinical trial data demonstrates that a complete clearance rate after application of imiquimod 3.75 % (treatment daily for 2 weeks, followed by 2 weeks without treatment, and then another 2 weeks with daily treatment) was 35.6 % and the partial clearance rate was 59.4 % [48]. Similar results have been seen with a regimen 3/3/3 (treatment daily for 3 weeks, followed by 3 weeks without treatment, and then another 3 weeks with daily treatment) with imiquimod 2.5 and 3.75 % [49]. Although most subjects experienced LSRs (up to 55 % of which were considered severe in the 3/3/3 protocol group), patient adherence rates exceeded 90 % in the trials [48, 49].

3.9.7 Resiquimod (Emerging Therapy)

Resiquimod is an investigational toll-like receptor 7 and 8 antagonist. Resiquimod's immunomodulatory effects are comparable to imiquimod, but it has greater potency in inducing cytokine expression [50, 51]. A phase 2 dose-ranging study evaluated the safety and efficacy of four different concentrations of resiquimod gel (0.01, 0.03, 0.06, and 0.1 %), applied once daily three times per week for 4 weeks [52]. Complete clearance rates after one course of treatment ranged from 40 % (0.01 % concentration) to 74.2 % (0.03 % concentration). After an 8-week treatment-free interval, patients with remaining lesions received a second course of treatment. Overall complete clearance rates ranged from 77.1 % (0.01 % concentration) to 90.3 % (0.03 % concentration). The most common adverse events were application-site reactions. In the dose-ranging study higher concentrations were associated with a greater incidence of adverse events and more severe adverse events. The lower concentrations (0.01 and 0.03 %) were better tolerated.

3.9.8 Ingenol Mebutate

Ingenol mebutate is the most recent option for the non-hyperkeratotic, non-hypertrophic AK treatment. Ingenol mebutate is a novel drug that appears to have two distinct and complementary mechanisms of action: initial rapid lesion necrosis within hours of application followed by specific neutrophil-mediated, antibody-dependent cellular cytotoxicity within days [53].

Ingenol mebutate gel is available in two strengths: 150 mcg/g, administered once daily for three consecutive days to the face and/or scalp, and 500 mcg/g, administered once daily for two consecutive days to the trunk and/or extremities. A pooled analysis of two phase 3 studies of ingenol mebutate 150 mcg/g for the face/scalp indicated that ingenol mebutate shows a complete clearance rate of 42.2 % versus 3.7 % for placebo ($p < 0.001$) [54]. A pooled analysis of two additional phase 3 studies of the 500 mcg/g concentration for the trunk/extremities revealed similar efficacy, with a complete clearance rate of 34.1 % with ingenol mebutate versus 4.7 % with placebo ($p < 0.001$) [54].

LSRs were the most common adverse events in the phase 3 studies [54]. For the 150 mcg/g concentration, LSRs peaked at day 4 following treatment initiation, rapidly decreased by day 8, and then continued to decrease until returning to baseline around day 29. For the 500 mcg/g concentration, LSRs peaked between days 3 and 8 and then followed a similar pattern as with the 150 mcg/g concentration, returning to baseline by about day 29. Fewer than 2 % of subjects who received ingenol mebutate experienced more serious adverse events. More than 98 % of patients in the four trials completed the treatment protocol, thus showing adherence rates similar to those expected with physician-directed treatments [54].

One hundred seventy-one patients who had achieved complete clearance by day 57 in the ingenol mebutate phase 3 trials completed a 12-month observational follow-up study [55]. At 12 months, there was a 46 % sustained clearance rate (face and scalp lesions) and an 87 % reduction in the number of AK lesions as compared to baseline.

A study that investigated the potential for systemic absorption of ingenol mebutate found that no systemic exposure of ingenol mebutate or its metabolites was detected in any sample (lower limit of quantification = 0.1 ng/mL) [56].

3.9.9 Photodynamic Therapy (PDT)

PDT involves the irradiation of AK lesions with light to cause cell death. Prior to light exposure, a photosensitizing agent is applied; neoplastic cells accumulate more of the agent than normal cells and are thus subject to greater thermal and chemical effects. The most frequently used photosensitizing agents are 5-aminolevulinic acid (ALA) and its methyl ester MAL. MAL-PDT is approved for treatment of thin or non-hyperkeratotic AKs on the face or scalp. ALA-PDT is approved for treatment of mild AKs with a maximum diameter of 1.8 cm on the face and hairless regions of the scalp. In addition to topical creams, an ALA patch is also available and demonstrates similar efficacy as the creams. Treatment protocols for PDT are not yet standardized; incubation times, wavelength, and dose differ in both trial and practice [57–61].

Studies of ALA-PDT and MAL-PDT reveal similar efficacy. One study results of ALA-PDT range between 66 % lesion clearance at 8 weeks (following single treatment) and 85–89 % at 16 weeks (following retreatment) [62, 63]. A study of MAL-PDT demonstrated complete (lesion) response rates of up to 89 % with retreatment [64]. Pretreatment curettage is often used in conjunction with PDT and probably enhances the efficacy rates. PDT is associated with pain (more significant with ALA) and hypersensitivity to light. However, PDT can be used over large areas in a single session and has been associated with favorable cosmetic results. A recent study demonstrated that MAL-PDT was associated with reduced keratinocyte atypia on photodamaged skin (supporting its efficacy in field cancerization) as well as an increase of new collagen deposition (perhaps explaining its beneficial cosmetic effect) [65].

In patients with thin AK lesions in large field-cancerized areas, daylight-mediated PDT may provide an effective and less painful treatment option [66]. Several small randomized clinical studies of daylight-mediated PDT for treatment of mostly thin AK lesions on the face and scalp have demonstrated 3-month lesion response rates of 75–79 %, with significantly less pain than reported with conventional PDT [67–69]. This treatment approach is still in development.

3.9.10 Radiotherapy

Radiotherapy is an effective approach for treatment of AK and field cancerization in patients who require treatment of a large field with a multiplicity of lesions or in patients with lesions that have not been responsive to other treatments [70–72].

Radiotherapy allows irradiation of large fields (the size of two outstretched hands) of damaged skin at each session and is most commonly used for treatment of the face and balding scalp. Recommended treatment is six sessions over 3 weeks, although some case reports have reported more sessions [71]. Cosmetic outcomes are typically excellent, and effects of treatment last up to two decades. Radiotherapy treatment for cutaneous neoplasms on the trunk and limbs has been associated with poorer cosmetic outcomes [73], but radiotherapy may be used to treat the lower arms and legs if indicated.

Grenz ray therapy is the preferred modality, as soft X-ray therapy may induce permanent alopecia. Side effects and adverse events are typically limited to some mild discomfort and reddening of the skin for 2 weeks following the treatment. Because there is a small increased risk for development of a secondary malignancy due to treatment, radiotherapy is contraindicated for treatment of AK in immunosuppressed patients. In addition, radiotherapy is best reserved for older patients (60 years +) in order to maximize the typically long-term results of treatment while minimizing the risk for secondary malignancy, which also has a typically long-term latency period.

3.9.11 Other Therapies

Other treatments for AK are available, but the evidence behind their use is less robust in comparison to effective options already presented. We briefly review these other treatment options.

Excision of AK lesions is not a first-line treatment approach. Shave or punch excision is occasionally used to treat individual lesions, typically to obtain a specimen for histologic examination in cases of suspected invasive SCC [74].

Skin grafting may have some benefit in high-risk patients with severely actinically damaged skin. A retrospective study of 11 kidney transplant patients who underwent surgical resurfacing of the entire dorsum of the hand as a treatment for multiple skin cancers demonstrated no recurrences of skin cancer over a mean follow-up time of 4.7 years [75].

Topical retinoids have been studied for treatment of AK. Recent results from a large randomized chemoprevention trial in high-risk patients demonstrated no differences in NMSC development or AK counts between the tretinoin group and the control group [76].

Skin resurfacing with chemical peels or lasers has shown some good results. A small, randomized, prospective study comparing carbon dioxide (CO_2) laser resurfacing, 30 % trichloroacetic acid (TCA) peels, and 5-FU administration (3 weeks) demonstrated similar efficacy results among the three treatment groups [77]. The results vary strongly depending on the agent used of chemical peeling and on skill and technique of the physician using a laser. Small studies have reported some benefits from dermabrasion for treatment of AK. But these study results are not compelling, and there are side effects, including bleeding and scarring.

Table 3.3 summarizes the available treatments for AK discussed throughout this section and their efficacy in the treatment of field cancerization. Figure 3.2 presents the REAKT Working Group's assessment of each available treatment within the context of important considerations related to selecting the optimum treatment for specific patients.

Table 3.3 Summary of treatments for actinic keratosis and efficacy in the treatment of field cancerization

Treatment	LD/FD	Evidence of treatment benefits	OCEBM LOE	Comments
Sunscreen	FD	Use of sunscreen improves lesion remission and reduces lesion progression	2	Use is encouraged adjunctively for all patients May be used as sole treatment in some patients Should be applied to all sun-exposed areas
Curettage/ electrodessication	LD	Undocumented	N/A	May be beneficial in hyperkeratotic lesions and in combination with field therapy Localized use preferred over field application
Cryotherapy	LD	Some field cancerization benefit reported in a review of charts from a single practice where patients were treated with a cryopeeling technique	4	Widely used lesion-directed treatment Physician-directed treatment Approach is not standardized, leading to wide range of outcomes Localized use preferred over field application
5-Fluorouracil	FD	Complete clearance rates for 5 % 5-FU 42–96 %, 4 weeks posttreatment Sustained clearance rate at 12 months: 33 % (one RCT) Complete clearance rate for 0.5 % 5-FU + SA at 8 weeks following treatment: 55.4 %	1	Treatment of large areas possible with occlusion (Unna boot). This use is physician directed
Diclofenac	FD	Complete clearance rate 30 days following treatment: approximately 40 % (meta-analysis of 3 RCTs with treatment duration either 60 or 90 days)	1	Good cosmesis Larger areas can be treated depending on side effects and patient tolerance

Table 3.3 (continued)

Treatment	LD/FD	Efficacy in treatment of field cancerization		Comments
		Evidence of treatment benefits	OCEBM LOE	
Imiquimod	FD	Complete clearance rates after 16-week course: 48.3–57.1 %	1	Unmasking of subclinical lesions
		Complete clearance rates after 4-week short-course treatment: 26.8 % after one course; 53.7 % after 2 courses		Systemic reactions rarely
				Larger areas can be treated depending on side effects and patient tolerance
Resiquimod (currently in phase 3)	FD	Complete clearance rates 8 weeks following treatment	3	Treatment aimed at biological response (inflammation). Inflammation may be early or late
		After one course of treatment: 40–74.2 % (dose dependent)		Larger areas can be treated depending on side effects and patient tolerance
		After second course of treatment: 77.1–90.3 % (dose dependent)		
Ingenol mebutate	FD	Complete clearance rates 57 days following treatment	1	Strong local reaction with short administration time
		37–47 % (face)		Larger areas can be treated depending on side effects and patient tolerance
		28–42 % (body)		
		Sustained clearance rates at 12 months following treatment (patients who had achieved complete clearance at 57 days)		
		46.1 % (face)		
		44 % (body)		
Topical retinoids	FD	Varied efficacies reported. Recent RCT reported no observed difference in lesion counts between topical tretinoin and placebo	2	Not recommended due to low efficacy
ALA/MAL + PDT	LD and FD	Lesion clearance rates range from 66 to 89 % depending on photosynthesizing agent and treatment regimen. Small studies indicate benefit for treatment of field cancerization	3	Physician-directed treatment
				Pain is a consideration and will limit the size of treatment field depending on patient preference and previous experience
				Daylight PDT in development
Radiotherapy (Grenz ray)	FD	13 out of 16 patients had complete clearance 2 weeks following treatment completion	4	Physician-directed treatment
				Recommended that its use be limited to patients over 60 years of age
				1 treatment cycle per field per lifetime
				Grenz ray is recommended. Soft X-ray may induce alopecia
				Larger areas can be treated depending on side effects and patient tolerance
Excision	LD	Undocumented	N/A	Not a first-line treatment
				Appropriate only for localized use. Typically reserved for lesions highly suspicious for invasive SCC
Skin grafting	FD	11 out of 11 patients had complete clearance out to 4.7 years	4	Rarely used; may be helpful in singular cases involving areas of pronounced field cancerization, such as the back of the hands

(continued)

Table 3.3 (continued)

Treatment	LD/FD	Efficacy in treatment of field cancerization		
		Evidence of treatment benefits	OCEBM LOE	Comments
Chemical peels	FD	AK lesion reduction of up to 89 % reported	3	May be helpful in select patients
				Larger areas can be treated depending on side effects and patient tolerance
Laser	FD	AK lesion reduction of up to 92 % reported	3	May be helpful in select patients
				Larger areas can be treated depending on side effects and patient tolerance
Dermabrasion	FD	Some sustained benefit observed in small case series	4	May be helpful in select patients
				Larger areas can be treated depending on side effects and patient tolerance

Note: The level of evidence has been noted based on evidence of each treatment's efficacy for field cancerization. Treatment comments and recommendations for use are based on a consideration of available evidence as of the article submission date regarding treatment of field cancerization, in conjunction with the subjective opinions of the authors based on their collective practical experiences. It is not the intention of the REAKT Working Group to preferentially promote the use of one modality or product over another except within the context of evidence and experience that supports better efficacy for a patient's unique presentation

3.10 Combination Therapy: Concomitant and Sequential Approaches

Combination therapy may be especially helpful when treating patients with many lesions. Although lesion-directed therapy is not recommended for treatment of field cancerization, in some patients judicious use of lesion-directed therapy in combination with field-directed therapy may prove to be the most beneficial approach. Although the potential benefits of combination therapy are significant, there are no guidelines or standardized treatment protocols for use of various modalities or topical agents in combination. Combination therapy is also presenting added risks for synergistic adverse events, with potential for increased treatment-related pain and LSRs.

3.10.1 PDT in Combination

One study has demonstrated that sequential therapy with ALA-PDT + imiquimod 5 % provides a better response than either therapy alone, with "significantly less intense local reactions," and greater patient satisfaction than imiquimod 5 % monotherapy [78].

Studies have also investigated sequential treatment strategies using topicals (tazarotene, 5 % 5-FU or diclofenac) as the initial therapy, followed by PDT. These small studies indicated enhanced results over PDT alone and significantly reduce lesion count [79–81].

3.10.2 Cryotherapy in Combination

A number of studies have investigated the use of cryotherapy in combination with other therapies. In two studies, patients with AK were treated with cryotherapy followed by application of imiquimod 3.75 %, imiquimod 5 %, or placebo cream. The results demonstrated that the use of imiquimod 3.75 % post-cryotherapy resulted in subject complete clearance rates of 60 % versus 30 % in subjects who received placebo ($p < 0.001$) and also imiquimod 5 % showed an improved efficiency [82, 83].

Similarly, another study found that cryotherapy followed by application of diclofenac for

Fig. 3.2 Summary of treatment-related considerations for actinic keratosis and field cancerization. The choice of therapeutic modality should be personalized based on physician assessment and patient preference. In practice, displaying options on a two-dimensional grid may provide orientation for such a joint decision-making. Possible pairings of characteristics separate treatment by (**a**) convenience of application versus side effects, (**b**) duration of remission versus duration of therapy, and (**c**) efficacy versus adherence. Treatments have been assessed according to the subjective opinions of the authors based on their collective practical experiences and not necessarily supported by objective data. Treatments are listed in alphabetical order

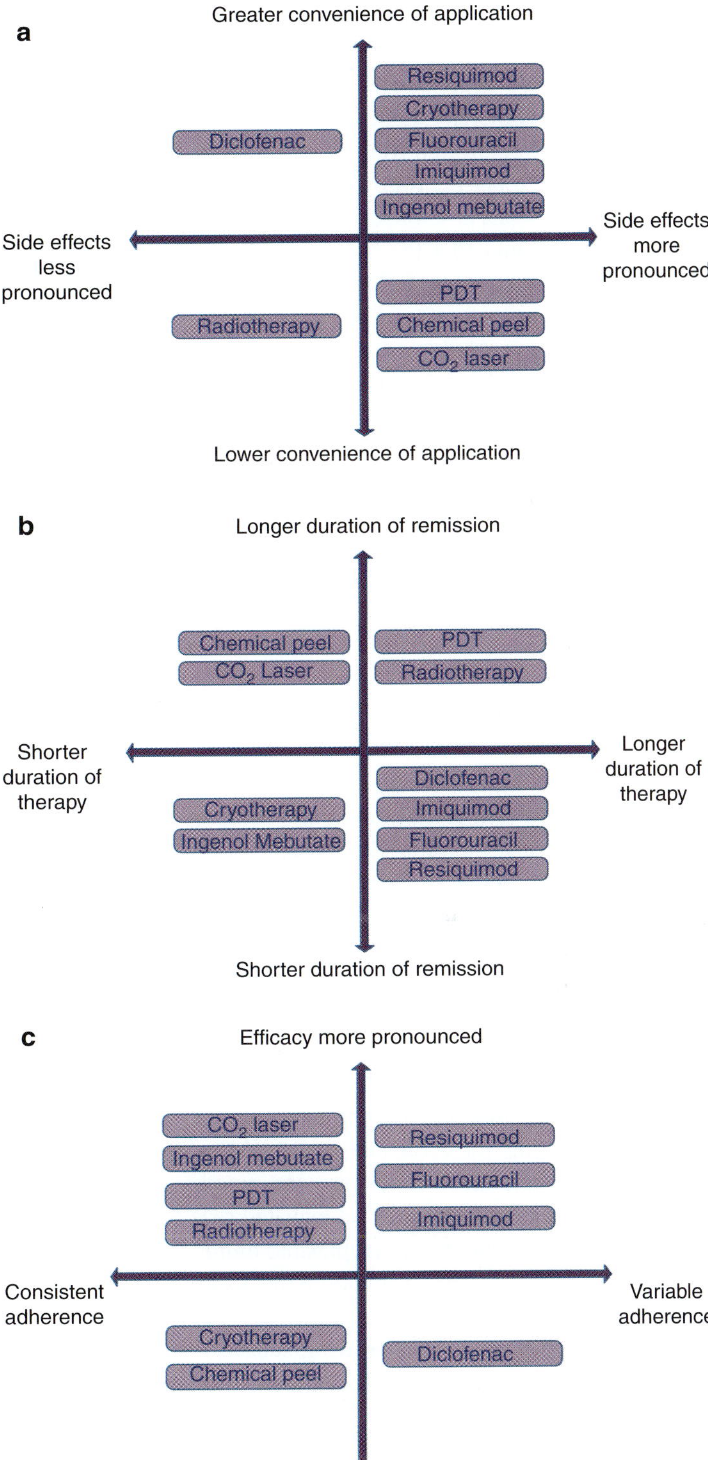

90 days was significantly more effective at clearing lesions than cryotherapy alone: 64 % achieved complete clearance with sequential therapy versus 32 % with cryotherapy alone [84].

A randomized controlled trial of the effect of treatment with 0.5 % 5-FU followed by cryotherapy to residual lesions at 4 weeks following treatment initiation found that the combination was significantly more effective in lowering 6-month lesion count when compared to cryotherapy alone [85].

Studies comparing a sequential treatment regimen of cryotherapy followed by field treatment with ingenol mebutate gel versus cryotherapy followed by vehicle gel for treatment of AKs demonstrated a significantly higher complete clearance rate following sequential treatment with cryotherapy + ingenol mebutate (60.5 % vs. 49.4 %; $p=0.04$) [86, 87].

3.10.3 Combining Topical Therapies

Combinations of topical therapies may also be beneficial. Studies testing the combination of two established topicals, imiquimod 5 % and 5-FU, have shown to be relatively faster and more convenient than either therapy alone [88, 89].

3.11 Management Considerations for the Immunocompromised

Patients who are immunocompromised require diligent monitoring for AKs and other NMSC and aggressive treatment if lesions are noted. Patients with CLL are at significant elevated risk for development of cutaneous neoplasms; multiple instances or aggressive forms of skin cancer could raise suspicion of CLL.

OTR are an important and growing subset of patients at increased risk for the development of NMSC with unusual presentation and aggressive progression rates. OTR have next to the same risk factors as the general population, the added burden of immunosuppressive therapy. Up to 40 % of OTR patients develop premalignant tumors within the first 5 years of immunosuppression [90, 91].

The increased risk of skin cancer may result from decreased immunosurveillance as well as drug-specific properties [92]. Azathioprine (AZA), for example, has a photosensitivity effect compared to mycophenolate (MMF). In a Swiss study results revealed that changing from AZA to MMF did reduce skin photosensitivity to UVA, but not UVB, in the patient population tested (primarily skin types II and III) [93].

The use of calcineurin inhibitors has also been associated with an increased risk for NMSC. One study noted a 2.8 times greater risk of NMSC when cyclosporine was added to an immunosuppressive protocol of AZA and prednisolone [94]. Another study found that replacing calcineurin inhibitors with sirolimus reduced the incidence of SCC and lengthened the time to onset, although adverse events were significantly greater with sirolimus therapy [92].

Other studies have found no specific connection between types of immunosuppressive therapy and NMSC risk, and it is possible that the level of immunosuppression is a more critical factor than the type [95].

The immunosuppressed population requires specific targeted surveillance to ensure early diagnosis and management of skin cancers. Therefore, we recommend that OTR and other patients who are immunocompromised receive yearly comprehensive screening to ensure early diagnosis of SCC in situ and timely and aggressive treatment to limit progression. Concern has been raised about the safety of immune stimulators such as imiquimod. However, there is now a body of evidence suggesting that these substances are safe in OTR [96].

References

1. Marks R, Foley P, Goodman G, Hage BH, Selwood TS. Spontaneous remission of solar keratoses: the case for conservative management. Br J Dermatol. 1986;115(6):649–55.
2. Anwar J, Wrone DA, Kimyai-Asadi A, Alam M. The development of actinic keratosis into invasive squamous cell carcinoma: evidence and evolving classification schemes. Clin Dermatol. 2004;22(3):189–96.
3. Roewert-Huber J, Stockfleth E, Kerl H. Pathology and pathobiology of actinic (solar) keratosis – an update. Br J Dermatol. 2007;157 Suppl 2:18–20.

4. Lucas RM, McMichael AJ, Armstrong BK, Smith WT. Estimating the global disease burden due to ultraviolet radiation exposure. Int J Epidemiol. 2008;37(3):654–67.

5. Frost CA, Green AC. Epidemiology of solar keratoses. Br J Dermatol. 1994;131(4):455–64.

6. Traianou A, Ulrich M, Apalla Z, et al. Risk factors for actinic keratosis in eight European centres: a case-control study. Br J Dermatol. 2012;167 Suppl 2:36–42.

7. Marks R, Rennie G, Selwood TS. Malignant transformation of solar keratoses to squamous cell carcinoma. Lancet. 1988;1(8589):795–7.

8. Mittelbronn MA, Mullins DL, Ramos-Caro FA, Flowers FP. Frequency of pre-existing actinic keratosis in cutaneous squamous cell carcinoma. Int J Dermatol. 1998;37(9):677–81.

9. Werner RN, Sammain A, Erdmann R, Hartmann V, Stockfleth E, Nast A. The natural history of actinic keratosis: a systematic review. Br J Dermatol. 2013;169(3):502–18.

10. Green A, Williams G, Neale R, et al. Daily sunscreen application and betacarotene supplementation in prevention of basal-cell and squamous-cell carcinomas of the skin: a randomised controlled trial. Lancet. 1999;354(9180):723–9.

11. Ulrich C, Jürgensen JS, Degen A, et al. Prevention of non-melanoma skin cancer in organ transplant patients by regular use of a sunscreen: a 24 months, prospective, case-control study. Br J Dermatol. 2009;161 Suppl 3:78–84.

12. Kadakia KC, Barton DL, Loprinzi CL, et al. Randomized controlled trial of acitretin versus placebo in patients at high-risk for basal cell or squamous cell carcinoma of the skin (North Central Cancer Treatment Group Study 969251). Cancer. 2012;118(8):2128–37.

13. Endrizzi BT, Lee PK. Management of carcinoma of the skin in solid organ transplant recipients with oral capecitabine. Dermatol Surg. 2009;35(10):1567–72.

14. Jirakulaporn T, Endrizzi B, Lindgren B, Mathew J, Lee PK, Dudek AZ. Capecitabine for skin cancer prevention in solid organ transplant recipients. Clin Transplant. 2011;25(4):541–8.

15. Hofbauer GF, Anliker M, Arnold A, et al. Swiss clinical practice guidelines for skin cancer in organ transplant recipients. Swiss Med Wkly. 2009;139(29–30):407–15.

16. Peris K, Micantonio T, Piccolo D, Fargnoli MC. Dermoscopic features of actinic keratosis. J Dtsch Dermatol Ges. 2007;5(11):970–6.

17. Zalaudek I, Giacomel J, Schmid K, et al. Dermatoscopy of facial actinic keratosis, intraepidermal carcinoma, and invasive squamous cell carcinoma: a progression model. J Am Acad Dermatol. 2012;66(4):589–97.

18. Wennberg AM, Stenquist B, Stockfleth E, et al. Photodynamic therapy with methyl aminolevulinate for prevention of new skin lesions in transplant recipients: a randomized study. Transplantation. 2008;86(3):423–9.

19. Wulf HC, Pavel S, Stender I, Bakker-Wensveen CA. Topical photodynamic therapy for prevention of new skin lesions in renal transplant recipients. Acta Derm Venereol. 2006;86(1):25–8.

20. Chen SC, Hill ND, Veledar E, Swetter SM, Weinstock MA. Reliability of quantification measures of actinic keratosis. Br J Dermatol. 2013;169(6):1219–22.

21. Elliott R. Non-adherence to medicines: not solved but solvable. J Health Serv Res Policy. 2009;14(1):58–61.

22. Darlington S, Williams G, Neale R, Frost C, Green A. A randomized controlled trial to assess sunscreen application and beta carotene supplementation in the prevention of solar keratoses. Arch Dermatol. 2003;139(4):451–5.

23. Thompson SC, Jolley D, Marks R. Reduction of solar keratoses by regular sunscreen use. N Engl J Med. 1993;329(16):1147–51.

24. Ferrandiz L, Ruiz-de-Casas A, Trakatelli M, et al. Assessing physicians' preferences on skin cancer treatment in Europe. Br J Dermatol. 2012;167 Suppl 2:29–35.

25. Thai KE, Fergin P, Freeman M, et al. A prospective study of the use of cryosurgery for the treatment of actinic keratoses. Int J Dermatol. 2004;43(9):687–92.

26. Zouboulis CC. Cryosurgery in dermatology. Eur J Dermatol. 1998;8(7):466–74.

27. Chiarello SE. Cryopeeling (extensive cryosurgery) for treatment of actinic keratoses: an update and comparison. Dermatol Surg. 2000;26(8):728–32.

28. Krawtchenko N, Roewert-Huber J, Ulrich M, Mann I, Sterry W, Stockfleth E. A randomised study of topical 5% imiquimod vs. topical 5-fluorouracil vs. cryosurgery in immunocompetent patients with actinic keratoses: a comparison of clinical and histological outcomes including 1-year follow-up. Br J Dermatol. 2007;157 Suppl 2:34–40.

29. Gupta AK. The management of actinic keratoses in the United States with topical fluorouracil: a pharmacoeconomic evaluation. Cutis. 2002;70(2 Suppl):30–6.

30. Loven K, Stein L, Furst K, Levy S. Evaluation of the efficacy and tolerability of 0.5% fluorouracil cream and 5% fluorouracil cream applied to each side of the face in patients with actinic keratosis. Clin Ther. 2002;24(6):990–1000.

31. Jorizzo J, Stewart D, Bucko A, et al. Randomized trial evaluating a new 0.5% fluorouracil formulation demonstrates efficacy after 1-, 2-, or 4-week treatment in patients with actinic keratosis. Cutis. 2002;70(6):335–9.

32. Weiss J, Menter A, Hevia O, et al. Effective treatment of actinic keratosis with 0.5% fluorouracil cream for 1, 2, or 4 weeks. Cutis. 2002;70(2 Suppl):22–9.

33. Stockfleth E, Kerl H, Zwingers T, Willers C. Low-dose 5-fluorouracil in combination with salicylic acid as a new lesion-directed option to treat topically actinic keratoses: histological and clinical study results. Br J Dermatol. 2011;165(5):1101–8.

34. Rundhaug JE, Fischer SM. Cyclo-oxygenase-2 plays a critical role in UV-induced skin carcinogenesis. Photochem Photobiol. 2008;84(2):322–9.

35. Fecker LF, Stockfleth E, Nindl I, Ulrich C, Forschner T, Eberle J. The role of apoptosis in therapy and prophylaxis of epithelial tumours by nonsteroidal anti-inflammatory drugs (NSAIDs). Br J Dermatol. 2007;156 Suppl 3:25–33.
36. Wolf JE, Taylor JR, Tschen E, Kang S. Topical 3.0% diclofenac in 2.5% hyaluronan gel in the treatment of actinic keratoses. Int J Dermatol. 2001;40(11):709–13.
37. Ulrich C, Hackethal M, Ulrich M, et al. Treatment of multiple actinic keratoses with topical diclofenac 3% gel in organ transplant recipients: a series of six cases. Br J Dermatol. 2007;156 Suppl 3:40–2.
38. Ulrich C, Johannsen A, Röwert-Huber J, Ulrich M, Sterry W, Stockfleth E. Results of a randomized, placebo-controlled safety and efficacy study of topical diclofenac 3% gel in organ transplant patients with multiple actinic keratoses. Eur J Dermatol. 2010;20(4):482–8.
39. Korman N, Moy R, Ling M, et al. Dosing with 5% imiquimod cream 3 times per week for the treatment of actinic keratosis: results of two phase 3, randomized, double-blind, parallel-group, vehicle-controlled trials. Arch Dermatol. 2005;141(4):467–73.
40. Szeimies RM, Gerritsen MJ, Gupta G, et al. Imiquimod 5% cream for the treatment of actinic keratosis: results from a phase III, randomized, double-blind, vehicle-controlled, clinical trial with histology. J Am Acad Dermatol. 2004;51(4):547–55.
41. Lee PK, Harwell WB, Loven KH, et al. Long-term clinical outcomes following treatment of actinic keratosis with imiquimod 5% cream. Dermatol Surg. 2005;31(6):659–64.
42. Jorizzo J, Dinehart S, Matheson R, et al. Vehicle-controlled, double-blind, randomized study of imiquimod 5% cream applied 3 days per week in one or two courses of treatment for actinic keratoses on the head. J Am Acad Dermatol. 2007;57(2):265–8.
43. Alomar A, Bichel J, McRae S. Vehicle-controlled, randomized, double-blind study to assess safety and efficacy of imiquimod 5% cream applied once daily 3 days per week in one or two courses of treatment of actinic keratoses on the head. Br J Dermatol. 2007;157(1):133–41.
44. Benson E. Imiquimod: potential risk of an immunostimulant. Australas J Dermatol. 2004;45(2):123–4.
45. Patel U, Mark NM, Machler BC, Levine VJ. Imiquimod 5% cream induced psoriasis: a case report, summary of the literature and mechanism. Br J Dermatol. 2011;164(3):670–2.
46. Fanti PA, Dika E, Vaccari S, Miscial C, Varotti C. Generalized psoriasis induced by topical treatment of actinic keratosis with imiquimod. Int J Dermatol. 2006;45(12):1464–5.
47. Wolfe CM, Tafuri N, Hatfield K. Exacerbation of myasthenia gravis during imiquimod treatment. J Drugs Dermatol. 2007;6(7):745–6.
48. Swanson N, Abramovits W, Berman B, Kulp J, Rigel DS, Levy S. Imiquimod 2.5% and 3.75% for the treatment of actinic keratoses: results of two placebo-controlled studies of daily application to the face and balding scalp for two 2-week cycles. J Am Acad Dermatol. 2010;62(4):582–90.
49. Hanke CW, Beer KR, Stockfleth E, Wu J, Rosen T, Levy S. Imiquimod 2.5% and 3.75% for the treatment of actinic keratoses: results of two placebo-controlled studies of daily application to the face and balding scalp for two 3-week cycles. J Am Acad Dermatol. 2010;62(4):573–81.
50. Dockrell DH, Kinghorn GR. Imiquimod and resiquimod as novel immunomodulators. J Antimicrob Chemother. 2001;48(6):751–5.
51. Fujisawa H, Kondo S, Wang B, Shivji GM, Sauder DN. The role of CD4 molecules in the induction phase of contact hypersensitivity cytokine profiles in the skin and lymph nodes. Immunology. 1996;89(2):250–5.
52. Szeimies RM, Bichel J, Ortonne JP, Stockfleth E, Lee J, Meng TC. A phase II dose-ranging study of topical resiquimod to treat actinic keratosis. Br J Dermatol. 2008;159(1):205–10.
53. Rosen RH, Gupta AK, Tyring SK. Dual mechanism of action of ingenol mebutate gel for topical treatment of actinic keratoses: rapid lesion necrosis followed by lesion-specific immune response. J Am Acad Dermatol. 2012;66(3):486–93.
54. Lebwohl M, Swanson N, Anderson LL, Melgaard A, Xu Z, Berman B. Ingenol mebutate gel for actinic keratosis. N Engl J Med. 2012;366(11):1010–9.
55. Lebwohl M, Shumack S, Stein Gold L, Melgaard A, Larsson T, Tyring SK. Long-term follow-up study of ingenol mebutate gel for the treatment of actinic keratoses. JAMA Dermatol. 2013;149(6):666–70.
56. Jarret M, Katsamas J, Cawkill K, Henderson L, Welburn P, editors. A pharmacokinetic study using a highly sensitive and specific method to determine systemic exposure of ingenol mebutate and its two main metabolites, PEP 015 and PEP 025 in human whole blood after topical administration. Am Acad Dermatol. 2013;AB 156.
57. Braathen LR, Szeimies RM, Basset-Seguin N, et al. Guidelines on the use of photodynamic therapy for nonmelanoma skin cancer: an international consensus. International Society for Photodynamic Therapy in Dermatology, 2005. J Am Acad Dermatol. 2007;56(1):125–43.
58. Morton CA, Brown SB, Collins S, et al. Guidelines for topical photodynamic therapy: report of a workshop of the British Photodermatology Group. Br J Dermatol. 2002;146(4):552–67.
59. Morton CA, McKenna KE, Rhodes LE, British Association of Dermatologists Therapy Guidelines and Audit Subcommittee and the British Photodermatology Group. Guidelines for topical photodynamic therapy: update. Br J Dermatol. 2008;159(6):1245–66.
60. Morton CA, Szeimies RM, Sidoroff A, Braathen LR. European guidelines for topical photodynamic therapy part 1: treatment delivery and current indications – actinic keratoses, Bowen's disease, basal cell carcinoma. J Eur Acad Dermatol Venereol. 2013;27(5):536–44.

61. Morton CA, Szeimies RM, Sidoroff A, Braathen LR. European guidelines for topical photodynamic therapy part 2: emerging indications–field cancerization, photorejuvenation and inflammatory/infective dermatoses. J Eur Acad Dermatol Venereol. 2013;27(6):672–9.

62. Jeffes EW, McCullough JL, Weinstein GD, Kaplan R, Glazer SD, Taylor JR. Photodynamic therapy of actinic keratoses with topical aminolevulinic acid hydrochloride and fluorescent blue light. J Am Acad Dermatol. 2001;45(1):96–104.

63. Piacquadio DJ, Chen DM, Farber HF, et al. Photodynamic therapy with aminolevulinic acid topical solution and visible blue light in the treatment of multiple actinic keratoses of the face and scalp: investigator-blinded, phase 3, multicenter trials. Arch Dermatol. 2004;140(1):41–6.

64. Tarstedt M, Rosdahl I, Berne B, Svanberg K, Wennberg AM. A randomized multicenter study to compare two treatment regimens of topical methyl aminolevulinate (Metvix)-PDT in actinic keratosis of the face and scalp. Acta Derm Venereol. 2005;85(5):424–8.

65. Szeimies RM, Torezan L, Niwa A, et al. Clinical, histopathological and immunohistochemical assessment of human skin field cancerization before and after photodynamic therapy. Br J Dermatol. 2012;167(1):150–9.

66. Wiegell SR, Wulf HC, Szeimies RM, et al. Daylight photodynamic therapy for actinic keratosis: an international consensus: International Society for Photodynamic Therapy in Dermatology. J Eur Acad Dermatol Venereol. 2012;26(6):673–9.

67. Wiegell SR, Haedersdal M, Philipsen PA, Eriksen P, Enk CD, Wulf HC. Continuous activation of PpIX by daylight is as effective as and less painful than conventional photodynamic therapy for actinic keratoses; a randomized, controlled, single-blinded study. Br J Dermatol. 2008;158(4):740–6.

68. Wiegell SR, Haedersdal M, Eriksen P, Wulf HC. Photodynamic therapy of actinic keratoses with 8% and 16% methyl aminolaevulinate and home-based daylight exposure: a double-blinded randomized clinical trial. Br J Dermatol. 2009;160(6):1308–14.

69. Wiegell SR, Fabricius S, Stender IM, et al. A randomized, multicentre study of directed daylight exposure times of 1½ vs. 2½ h in daylight-mediated photodynamic therapy with methyl aminolaevulinate in patients with multiple thin actinic keratoses of the face and scalp. Br J Dermatol. 2011;164(5):1083–90.

70. Barta U, Gräfe T, Wollina U. Radiation therapy for extensive actinic keratosis. J Eur Acad Dermatol Venereol. 2000;14(4):293–5.

71. Dinehart SM, Graham M, Maners A. Radiation therapy for widespread actinic keratoses. J Clin Aesthet Dermatol. 2011;4(7):47–50.

72. Pipitone MA, Gloster HM. Superficial squamous cell carcinomas and extensive actinic keratoses of the scalp treated with radiation therapy. Dermatol Surg. 2006;32(5):756–9.

73. Caccialanza M, Piccinno R, Beretta M, Gnecchi L. Results and side effects of dermatologic radiotherapy: a retrospective study of irradiated cutaneous epithelial neoplasms. J Am Acad Dermatol. 1999;41(4):589–94.

74. Emmett AJ, Broadbent GD. Shave excision of superficial solar skin lesions. Plast Reconstr Surg. 1987;80(1):47–54.

75. van Zuuren EJ, Posma AN, Scholtens RE, Vermeer BJ, van der Woude FJ, Bouwes Bavinck JN. Resurfacing the back of the hand as treatment and prevention of multiple skin cancers in kidney transplant recipients. J Am Acad Dermatol. 1994;31(5 Pt 1):760–4.

76. Weinstock MA, Bingham SF, Digiovanna JJ, et al. Tretinoin and the prevention of keratinocyte carcinoma (Basal and squamous cell carcinoma of the skin): a veterans affairs randomized chemoprevention trial. J Invest Dermatol. 2012;132(6):1583–90.

77. Hantash BM, Stewart DB, Cooper ZA, Rehmus WE, Koch RJ, Swetter SM. Facial resurfacing for nonmelanoma skin cancer prophylaxis. Arch Dermatol. 2006;142(8):976–82.

78. Serra-Guillén C, Nagore E, Hueso L, et al. A randomized pilot comparative study of topical methyl aminolevulinate photodynamic therapy versus imiquimod 5% versus sequential application of both therapies in immunocompetent patients with actinic keratosis: clinical and histologic outcomes. J Am Acad Dermatol. 2012;66(4):e131–7.

79. Galitzer BI. Effect of retinoid pretreatment on outcomes of patients treated by photodynamic therapy for actinic keratosis of the hand and forearm. J Drugs Dermatol. 2011;10(10):1124–32.

80. Martin G. Prospective case-based assessment of sequential therapy with topical fluorouracil cream 0.5% and ALA-PDT for the treatment of actinic keratosis. J Drugs Dermatol. 2011;10(4):372–8.

81. Van der Geer S, Krekels GA. Treatment of actinic keratoses on the dorsum of the hands: ALA-PDT versus diclofenac 3% gel followed by ALA-PDT. A placebo-controlled, double-blind, pilot study. J Dermatolog Treat. 2009;20(5):259–65.

82. Jorizzo JL, Markowitz O, Lebwohl MG, et al. A randomized, double-blinded, placebo-controlled, multicenter, efficacy and safety study of 3.75% imiquimod cream following cryosurgery for the treatment of actinic keratoses. J Drugs Dermatol. 2010;9(9):1101–8.

83. Tan JK, Thomas DR, Poulin Y, Maddin F, Tang J. Efficacy of imiquimod as an adjunct to cryotherapy for actinic keratoses. J Cutan Med Surg. 2007;11(6):195–201.

84. Berlin JM, Rigel DS. Diclofenac sodium 3% gel in the treatment of actinic keratoses postcryosurgery. J Drugs Dermatol. 2008;7(7):669–73.

85. Jorizzo J, Weiss J, Furst K, VandePol C, Levy SF. Effect of a 1-week treatment with 0.5% topical fluorouracil on occurrence of actinic keratosis after cryosurgery: a randomized, vehicle-controlled clinical trial. Arch Dermatol. 2004;140(7):813–6.

86. Website Cg. A sequential treatment regimen of cryotherapy and Picato® for the treatment of actinic keratosis on the face and scalp. http://clinicaltrials.gov/ct2/show/NCT01541553?term=ingenol+mebutate+cryotherapy&rank=2. Accessed 4 Jun 2013.

87. Berman B, Goldenberg G, Hanke CW, et al. Efficacy and safety of ingenol mebutate 0.015% gel 3 weeks after cryosurgery of actinic keratosis: 11-week results. J Drugs Dermatol. 2014;13(2):154–60.

88. Ondo AL, Padilla RS, Miedler JD, et al. Treatment-refractory actinic keratoses successfully treated using simultaneous combination topical 5-fluorouracil cream and imiquimod cream: a case-control study. Dermatol Surg. 2012;38(9):1469–76.

89. Price NM. The treatment of actinic keratoses with a combination of 5-fluorouracil and imiquimod creams. J Drugs Dermatol. 2007;6(8):778–81.

90. Ulrich C, Christophers E, Sterry W, Meyer T, Stockfleth E. Skin diseases in organ transplant patients. Hautarzt. 2002;53(8):524–33.

91. Stockfleth E, Ulrich C, Meyer T, Christophers E. Epithelial malignancies in organ transplant patients: clinical presentation and new methods of treatment. Recent Results Cancer Res. 2002;160:251–8.

92. Euvrard S, Morelon E, Rostaing L, et al. Sirolimus and secondary skin-cancer prevention in kidney transplantation. N Engl J Med. 2012;367(4):329–39.

93. Hofbauer GF, Attard NR, Harwood CA, et al. Reversal of UVA skin photosensitivity and DNA damage in kidney transplant recipients by replacing azathioprine. Am J Transplant. 2012;12(1):218–25.

94. Jensen P, Hansen S, Møller B, et al. Skin cancer in kidney and heart transplant recipients and different long-term immunosuppressive therapy regimens. J Am Acad Dermatol. 1999;40(2 Pt 1):177–86.

95. Tessari G, Girolomoni G. Nonmelanoma skin cancer in solid organ transplant recipients: update on epidemiology, risk factors, and management. Dermatol Surg. 2012;38(10):1622–30.

96. Ulrich C, Bichel J, Euvrard S, et al. Topical immunomodulation under systemic immunosuppression: results of a multicentre, randomized, placebo-controlled safety and efficacy study of imiquimod 5% cream for the treatment of actinic keratoses in kidney, heart, and liver transplant patients. Br J Dermatol. 2007;157 Suppl 2:25–31.

Personalized Treatment in Cutaneous T-Cell Lymphoma (CTCL)

4

Jan P. Nicolay and Claus-Detlev Klemke

Contents

J.P. Nicolay, MD, MSc (✉) • C.-D. Klemke, MD
Klinik für Dermatologie, Venerologie und
Allergologie, Universitätsmedizin Mannheim,
Mannheim 68167, Germany
e-mail: jan.nicolay@umm.de

4.1   Introduction

Tumor therapy more and more focuses on individualized therapeutic regimens, as they allow for a maximum of efficacy in a single patient while simultaneously minimizing the risk of adverse events. Cutaneous T-cell lymphoma (CTCL) is especially suited for the development of such individualized therapeutic approaches due to its typical characteristics.

The term CTCL was introduced in the 1970s with the first reported staging classification [7]. During the following decades, the introduction of immunohistochemistry allowed a more detailed description of cutaneous lymphomas. The histo-immunohistochemical findings were correlated with the clinical presentation and follow-up of patients with cutaneous lymphomas. This led to the development of a first separate classification of cutaneous lymphomas [46]. Today, cutaneous lymphomas are classified according to the WHO/EORTC classification [45]. This classification acknowledges the individual clinical picture and prognosis of each cutaneous lymphoma entity. Many cutaneous lymphomas run an indolent course. However, they have to be distinguished from more aggressive forms of cutaneous lymphomas. A correct diagnosis and classification is the basis for treatment decisions. Furthermore, staging classifications for cutaneous lymphomas have been developed [23, 31]. An increased incidence of cutaneous lymphomas was described for the last decades in a large US study [3].

T. Bieber, F. Nestle (eds.), *Personalized Treatment Options in Dermatology*,
DOI 10.1007/978-3-662-45840-2_4, © Springer-Verlag Berlin Heidelberg 2015

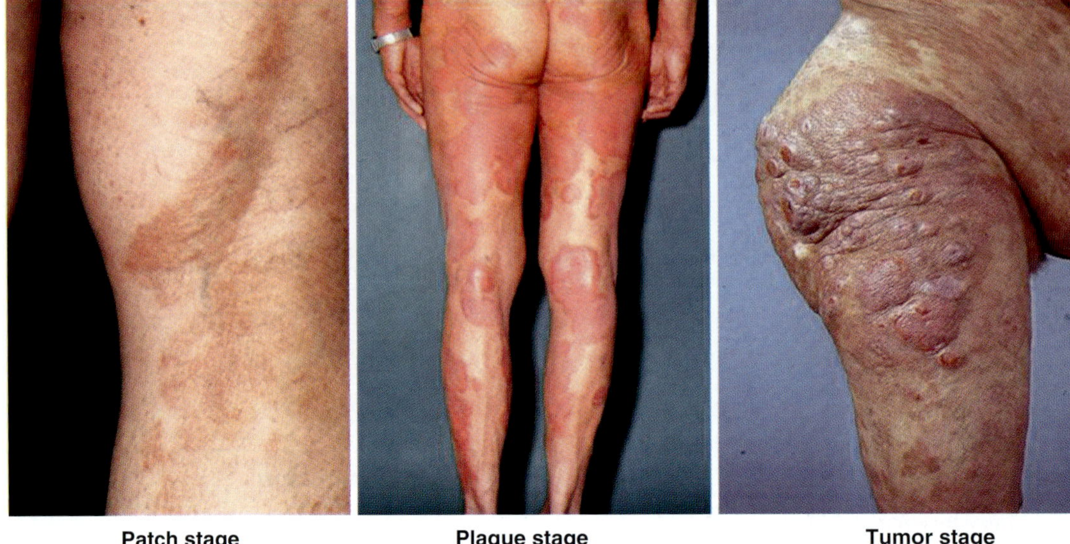

Fig. 4.1 The clinical stages of mycosis fungoides

A significant influence on the quality of life was noted in a number of studies. The leading symptom is itching. Many patients are worried about having a serious disease which is possibly life-threatening [11].

The most common form of CTCL is mycosis fungoides (MF), a generally indolent variant with restriction to skin manifestations. It runs a slowly progressive course over years up to decades in individual patients. Three clinical stages have been described: patch, plaque, and tumor stage (Fig. 4.1). MF is characterized by a monoclonal proliferation of CD4+ T cells (Fig. 4.2). The second most common group of CTCL is primary cutaneous CD30-positive lymphoproliferative disorders like lymphomatoid papulosis and primary cutaneous anaplastic large cell lymphoma. Both types have an indolent clinical course. Sézary syndrome is an aggressive and leukemic form that beyond skin manifestation shows blood and lymph node involvement. All types of cutaneous lymphomas are summarized in Table 4.1.

CTCL challenges both basic and clinical research for three reasons: first, its pathogenesis is widely unknown, although evidence on altered signaling or metabolic pathways as well as changes in the microenvironment increases. Second, quick and precise diagnosis is complicated by the lack of unique diagnostic markers defining CTCL and demarcating it from other skin diseases. Third, the disease is not curable by now. Existing CTCL treatment only prolongs or delays the disease progression and shows high relapse rates. Hence, there is an urgent need to further investigate the mechanism of CTCL development in order to develop new therapeutic approaches.

4.2 New Insights into CTCL Pathogenesis

The development of individualized therapeutic approaches requires knowledge on the pathogenesis of a disease. Information is needed on possible alterations in signaling or metabolic pathways, in microenvironment or protein activities in a specific patient. Identifying any cellular or molecular changes that might explain the development of the disease is essential, as every difference between a malignant and a healthy cell represents a possible therapeutic target. In recent years, a wide variety of altered molecular structures or pathways have been identified that might be therapeutically targeted. Each of these altered target structures affects only a more or less small percentage of CTCL patients, which underlines the need for individualized approaches in identifying target structures for cancer therapy. The development of such therapies fills a gap

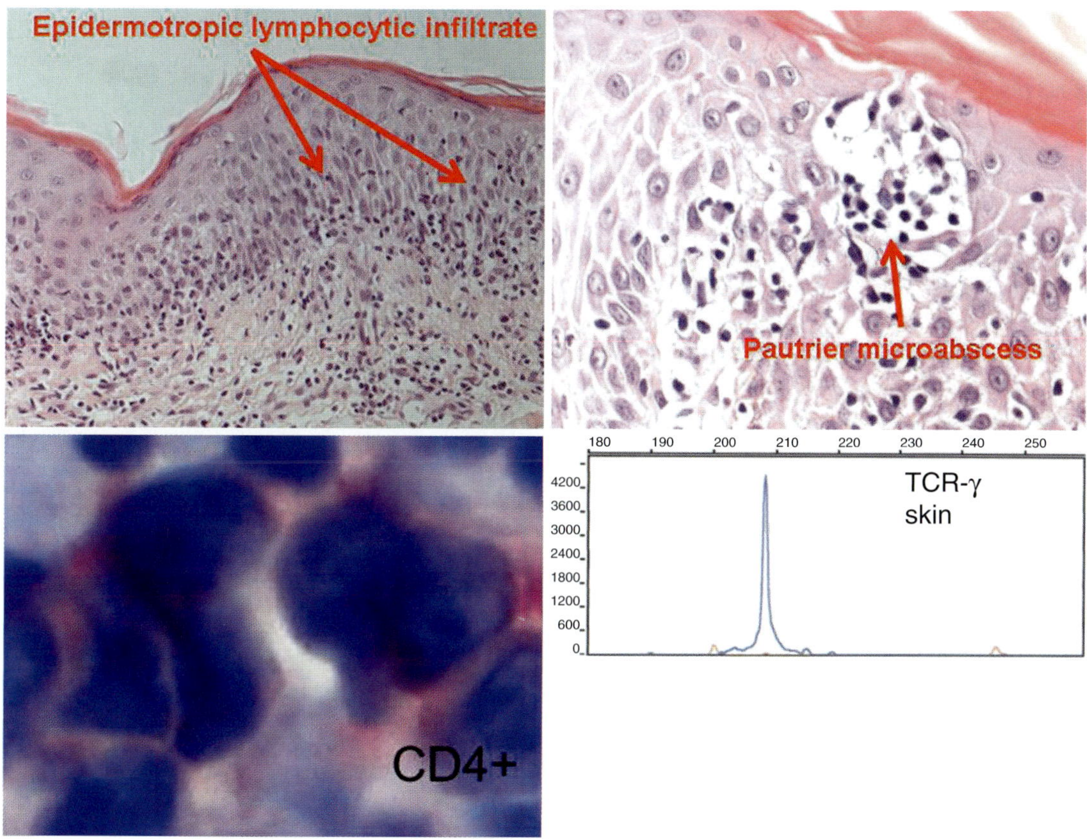

Fig. 4.2 Histopathological and molecular diagnosis of mycosis fungoides

Table 4.1 WHO classification of cutaneous lymphomas

Cutaneous T-cell and NK-cell lymphomas	Cutaneous B-cell lymphomas
Mycosis fungoides (MF)	Primary cutaneous follicular B-cell lymphoma (PCFCL)
Mycosis fungoides variants and subtypes	Primary cutaneous marginal zone B-cell lymphoma (PCMZL)
Folliculotropic MF	Primary cutaneous diffuse large cell B-cell lymphoma – leg type (PCBLT)
Pagetoid reticulosis Granulomatous slack skin	Primary cutaneous diffuse large cell B-cell lymphoma, others
Sézary syndrome (SS)	Primary cutaneous intravascular large cell B-cell lymphoma
Adult T-cell leukemia/lymphoma	

Primary cutaneous CD30+ lymphoproliferative diseases
  Primary cutaneous anaplastic large cell lymphoma (PCALCL)
  Lymphomatoid papulosis (LyP)
	Hematological precursor neoplasms CD4+, CD56+ hematodermic neoplasm (plasmacytoid dendritic cell neoplasm)

Subcutaneous panniculitis-like T-cell lymphoma (SPTCL)	
Extranodal NK/T-cell lymphoma, nasal type	
Primary cutaneous γ/δ T-cell lymphoma	
Primary cutaneous aggressive epidermotropic CD8+ T-cell lymphoma (provisional)	
Primary cutaneous small- to medium-sized pleomorphic T-cell lymphoma (provisional)	
Peripheral T-cell lymphoma, not otherwise specified	

in the therapeutic spectrum of CTCL that at the moment consists mainly of general therapeutic concepts.

4.2.1 Apoptosis Resistance

The malignant T-cell population in CTCL is characterized by a phenotype of resting, $CD3^+CD4^+CD7^-CD45RO^+$-bearing Th2 memory cells. The lifespan of a peripheral T cell is normally limited to several days under physiologic conditions. Upon activation, a cell death program, the activation-induced cell death (AICD), is enabled and even decreases this lifespan. CTCL cells have been found to return to a resting state decreasing their turnover and rendering them insensitive towards cell death stimuli. They evade AICD that is triggered by the death receptor CD95 by their lack of phospholipase-γ1 [24]. This enzyme is needed to process the TCR stimulation signal intracellularly that leads to formation of CD95 ligand. This ligand activates CD95 in an autocrine way leading to induction of AICD (Fig. 4.3). Due to this mechanism and their resistance towards intrinsic and extrinsic cell death stimuli, the accumulation of CTCL cells in the skin and subsequently in the lymph nodes rather derives from an acquired resistance towards cell death than from an increased proliferation rate. This cell death resistance is a very typical characteristic of CTCL cells that originates from alterations in several signaling pathways. Restoring sensitivity towards cell death contains a powerful therapeutic potential in fighting CTCL.

The nuclear factor κB (NFκB) represents one important trigger structure that can turn a cell resistant to cell death stimuli. Different alterations in this complex pathway have been described in CTCL cell lines and primary patient cells. These alterations lead to a constitutive activation in the NFκB pathway in the nucleus which impairs cell death signaling. The exact reason for this activation is unknown, but enhanced levels of single NFκB subunits like p50 as well as increased DNA binding of NFκB components found in CTCL cells explain it at least in part. This insight into CTCL pathogenesis has led to great ambition in medically reverting NFκB activation and thus inducing apoptosis in the CTCL cells [21, 36].

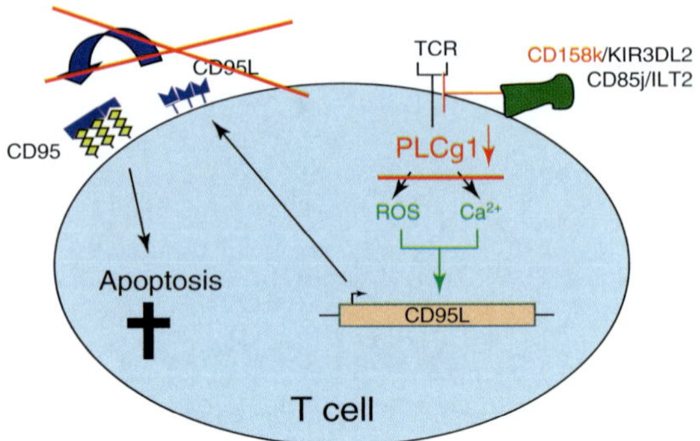

Fig. 4.3 Modified TCR signaling is responsible for AICD resistance in CTCL

NFκB activity can be targeted directly and indirectly via either inhibiting NFκB components themselves or other molecules crosstalking with the NFκB pathway. NFκB activation is sensitively regulated by phosphorylation and dephosphorylation of single components. The kinases in this interplay are well characterized. Recently, the phosphatases involved in antagonizing the kinase activity have come into focus more closely. The phosphatase PP4R1 connects the inhibitory phosphatase PP4c with the IKK complex within the NFκB signal, so that NFκB signaling is inactivated by PP4c. PP4R1 is hardly expressed in malignant T cells of many CTCL patients, so that PP4c cannot bind to the IKK complex and thus block its signaling (Fig. 4.4). This results in a constitutive activation of the NFκB pathway [6]. This phosphatase activity might represent an interesting therapeutic target for an individualized approach, but by now no substance exists that would interfere with the mentioned mechanism.

Another pathway that is related to the NFκB pathway and can also, independently of NFκB, lead to enhanced survival signals in T cells is the MAPK pathway. This signaling cascade has also been recently found relevant for CTCL pathogenesis and represents another structure for individualized CTCL patient care for several reasons. Both in CTCL cell lines and in isolated T cells of about 5 % of CTCL patients single nucleotide mutations in the n-ras (Q61K) and k-ras (G13D) genes were detected. These mutations lead to an excessive activation of the gene products N-Ras and K-Ras within the MAPK pathway and thus to decreased cellular susceptibility towards cell death signals [22]. As the MAPK and the NFκB

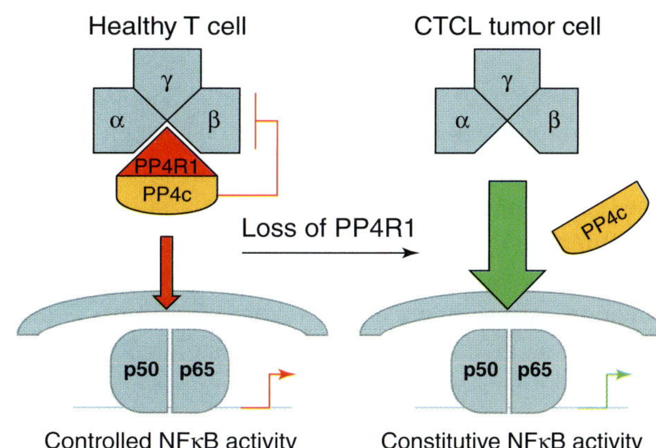

Fig. 4.4 Scheme of NFkB phosphatase signaling in healthy and CTCL T cells

pathway communicate, enhanced MAPK activity also results in increased constitutive NFκB activity.

4.2.2 Altered T-Cell Functions

Besides cell death resistance, other T-cell functions have been found impaired in CTCL cells on a molecular level recently. In parallel to other malignancies like melanoma, the expression of the cell surface protein programmed death-1 (PD-1) is pathologically increased in some types of CTCL [9, 20]. Similar to the surface protein CTLA-4 PD-1 inhibits effector T-cell function and thus possibly leads to suppression of an antitumor immune response. However, the exact significance of PD-1 overexpression is not clarified in the context of CTCL pathogenesis. Nevertheless, PD-1 can already be targeted medically; respective studies are in the clinical phase in melanoma patients. So this overexpression in CTCL contributes to the spectrum of targets for individualized approaches in CTCL therapy.

In addition, a wide variety of molecules influencing cellular transcription patterns have been found altered in CTCL. For example, the transcription factor E2A is genetically deleted in about 70 % of patients with Sézary syndrome. This loss results in increased proliferation rates and cell cycle progression via derepression of the proto-oncogene MYC and the cell cycle regulator CDK6 [38]. The transcription factor E2A also communicates in a synergistic with the Ras pathway that also enhances CTCL cell survival. Transcriptional activity is further pathologically

influenced by signal transducer of transcription (STAT) protein family members in CTCL. STAT3 shows constitutional activation in Sézary syndrome, at least in part due to autocrine IL-21 stimulation [42]. STATs trigger the expression of certain miRNAs like miRNA155 and miRNA21 in CTCL [26, 43] which themselves induce resistance towards cell death stimuli.

A unique target for T-cell-directed therapy in CTCL is found in the T-cell receptor (TCR). The monoclonal, malignant T-cell population bears a specific TCR composition that differs from the TCR repertoire that is formed by the nonmalignant cell population. So far, one primary limitation in this approach lies within the detection of the monoclonal TCR. In recent years, the detection methodology has largely improved including highly sensitive PCR and high-throughput deep sequencing techniques [44].

4.2.3 CTCL Tumor Microenvironment

Basic cancer research has mainly focused on the tumor cell itself. Since the first description of the hallmarks of cancer by Hanahan and Weinberg in 2000, it became more important to investigate the microenvironment of each tumor [17]. Today, it is known that tumor cells interact with their microenvironment in order to avoid immune destruction and to induce tumor-promoting inflammation [18]. The interaction of CTCL tumor cells with inflammatory cells in the skin is also important for the understanding of CTCL pathogenesis. In many CTCL skin lesions, the minority of skin-infiltrating cells represent CTCL tumor cells. The majority of lesional cells are reactive immune cells – mainly lymphocytes. Only in the rare case of progressive advanced disease the tumor cells become more prominent than the reactive cells. Therefore, CTCL basic research has so far mainly focused on the CTCL tumor cell microenvironment.

Tumor-infiltrating inflammatory cells are known to stimulate tumor cell growth, to induce angiogenesis in tumors, and to promote tumor invasion as evidenced by a dense inflammatory infiltrate at the marginal zones of a tumor. Immune progenitor cells (CD11b+, Gr1+) are able to suppress cytotoxic T and NK cells directed against the tumor. Rabenhorst et al. investigated the role of mast cells in the pathogenesis of CTCL [32]. They observed a better outcome in CTCL patients with less mast cells in the CTCL lesion (<100 mast cells/mm^2) than those with a denser cutaneous mast cell infiltrate (>100 mast cells/mm^2). Their in vitro experiments identified a stimulation of CTCL tumor cell growth by incubation with a mast cell supernatant. They concluded a growth promotion of CTCL tumor cells by mast cells.

In 1990, Reinhold et al. isolated suppressive lymphocytes from MF skin lesions in contrast to non-suppressive MF tumor cells [33]. Five years later, these suppressive cells were termed regulatory T cells (Treg) [35]. Treg are CD4+ lymphocytes with suppressive properties in order to terminate immune responses and to avoid autoimmunity. They are characterized by expression of the transcription factor FOXP3. Elimination of these important immune regulatory cells leads to severe autoimmune conditions in mice and humans. Immunohistochemical studies of CTCL skin samples revealed a significant decrease of FOXP3+ cells in biopsies from Sézary syndrome in contrast to MF lesions [25]. Other studies correlated low numbers of FOXP3+ cells with advanced disease in MF or CD30+ cutaneous lymphoma patients (summarized in [28]). The physiological target of suppression by Treg is the CD4+ lymphocyte. The abovementioned findings in CTCL lead to the hypothesis that Treg are capable of suppressing CTCL tumor cells in the early stages. The property is lost in advanced disease or aggressive forms of CTCL (e.g., Sézary syndrome) (Fig. 4.5).

In a subgroup of Sézary patients, the CTCL tumor cells themselves are FOXP3+ [19, 27]. FOXP3 might serve as a tumor suppressor in wt

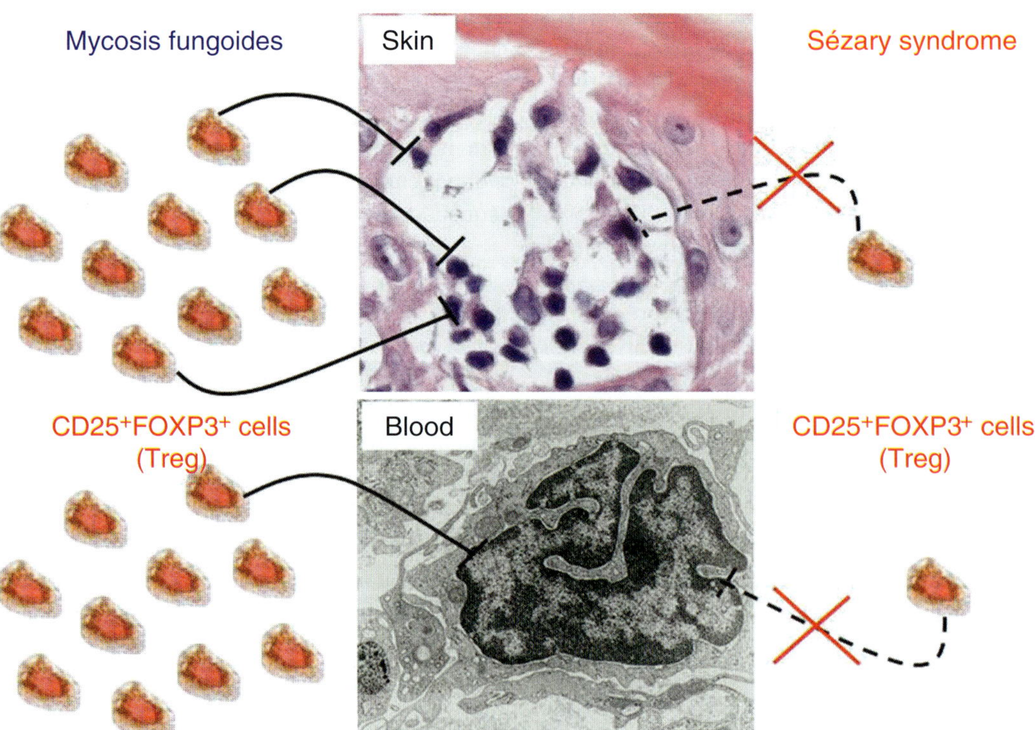

Fig. 4.5 The number of Treg correlates with an indolent course in CTCL

expression. However, the expression of FOXP3 splice variants might be a pro-survival factor for tumor cells [50, 51].

4.3 Personalized Aspects in Established CTCL Therapies

4.3.1 Standard of Care/Treatment Guidelines

Treatment of CTCL patients is entity specific due to the very different clinical courses of the different types of CTCL (see Fig. 4.1 and Table 4.1). And treatment should be stage-adapted to avoid too aggressive therapies. Most patients run an indolent course and require treatment for years up to decades. Therefore, the therapeutic effect needs to be balanced against possible side effects. The treatment guidelines of the German dermato-oncology group recommend skin-directed therapies for indolent forms and early stages [37]. Skin-directed therapies include topical corticosteroids, UV-based treatments like PUVA or UVB311 nm and radiotherapy. In more advanced disease or nonresponders, systemic treatments are added to the skin-directed treatment. First-line systemic treatments are interferon-α and the rexinoid bexarotene. In erythrodermic patients, extracorporeal photopheresis is given additionally or as monotherapy. For second-line treatments of CTCL, either cytotoxic monotherapies like low-dose methotrexate, gemcitabine, or liposomal doxorubicin or antibodies like denileukin diftitox are applied. Other options include the use of HDAC inhibitors like vorinostat and romidepsin or total skin electron beam irradiation. In the majority of CTCL patients, the disease can be well controlled with the mentioned standard treatments. However, even within one type of CTCL, individual patients might behave very differently requiring personalized treatment approaches.

4.3.2 Individualized Management of Bexarotene Therapy

Although being a standard therapy bexarotene treatment requires an elaborate personalized therapeutic regimen. Its characteristic side effects are often misunderstood and may lead physicians to wrong interpretations and decisions. Mainly these side effects include central hypothyroidism and hyperlipidemia, which are observed in almost 100 % of patients [1]. The occurrence of these side effects can be explained by the molecular mechanism of the bexarotene effect. This compound mainly affects nuclear retinoid X receptors (RXR) and thus influences apoptosis. RXR are in combination with retinoic acid receptors (RAR) involved in the regulation of thyroid function and lipid metabolism. So intriguingly, hypothyroidism and hyperlipidemia rather reflect bexarotene being active and effective in a patient than displaying a reason for discontinuation of treatment. Both bexarotene effectiveness in suppression of CTCL symptoms and the occurrence of these side effects show great interindividual differences, but so far there are no known correlations with any individual parameters that would allow any predictions about effectiveness and severity of side effects in a certain patient. Therefore, the side effect management has to be tuned individually in accordance with their characteristic and severity. All patients need an accompanying medication with thyroxin, whereas the dosage may vary between 50 and 200 μg/day depending on the blood values of thyroxin and triiodothyronine. The dramatically suppressed TSH that necessarily occurs during bexarotene therapy reflects the central character of the hypothyroidism and may in combination with the normal values of thyroxin and triiodothyronine under substitution not be mistaken for a constellation of peripheral hyperthyroidism. The individualized management of hyperlipidemia is more sophisticated. First-line therapy would include fibrates in therapeutic doses. In case of insufficiency of this therapy, it can be combined with esterified fish oils that are FDA approved under the brand name Lovaza® or Omacor® to lower very high triglyceride blood levels. In case of myopathies or signs of rhabdomyolysis under fibrate therapy, it can be replaced by atorvastatin 10 mg/day that influences both triglyceride and cholesterol levels with a milder side effect spectrum [1, 14, 39]. Obviously dose adjustments have to be considered in accordance with efficacy and risk of the treatment. In our experience, not many patients tolerate the maximum dose aimed for, which is not necessarily a problem. Most patients who respond at all to bexarotene show already good response rates at moderate doses, so that tapering down the dose to the lowest level of response is obviously the most reasonable method to manage side effects. It has to be emphasized that bexarotene needs up to 6 months to show a clinical therapeutic effect.

4.3.3 Individualized Management of Interferon Therapy

The handling of interferon therapy with respect to side effect management or concurrent medication is less difficult and requires less experience and consideration of mechanistic interaction. In terms of concurrent medication, the most common side effects that have to be individually dealt with are flulike inflammatory responses and depressive disorders.

The first one can in almost all cases easily be treated by nonsteroidal anti-inflammatory drugs (NSAID) like paracetamol 500 mg 1 h before and 1 h after the injection of interferon. The management of depressive disorder in interferon therapy includes two different possibilities. Either interferon can be reduced to the lowest possible effective dose, although that often does not reduce depression sufficiently. The alternative would be a medical symptom suppression. This can be reached by cotreatment with different antidepressants. Selective serotonin reuptake inhibitors (SSRI), tricyclic antidepressants (TCA), and mirtazapine can be equally effective depending on the individual patient's tolerance and response [2]. Interestingly different antidepressant drugs are effective in suppression of pruritus that is often an agonizing symptom of CTCL [15]. These drugs include mirtazapine and amitriptyline. Therefore, we would first line recommend a depression management upon interferon therapy with mirtazapine due to its lowest side effect profile and its proven effectiveness for pruritus control in CTCL [12].

4.4 New Individualized Therapeutic Options in Clinical Trials

4.4.1 Anti-CCR4 Therapy

In recent years, cytokines and chemokines have gained increasing interest in the therapy of hematological malignancies. They conduct important immune modulating signaling functions in T cells and thus represent powerful potential to impede malignant T-cell functions. Among other functions, T-cell migration is influenced. Especially the chemokine receptor CCR4 has been found to be associated with a skin-homing T-cell phenotype [8]. In accordance with this finding, CTCL cells show an increased CCR4 expression driving them into the skin [13]. Indeed, targeting of CCR4 in CTCL has shown therapeutic potential in vitro and in vivo and thus might become a standard therapeutic option in fighting this disease [10, 16]. Yet, the percentage of CCR4$^+$ cells shows a strong interindividual variation. Ferenczi et al. show a range between 31.5 and 80 % of CCR4$^+$ cells in the peripheral blood of Sézary syndrome patients ($n=11$) and 39.2 and 95 % within skin lesions ($n=7$). Unfortunately, no predictive markers are known so far that correlate with the number of CCR4$^+$ cells in an individual patient and thus with the chance of therapeutic success when treating with an anti-CCR4 antibody.

In order to solve these questions, the randomized multicenter phase 3 study NCT01728805 compares therapy with the anti-CCR4-mAB KW-0761 (Mogamulizumab) to vorinostat as a standard treatment. Progression-free survival, response, quality of life, and pruritus are assessed. Thus, planned in 2015, the study will deliver information, if anti-CCR4 treatment will be effective in a wide population of CTCL patients or if perhaps patient stratification is necessary prior to therapy. Therefore, targeting CCR4 might in any case be an effective treatment option in individual CTCL patients, who show a high expression of CCR4 on their malignant T cells or an "addiction" of their cells to CCR4 signaling.

4.4.2 Anti-CD30 Therapy

The abovementioned anti-CCR4 study excludes patients with transformed CTCL. These patients might benefit from another clinical study. Cellular transformation in CTCL represents an event accompanied by tumor progression, a higher risk of systemic involvement and thus a decline in prognosis. Upon transformation, CTCL cells start the expression of the surface marker CD30. This protein belongs to the TNF receptor superfamily and can mediate signal transduction via TRAFs that leads to the activation of NFκB and cell death resistance. CD30 is highly expressed in a variety of nodal and systemic lymphoma subsets, including Hodgkin lymphoma and anaplastic large cell lymphoma. Treatment of systemic lymphoma patients with a CD30-mAB alone showed limited success. Therefore, the antibody was bound to different cytostatic substances. Indeed, brentuximab vedotin, an antibody-drug conjugate that selectively delivers monomethyl auristatin E, an antimicrotubule agent, into CD30-expressing cells, showed very promising study results that even led to the approval of this drug for the therapy of patients with relapsed Hodgkin lymphoma and anaplastic large cell lymphoma [30, 47, 48].

At the moment, the randomized phase 3 trial NCT01578499 of brentuximab vedotin (SGN-35) versus physician's choice (methotrexate or bexarotene) addresses the question if brentuximab vedotin is also effective in CD30-transformed CTCL. Response to therapy, progression-free survival, and tumor burden of the skin are evaluated. The study obviously only includes the small subgroup of CTCL patients whose malignant cell population expresses CD30. Similar to the abovementioned anti-CCR4 treatment brentuximab vedotin might be effective only in a subgroup of enrolled patients. Individualized stratification of eligible patients might make a correlation of CD30 expression levels on the malignant cell population and therapeutic success necessary. On the other hand, the coupling to auristatin E could make it an effective drug even in case only very few CD30 molecules are expressed, as the drug itself has cytotoxic activity and does, in contrast to the anti-CCR4-mAB, not need the involvement of the immune system in killing the opsonized CTCL cells. Indeed, in Hodgkin's disease, there is evidence that brentuximab vedotin is effective even in case very few or no CD30 molecules are expressed on the malignant cell population. The exact mechanisms for that are still to be elucidated, but most probably influences on the tumor microenvironment and subsequent antitumor immunologic effects are responsible for this effect [34, 40].

4.5 Experimental/Future Individualized Therapies

4.5.1 Restoring Apoptosis Sensitivity

As described above, cell death resistance is one major feature of CTCL cell that complicates therapy. Different, partly interacting pathways have been described that are involved in this process (see also 4.2.1). Due to their crosstalk, it is crucial to identify essential switch points within the signaling. Ideally, inhibition of such a switch point would impede a certain pathway without allowing for another redundant pathway to take over the respective signal and function of the impaired pathway. Alternatively, a far downstream signal of one pathway or even a common end signal of different pathways can be targeted. Good candidate molecules fulfilling these conditions can be found within the NFκB pathway. Unfortunately, by now possible candidate drugs either showed too little therapeutic efficacy already on a preclinical level or were not suitable for treatment of human patients due to their high degree of toxicity [21, 36]. Recently, new nontoxic direct NFκB inhibitors have been identified and successfully tested preclinically. Yet, their exact molecular targets within the NFκB pathway are unclear. In addition, clinical studies will have to prove them effective in the treatment of CTCL.

For the crosstalking MAPK pathway that is also involved in apoptosis resistance of CTCL cells, there are already well-established inhibiting drugs that are already in clinical use for treatment of other malignant diseases. For example, the multikinase inhibitor sorafenib could be a promising therapeutic approach, at least for patients whose malignant T cells bear a K-Ras or N-Ras mutation. In vitro data hints towards sorafenib being able to induce apoptosis in CTCL cells. Interestingly inhibitors of b-Raf or other Ras/Raf proteins like U0126 and PLX4720 do not show any cell death-inducing properties. In addition, sorafenib can sensitize cells towards cell death stimulation by other drugs. Therefore, it is rather a candidate for combination therapy with other drugs that are limited in dosage by toxicity or side effects by enhancing the effects of these substances.

Another interesting therapeutic approach for targeting apoptosis resistance in CTCL includes the antiapoptotic members of the Bcl-2 protein family like Bcl-2, Bcl-xL, and Mcl-1. In CTCL, genetic and functional alterations of the protein Bcl-2 have been described [29]. This protein inhibits cytochrome c externalization from the mitochondria during apoptosis and thus blocks apoptosis signaling on a crucial step. Inhibitors or Bcl-2 like ABT-737, ABT-263, and the most recently developed ABT-199 are already in clinical testing or even clinical use for different other hematologic malignancies like multiple myeloma and chronic lymphocytic leukemia (http://clinicaltrials.gov/ct2/results?term=ABT199). Similar to sorafenib, Bcl-2 inhibitors are rarely used as single treatment. Their ability to block cell death evasion via Bcl-2 upon drug-induced apoptosis stimulation makes them ideal combination therapy partners for cytotoxic substances. Therefore, they rather represent cell death enhancers than cell death inducers in most malignant cells. In CTCL cells, it is unclear whether they depend on Bcl-2 function with respect to survival or whether Bcl-2 signaling is just switched on upon cellular stress. A dependence of CTCL cell survival on constitutive Bcl-2 function would make the Bcl-2 inhibitors even promising candidates for monotherapy. Yet, the described heterogeneity in alterations in Bcl-2 function found in CTCL cells from different patients would make a stratification

necessary, as this therapy would just exert its action in an eligible subgroup of patients with high Bcl-2 levels and Bcl-2 "addiction" of their cells.

Curcumin is a drug that at least in vitro combines the inhibition of different essential pathways involved in cell death resistance of CTCL cells. For curcumin, a downregulation of survivin, of Bcl-2, and of STAT-3 on mRNA level and a reduction of NFκB and STAT-3 function via inhibition of phosphorylation has been described [49]. These effects would induce cell death by several different and independent pathways and would simultaneously inhibit survival signals that could counteract this cell death induction. Despite these very promising in vitro data, no clinical data exists yet that would give evidence if these effects also hold true in patients and their malignant cells – neither in the general collective nor in special subpopulations. It is not known either if these effects can be reached by reasonable and nontoxic doses of this drug.

In some patients, nonsteroidal anti-inflammatory drugs (NSAID) might be a therapeutic option that could support or enhance therapeutic effects of CTCL standard treatment. NSAID have been shown to induce apoptosis in CTCL cells. Although the exact target or involved mechanisms for this finding are not completely elucidated, an involvement of Mcl-1 downregulation, an antiapoptotic Bcl-2 family member, could be identified [5]. So far, no systematic clinical testing of these in vitro and ex vivo results has been performed in order to confirm a possible therapeutic action of NSAID in CTCL patients. There is also no published data on a possible correlation between a favorable prognosis or milder CTCL symptom occurrence and systemic NSAID intake in CTCL patients, as many people take them anyway for other indications.

4.5.2 Targeting Impaired T-Cell Functions (Beyond Apoptosis)

Besides direct apoptosis induction, a wide variety of T-cell functions that are altered in CTCL cells compared to healthy T cells are within the focus of defining new individualized therapies for fighting CTCL.

The protein PD-1, which suppresses antitumor response and is overexpressed in CTCL, can be targeted medically. Different monoclonal antibodies against PD-1 have been developed. One of them, nivolumab, has already shown promising clinical phase II results in the treatment of small cell lung cancer, melanoma, and renal cell cancer. Colon and pancreatic cancer that were also tested did not respond [4, 41]. Unfortunately for lymphoma, especially CTCL, no data exists on a possible effect of anti-PD1 therapy. For CTCL, besides an anti-PD-1 antibody, a conjugate of the antibody to a cytostatic drug might be a promising new therapeutic approach in parallel to brentuximab vedotin in CD30+ lymphoma.

From the pharmacologic point of view, the perfect individualized therapy in CTCL would be a monoclonal antibody against the specific and monoclonal TCR of the CTCL cell population, as it would specifically exert maximal therapeutic effect on the malignant population while leaving the rest of the T cells or other tissues unaffected. Techniques in identifying the monoclonal TCR have improved a lot, so that this identification should be possible in all cases now. A problem in this approach that so far impaired all attempts in this field lies in the very high cost. Performing high-sensitivity PCR and deep sequencing for identifying the clonal TCR alone is very expensive. In addition, every patient would need an antibody generated for just one person. So far, nothing is known about possible TCR loci that preferred for monoclonal expansion, so that one has to consider a random interindividual distribution of clonal TCR in the CTCL patient collective. Therefore, as long as such an anti-TCR-mAB therapy is connected to such high cost, it can at best be considered in experimental or strictly selected single individuals.

A wide variety of other molecules that are involved in T-cell development and signaling could be possible targets in CTCL therapy in the future. These include transcription factors like E2A; cytokines and chemokines like IL-2, IL32, IL17F, and IL31; and different miRNAs (see also 4.2.2). At the moment, therapeutic strategies against these targets would collapse as neither small molecules nor safely clinically usable antibodies exist to interfere with these structures. Nonetheless, recent research in CTCL pathogenesis and therapy showed a wide number of new therapeutic approaches and pushed them quickly into clinical settings. Therefore, there is good hope that the pipeline of new individualized or general therapies in fighting CTCL will not run dry, as there is constant need of new therapies in this so far incurable disease.

References

1. Abbott RA, Whittaker SJ, Morris SL, Russell-Jones R, Hung T, Bashir SJ, Scarisbrick JJ. Bexarotene therapy for mycosis fungoides and Sezary syndrome. Br J Dermatol. 2009;160:1299–307.
2. Baraldi S, Hepgul N, Mondelli V, Pariante CM. Symptomatic treatment of interferon-alpha-induced depression in hepatitis C: a systematic review. J Clin Psychopharmacol. 2012;32:531–43.
3. Bradford PT, Devesa SS, Anderson WF, Toro JR. Cutaneous lymphoma incidence patterns in the United States: a population-based study of 3884 cases. Blood. 2009;113:5064–73.
4. Brahmer JR, Tykodi SS, Chow LQ, Hwu WJ, Topalian SL, Hwu P, Drake CG, Camacho LH, Kauh J, Odunsi K, et al. Safety and activity of anti-PD-L1 antibody in patients with advanced cancer. N Engl J Med. 2012;366:2455–65.
5. Braun FK, Al-Yacoub N, Plotz M, Mobs M, Sterry W, Eberle J. Nonsteroidal anti-inflammatory drugs induce apoptosis in cutaneous T-cell lymphoma cells and enhance their sensitivity for TNF-related apoptosis-inducing ligand. J Invest Dermatol. 2012;132:429–39.
6. Brechmann M, Mock T, Nickles D, Kiessling M, Weit N, Breuer R, Muller W, Wabnitz G, Frey F, Nicolay JP, et al. A PP4 holoenzyme balances physiological and oncogenic nuclear factor-kappa B signaling in T lymphocytes. Immunity. 2012;37:697–708.
7. Bunn Jr PA, Lamberg SI. Report of the committee on staging and classification of cutaneous T-cell lymphomas. Cancer Treat Rep. 1979;63:725–8.
8. Campbell JJ, Haraldsen G, Pan J, Rottman J, Qin S, Ponath P, Andrew DP, Warnke R, Ruffing N, Kassam N, et al. The chemokine receptor CCR4 in vascular recognition by cutaneous but not intestinal memory T cells. Nature. 1999;400:776–80.
9. Cetinozman F, Jansen PM, Willemze R. Expression of programmed death-1 in primary cutaneous CD4-positive small/medium-sized pleomorphic T-cell lymphoma, cutaneous pseudo-T-cell lymphoma, and other types of cutaneous T-cell lymphoma. Am J Surg Pathol. 2012;36:109–16.

10. Chang DK, Sui J, Geng S, Muvaffak A, Bai M, Fuhlbrigge RC, Lo A, Yammanuru A, Hubbard L, Sheehan J, et al. Humanization of an anti-CCR4 antibody that kills cutaneous T-cell lymphoma cells and abrogates suppression by T-regulatory cells. Mol Cancer Ther. 2012;11:2451–61.

11. Demierre MF, Gan S, Jones J, Miller DR. Significant impact of cutaneous T-cell lymphoma on patients' quality of life: results of a 2005 National Cutaneous Lymphoma Foundation Survey. Cancer. 2006;107:2504–11.

12. Demierre MF, Taverna J. Mirtazapine and gabapentin for reducing pruritus in cutaneous T-cell lymphoma. J Am Acad Dermatol. 2006;55:543–4.

13. Ferenczi K, Fuhlbrigge RC, Pinkus J, Pinkus GS, Kupper TS. Increased CCR4 expression in cutaneous T cell lymphoma. J Invest Dermatol. 2002;119:1405–10.

14. Gniadecki R, Assaf C, Bagot M, Dummer R, Duvic M, Knobler R, Ranki A, Schwandt P, Whittaker S. The optimal use of bexarotene in cutaneous T-cell lymphoma. Br J Dermatol. 2007;157:433–40.

15. Gupta MA, Guptat AK. The use of antidepressant drugs in dermatology. J Eur Acad Dermatol Venereol. 2001;15:512–8.

16. Han T, Abdel-Motal UM, Chang DK, Sui J, Muvaffak A, Campbell J, Zhu Q, Kupper TS, Marasco WA. Human anti-CCR4 minibody gene transfer for the treatment of cutaneous T-cell lymphoma. PLoS One. 2012;7:e44455.

17. Hanahan D, Weinberg RA. The hallmarks of cancer. Cell. 2000;100:57–70.

18. Hanahan D, Weinberg RA. Hallmarks of cancer: the next generation. Cell. 2011;144:646–74.

19. Heid JB, Schmidt A, Oberle N, Goerdt S, Krammer PH, Suri-Payer E, Klemke CD. FOXP3+CD25- tumor cells with regulatory function in Sezary syndrome. J Invest Dermatol. 2009;129:2875–85.

20. Kantekure K, Yang Y, Raghunath P, Schaffer A, Woetmann A, Zhang Q, Odum N, Wasik M. Expression patterns of the immunosuppressive proteins PD-1/CD279 and PD-L1/CD274 at different stages of cutaneous T-cell lymphoma/mycosis fungoides. Am J Dermatopathol. 2012;34:126–8.

21. Kiessling MK, Klemke CD, Kaminski MM, Galani IE, Krammer PH, Gulow K. Inhibition of constitutively activated nuclear factor-kappaB induces reactive oxygen species- and iron-dependent cell death in cutaneous T-cell lymphoma. Cancer Res. 2009;69:2365–74.

22. Kiessling MK, Oberholzer PA, Mondal C, Karpova MB, Zipser MC, Lin WM, Girardi M, Macconaill LE, Kehoe SM, Hatton C, et al. High-throughput mutation profiling of CTCL samples reveals KRAS and NRAS mutations sensitizing tumors toward inhibition of the RAS/RAF/MEK signaling cascade. Blood. 2011;117:2433–40.

23. Kim YH, Willemze R, Pimpinelli N, Whittaker S, Olsen EA, Ranki A, Dummer R, Hoppe RT. TNM classification system for primary cutaneous lymphomas other than mycosis fungoides and Sezary syndrome: a proposal of the International Society for Cutaneous Lymphomas (ISCL) and the Cutaneous Lymphoma Task Force of the European Organization of Research and Treatment of Cancer (EORTC). Blood. 2007;110:479–84.

24. Klemke CD, Brenner D, Weiss EM, Schmidt M, Leverkus M, Gulow K, Krammer PH. Lack of T-cell receptor-induced signaling is crucial for CD95 ligand up-regulation and protects cutaneous T-cell lymphoma cells from activation-induced cell death. Cancer Res. 2009;69:4175–83.

25. Klemke CD, Fritzsching B, Franz B, Kleinmann EV, Oberle N, Poenitz N, Sykora J, Banham AH, Roncador G, Kuhn A, et al. Paucity of FOXP3+ cells in skin and peripheral blood distinguishes Sezary syndrome from other cutaneous T-cell lymphomas. Leukemia. 2006;20:1123–9.

26. Kopp KL, Ralfkiaer U, Gjerdrum LM, Helvad R, Pedersen IH, Litman T, Jonson L, Hagedorn PH, Krejsgaard T, Gniadecki R, et al. STAT5-mediated expression of oncogenic miR-155 in cutaneous T-cell lymphoma. Cell Cycle. 2013;12:1939–47.

27. Krejsgaard T, Gjerdrum LM, Ralfkiaer E, Lauenborg B, Eriksen KW, Mathiesen AM, Bovin LF, Gniadecki R, Geisler C, Ryder LP, et al. Malignant Tregs express low molecular splice forms of FOXP3 in Sezary syndrome. Leukemia. 2008;22:2230–9.

28. Krejsgaard T, Odum N, Geisler C, Wasik MA, Woetmann A. Regulatory T cells and immunodeficiency in mycosis fungoides and Sezary syndrome. Leukemia. 2012;26:424–32.

29. Mao X, Orchard G, Lillington DM, Child FJ, Vonderheid EC, Nowell PC, Bagot M, Bensussan A, Russell-Jones R, Young BD, et al. BCL2 and JUNB abnormalities in primary cutaneous lymphomas. Br J Dermatol. 2004;151:546–56.

30. Oki Y, Younes A. Brentuximab vedotin in systemic T-cell lymphoma. Expert Opin Biol Ther. 2012;12:623–32.

31. Olsen E, Vonderheid E, Pimpinelli N, Willemze R, Kim Y, Knobler R, Zackheim H, Duvic M, Estrach T, Lamberg S, et al. Revisions to the staging and classification of mycosis fungoides and Sezary syndrome: a proposal of the International Society for Cutaneous Lymphomas (ISCL) and the cutaneous lymphoma task force of the European Organization of Research and Treatment of Cancer (EORTC). Blood. 2007;110:1713–22.

32. Rabenhorst A, Schlaak M, Heukamp LC, Forster A, Theurich S, von Bergwelt-Baildon M, Buttner R, Kurschat P, Mauch C, Roers A, et al. Mast cells play a protumorigenic role in primary cutaneous lymphoma. Blood. 2012;120:2042–54.

33. Reinhold U, Pawelec G, Fratila A, Leippold S, Bauer R, Kreysel HW. Phenotypic and functional characterization of tumor infiltrating lymphocytes in mycosis fungoides: continuous growth of CD4+ CD45R+ T-cell clones with suppressor-inducer activity. J Invest Dermatol. 1990;94:304–9.

34. Rothe A, Sasse S, Goergen H, Eichenauer DA, Lohri A, Jager U, Bangard C, Boll B, von Bergwelt

Baildon M, Theurich S, et al. Brentuximab vedotin for relapsed or refractory CD30+ hematologic malignancies: the German Hodgkin Study Group experience. Blood. 2012;120:1470–2.

35. Sakaguchi S, Sakaguchi N, Asano M, Itoh M, Toda M. Immunologic self-tolerance maintained by activated T cells expressing IL-2 receptor alpha-chains (CD25). Breakdown of a single mechanism of self-tolerance causes various autoimmune diseases. J Immunol. 1995;155:1151–64.

36. Sors A, Jean-Louis F, Pellet C, Laroche L, Dubertret L, Courtois G, Bachelez H, Michel L. Down-regulating constitutive activation of the NF-kappaB canonical pathway overcomes the resistance of cutaneous T-cell lymphoma to apoptosis. Blood. 2006;107:2354–63.

37. Stadler R, Assaf C, Klemke CD, Nashan D, Weichenthal M, Dummer R, Sterry W. Brief S2k guidelines - cutaneous lymphomas. J Dtsch Dermatol Ges. 2013;11(Suppl) 3:19–28; 20–30.

38. Steininger A, Mobs M, Ullmann R, Kochert K, Kreher S, Lamprecht B, Anagnostopoulos I, Hummel M, Richter J, Beyer M, et al. Genomic loss of the putative tumor suppressor gene E2A in human lymphoma. J Exp Med. 2011;208:1585–93.

39. Talpur R, Ward S, Apisarnthanarax N, Breuer-Mcham J, Duvic M. Optimizing bexarotene therapy for cutaneous T-cell lymphoma. J Am Acad Dermatol. 2002;47:672–84.

40. Theurich S, Malcher J, Wennhold K, Shimabukuro-Vornhagen A, Chemnitz J, Holtick U, Krause A, Kobe C, Kahraman D, Engert A, et al. Brentuximab vedotin combined with donor lymphocyte infusions for early relapse of Hodgkin lymphoma after allogeneic stem-cell transplantation induces tumor-specific immunity and sustained clinical remission. J Clin Oncol. 2013;31:e59–63.

41. Topalian SL, Hodi FS, Brahmer JR, Gettinger SN, Smith DC, McDermott DF, Powderly JD, Carvajal RD, Sosman JA, Atkins MB, et al. Safety, activity, and immune correlates of anti-PD-1 antibody in cancer. N Engl J Med. 2012;366:2443–54.

42. van der Fits L, Out-Luiting JJ, van Leeuwen MA, Samsom JN, Willemze R, Tensen CP, Vermeer MH. Autocrine IL-21 stimulation is involved in the maintenance of constitutive STAT3 activation in Sezary syndrome. J Invest Dermatol. 2012;132:440–7.

43. van der Fits L, van Kester MS, Qin Y, Out-Luiting JJ, Smit F, Zoutman WH, Willemze R, Tensen CP, Vermeer MH. MicroRNA-21 expression in CD4+ T cells is regulated by STAT3 and is pathologically involved in Sezary syndrome. J Invest Dermatol. 2011;131:762–8.

44. Weng WK, Armstrong R, Arai S, Desmarais C, Hoppe R, Kim YH. Minimal residual disease monitoring with high-throughput sequencing of T cell receptors in cutaneous T cell lymphoma. Sci Transl Med. 2013;5:214ra171.

45. Willemze R, Jaffe ES, Burg G, Cerroni L, Berti E, Swerdlow SH, Ralfkiaer E, Chimenti S, Diaz-Perez JL, Duncan LM, et al. WHO-EORTC classification for cutaneous lymphomas. Blood. 2005; 105:3768–85.

46. Willemze R, Kerl H, Sterry W, Berti E, Cerroni L, Chimenti S, Diaz-Perez JL, Geerts ML, Goos M, Knobler R, et al. EORTC classification for primary cutaneous lymphomas: a proposal from the Cutaneous Lymphoma Study Group of the European Organization for Research and Treatment of Cancer. Blood. 1997;90:354–71.

47. Younes A, Gopal AK, Smith SE, Ansell SM, Rosenblatt JD, Savage KJ, Ramchandren R, Bartlett NL, Cheson BD, de Vos S, et al. Results of a pivotal phase II study of brentuximab vedotin for patients with relapsed or refractory Hodgkin's lymphoma. J Clin Oncol. 2012;30:2183–9.

48. Younes A, Yasothan U, Kirkpatrick P. Brentuximab vedotin. Nat Rev Drug Discov. 2012;11:19–20.

49. Zhang C, Li B, Zhang X, Hazarika P, Aggarwal BB, Duvic M. Curcumin selectively induces apoptosis in cutaneous T-cell lymphoma cell lines and patients' PBMCs: potential role for STAT-3 and NF-kappaB signaling. J Invest Dermatol. 2010;130:2110–9.

50. Zuo T, Liu R, Zhang H, Chang X, Liu Y, Wang L, Zheng P. FOXP3 is a novel transcriptional repressor for the breast cancer oncogene SKP2. J Clin Invest. 2007;117:3765–73.

51. Zuo T, Wang L, Morrison C, Chang X, Zhang H, Li W, Liu Y, Wang Y, Liu X, Chan MW, et al. FOXP3 is an X-linked breast cancer suppressor gene and an important repressor of the HER-2/ErbB2 oncogene. Cell. 2007;129:1275–86.

Personalized Management of Atopic Dermatitis: Beyond Emollients and Topical Steroids

Thomas Bieber

Contents

T. Bieber, MD, PhD, MDRA
Department of Dermatology and Allergy,
Center of Translational Medicine, University of
Bonn, Sigmund Freud Str. 25, Bonn 53105, Germany
e-mail: Thomas.Bieber@ukb.uni-bonn.de

5.1 Introduction

Atopic dermatitis (eczema) is probably the most common inflammatory disease overall [1]. The incidence of atopic dermatitis has increased by about threefold in the last four decades, particularly in Western countries [2]. The disease affects between 15 and 20 % of the children and – depending on the studies – between 2 and 10 % of adults. One of the most important aspects of this disease relies in the considerable impact on the quality of life of patients and their relatives [3–5]. Therefore, due to its high prevalence and incidence, atopic dermatitis generates a substantial socioeconomic burden [6–17].

One of the key aspects of atopic dermatitis is its wide spectrum of clinical phenotype [18, 19]. There is a great discrepancy between the physician's perception, on the one hand, and the patient's perception or of their relatives, on the other hand. The physician usually sees the disease as a kind of screenshot situation and tends to prescribe some therapeutic management based on his own experience with this kind of particular diagnosis and situation. The parents and patients on the other hand have in mind a long and sometimes painful history of the disease with a strong impact on the quality of life. Moreover, the therapeutic management by the physician is more and more dictated by national or international guidelines, which usually do not consider the natural history of the disease. Instead, these guidelines concentrate on the treatment of individual flares

T. Bieber, F. Nestle (eds.), *Personalized Treatment Options in Dermatology*,
DOI 10.1007/978-3-662-45840-2_5, © Springer-Verlag Berlin Heidelberg 2015

and hardly consider the chronic and possibly life-long aspect of atopic dermatitis [20–28]. Thus, while the patient is always considering himself as a single individual requesting a tailored management, the physician will tend to apply a therapeutic approach according to the "one size fits for all" schema. Finally, there is a substantial gap between the wide heterogeneity of the clinical phenotype and the very limited choice of available and approved drugs for the management of atopic dermatitis despite the progress in our understanding of the genetic background and the pathophysiology of atopic dermatitis.

5.2 Pathophysiological Heterogeneity of Atopic Dermatitis

Atopic dermatitis is by definition a genetically complex disease where gene-gene and gene-environment interactions seem to play a key role. In most of the cases, typically starting during infancy, the disease can be divided into three main phases [1]:

- Phase 1: The initial infantile form where IgE sensitization is not yet detectable and where there is no evidence for allergic reactions. This phase could also be defined as non-IgE (formerly intrinsic)-associated form.
- Phase 2: The chronic inflammation catalyzes the emergence of IgE sensitization, and allergies – at the beginning particularly to food followed by environmental allergens – are known to play a role as provocation factors. This phase could also be defined as IgE (formerly extrinsic)-associated form.
- Phase 3: While the sensitization profile is expanding, other allergic diseases such as allergic rhinitis and asthma are developing. The atopic march is completed. In some cases (30 % of adult patients), the individuals develop an IgE sensitization towards self-proteins, typically derived from keratinocytes: atopic dermatitis has a strong autoimmune component.

Figure 5.1 schematically depicts the main factors involved in the pathophysiology of this disease with regard to the different phases of the natural history, i.e., the atopic march.

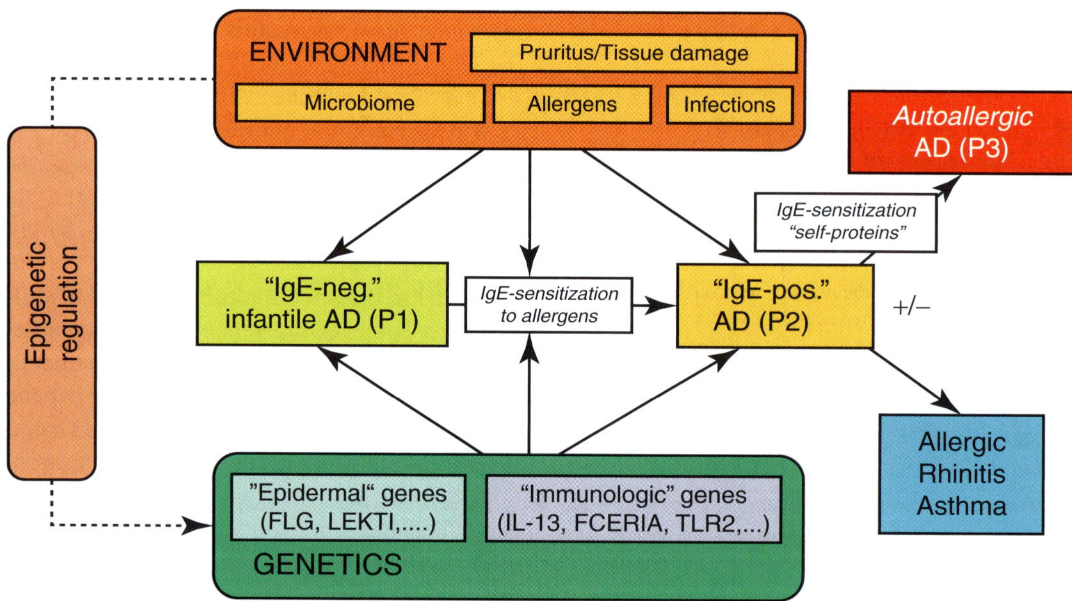

Fig. 5.1 The pathophysiological factors and the classical natural history of atopic dermatitis for a patient developing an atopic march (Adapted from Bieber [1])

5.2.1 Environmental Factors

A number of environmental factors have been analyzed in many epidemiological studies over the last three decades. Besides the exposition to highly variable factors like hard water or soaps [29–32] which may directly impact or worsen the well-accepted impaired epidermal barrier function, a number of more specific factors have been highlighted and which may play a crucial role in the sensitization phenomenon as well as in inducing skin inflammation.

5.2.1.1 Allergens

Although the exposition to allergens has been assumed during pregnancy [33–36] and conditioned by the mother's diet, the most evident exposition to allergen occurs directly after birth. Hereby, food allergens as well as environmental allergens (such as animal dander or pollens) are certainly to be considered with regard to the sensitization phenomenon [33, 35, 37]. However, there is more and more evidence that the disease starts initially without any kind of sensitization and that the latter is most probably started or enforced during the chronic course of the disease in early childhood [2, 38, 39]. This also means that the disease most probably starts as a nonallergic condition where the impaired epidermal barrier function plays a primary role in the induction of the inflammation. However, it is still not clear how genetic mutations or variants of relevant genes for the epidermal barrier function can solely lead to the underlying inflammatory condition. On the other hand, it has been speculated that the contact of foodstuff with the inflamed skin on the perioral region could contribute to the sensitization to food allergens, while the contact of food with the oral mucosa and the gastrointestinal tract would rather lead to tolerance mechanism [40]. This is even supported by recent epidemiological data strongly suggesting that an early introduction of food diversity may be protective against atopic dermatitis [35, 41, 42]. However, it is not clear which individuals may have greater benefit from this kind of strategy.

5.2.1.2 Microbiome and Infections

The role of *Staphylococcus aureus* and the products thereof has been supported by a number of in vitro and only few in vivo experiments [43, 44]. It is well accepted that the skin of patients with atopic dermatitis is heavily colonized with this bacterium and that the superantigens produced by staphylococci could amplify the inflammatory condition in an allergen-independent way [45, 46]. However, the use of antibiotics and antiseptics seems to only have a limited efficacy in controlling the flares of atopic dermatitis [47–49]. The overall role of bacteria on the skin in atopic dermatitis has more recently been highlighted by new insights in the diversity and complexity of the skin microbiome [50, 51]. Indeed, it appears that healthy skin is characterized by the colonization of at least 250–500 different bacteria, yeast, and viruses which all are involved in a continuous cross talk between themselves and the skin innate immune system [52–54]. Thus, healthy skin seems to be dependent on a balanced colonization, and a reduction of the diversity of the skin microbiome could be of pathophysiological relevance not only for atopic dermatitis [55], but also for other inflammatory skin conditions such as acne, rosacea, and psoriasis [56–58]. As the microbiome is now considered as our second genome, it introduces a new level of complexity that we are just starting to realize but far from being able to understand. We will have to increasingly consider the microbiome and its products in the context of an impaired epidermal barrier dysfunction since the latter allows a more facilitated interaction with our skin immune system and possibly the facilitated growth of pathogens.

5.2.1.3 Pruritus and Tissue Damage

Pruritus belongs to the main symptoms of atopic dermatitis, and it largely contributes to the impairment of the quality of life of the patients [59]. Besides this aspect, it has been shown that scratching may induce substantial tissue damage within the epidermal compartment, and this damage leads to the release of intracellular keratinocyte-derived compounds [60]. It has been assumed that these compounds are then captured by epidermal dendritic cells in the context of a microenvironment favoring a switch towards Th2, mainly provided by cytokines such as TSLP [61]. This constellation ultimately leads to the sensitization to keratinocyte-derived self-proteins to which the immune system mounts an IgE immune response [62–65]. While pruritus and scratching are not observed in the first weeks of the diseases in infancy, the first evidence for an IgE response to self-proteins is reported within the first year [66], where the chronic scratching activity has already been installed. However, it is still unclear why a number of children sensitized to self-proteins do not experience a more chronic course of the disease and the exposition to allergens like food and pollens still seems to represent the primary provocation factors in these sensitized individuals. On the other hand, a substantial proposition of adult patients with chronic and difficult to manage atopic dermatitis displays high amounts of IgE directed through self-proteins leading to the assumption that this particular population may have experienced a switch from an allergic to an auto-allergic form of atopic dermatitis (Phase 3) [1, 61].

5.2.2 Genetics of Atopic Dermatitis

The genetic background of atopic dermatitis is highly complex, but it can be schematically stratified in two main groups of genes possibly responsible for this disease (Fig. 5.1) [1]. This dichotomic view is mainly based on the fact that two main aspects learned from the pathophysiological understanding of atopic dermatitis have been put forward: an intrinsic defect in the epidermal barrier function on the one hand and a genetically driven dysfunction of the immune system leading to high tendency of IgE-mediated immune responses on the other hand.

5.2.2.1 Epidermal Genes

A number of different genes involved in the structure and regulation of the epidermal barrier functions have been proposed as candidates for the explanation of the impaired epidermal barrier function observed in atopic dermatitis. However, only two of them have reproducibly been investigated, and the functional consequences of mutations or single nucleotide polymorphisms (SNPs) of these genes have just started to be elucidated. Mutations of the gene encoding for filaggrin (FLG) have been shown to be relevant for the pathophysiology of ichthyosis vulgaris, the most common genodermatosis [67]. Similarly, genetic variants of the same gene have been shown to be associated with atopic dermatitis [68]. However, it should be noted that at least 50 different mutations or variants of filaggrin have been shown in different populations while the hot spots in European Caucasian populations seem to be different from those observed, for example, in Asian countries. Due to the relevance of filaggrin as a precursor molecule of the so-called natural moisturizing factor [69], this functional aspect is of primary interest for epidemiological studies which have supported the hypothesis that individuals carrying filaggrin mutations seem to have the highest risk to develop an early onset of atopic dermatitis followed by a severe and chronic form of the disease associated with other allergic diseases, i.e., an atopic march [38, 70–76].

Similarly, the protease-antiprotease system involved in the regulation of the epidermal barrier function has been scrutinized, and genetic variants of the gene encoding for the so-called LEKTI/SPINK5 gene has been shown to be associated with atopic dermatitis [77]. Interestingly, as is the case for filaggrin in ichthyosis vulgaris, mutations in LEKTI/SPINK5 are known to be at the origin of another genodermatosis associated with an impairment of the epidermal barrier function and the occurrence of an atopic dermatitis-like inflammation with high IgE levels: the Netherton syndrome [78]. A series of experiments performed in animal models where variants of the SPINK5 gene have been knocked in have shown that this genetic background can indeed induce an unspecific skin inflammation simply driven by an imbalance in the epidermal protease-antiprotease system [79–83]. As a consequence, this genetic background also induces a strong TSLP production by the epidermal keratinocytes and thereby prones the overall immune response towards Th2 profile. These observations could be relevant for the very initial infantile stage of atopic dermatitis (Phase 1) where an inflammatory condition is observed in the absence of any IgE sensitization context.

More recently, due to the progress in high-throughput technologies, a number of genome-wide association studies (GWAS) have been conducted in atopic dermatitis and have high-lighted some new candidate genes such as C11 of 30, or ACTL9, and KIF3A [84–88]. While the functional relevance of these genes is still not understood, it is clear however that the genetic background of atopic dermatitis is even more complex than initially suspected.

5.2.2.2 Immunological Genes

Since atopic dermatitis was initially considered primarily as an immunologically driven condition, many candidate gene approaches have been performed in the past and highlighted a number of relevant genes possibly involved in the context of the immunological mechanisms underlying the IgE sensitization as well as the skin inflammation. Interestingly, several candidate genes have been identified in the so-called cytokine cluster on chromosome 5q31-33 which encompasses key mediators such as IL4, IL5, and IL13 [89–91]. Similarly, genetic variants of the genes encoding for the receptor for IL4 [92, 93] have reproducibly been described as well as mutations in the promoter region for the gene and encoding for the chemokine CTACK/CCL27 and particularly the keratinocyte-derived cytokine TSLP which seems to play a key role in the pathophysiology of the disease [94–97]. The immunological aspects underlying atopic dermatitis have been reviewed recently [98] highlighting the move away from a uniform dogma involving mainly the Th1–Th2 balance towards a more complex network of many different T cells with a wide spectrum of cytokines such as IL-22 [99–102], IL-9 [103–105], and IL25 [106–109].

When it will come to establish a genomic profile supposed to be more or less characteristic for a subgroup of patients with atopic dermatitis, a various combination of different candidate genes will certainly be considered and will hopefully give us more information about the individual risk for the disease itself and the associated atopic march.

5.2.3 Epigenetics in Atopic Dermatitis

In the recent years, it became evident that the classical genetic background can be substantially modulated by mechanisms involving the methylation of genes and the acetylation/deacetylation of chromatin regions or microRNA sequences. Thus, since these mechanisms are under the significant influence of environmental factors such as foodstuff, exposition to pollutants, or potentially signals from the microbiome, epigenetic regulation could explain some contradictory results of a number of genetic studies reported in the field of allergic diseases. Only few studies have addressed the epigenetic regulation in atopic dermatitis [110–114], but it is expected that new knowledge in this field could provide important information with regard to new prevention strategies relevant for individualized prevention measures.

5.3 Heterogeneity of the Clinical Phenotype of Atopic Dermatitis

The clinical phenotype of atopic dermatitis displays a very wide spectrum of different aspects, and at least four levels of complexity can be distinguished, namely, (1) the age of onset, (2) the natural history, (3) the semiology of the lesions, and (4) the severity of the disease. These aspects are not independent but are usually related and sometimes strongly interacting.

5.3.1 Age of Onset of Atopic Dermatitis

As shown on Fig. 5.2, at least six different ages of onset can be identified [115]. It is currently far to be clear what the reasons for this high heterogeneity in the age of onset could be and whether genetic or more environmental factors could play a major role in the initiation of the study. Overall, it is interesting to note that the sensitization rate is the highest among people having started the disease before adulthood, while the classical late onset (between 20 and 60 years) seems to be a

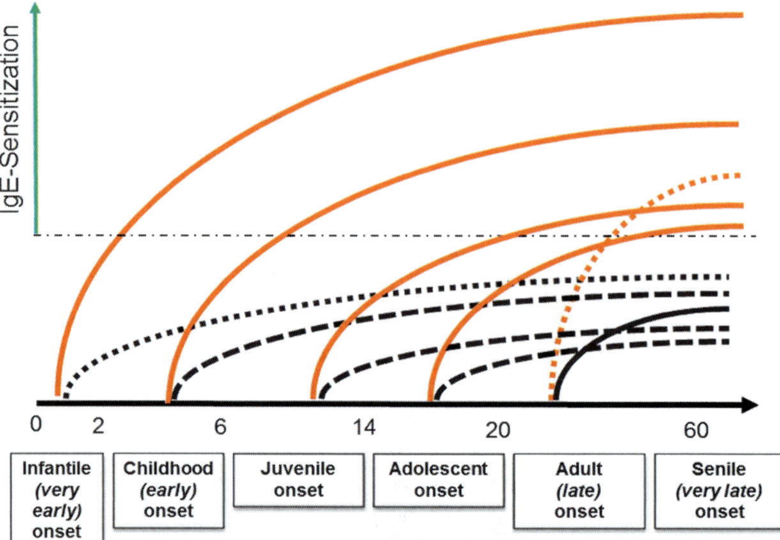

Fig. 5.2 The different types of onsets observed in atopic dermatitis (Adapted from [115]) and the risk of IgE sensitization

particular form which affects mainly females in which an IgE sensitization as well as other atopic diseases such as rhinitis or asthma are rarely seen [116–122]. Interestingly however, as it seems the case for psoriasis, we are currently assisting to the emergence of a very late onset (senile) of atopic dermatitis which is characterized by an average age of onset of more than 65 years, a rather severe form of atopic dermatitis typically as an erythrodermic variant, a male predominance (ratio M:F of 3:1), and a mean high total IgE level above 8,000 kU/l [123–126].

5.3.2 The Natural History of Atopic Dermatitis

Figure 5.1 depicts the classical natural history of a child with an infantile or childhood onset of atopic dermatitis in which the sensitization emerges during the chronic phase of the disease and potentially ending up with other atopic diseases affecting the airways, i.e., allergic rhinitis and allergic asthma. This natural history affects approximately 45 % of all patients, and they usually suffer from the more severe forms of the disease. On the other hand, it has been reported that approximately 60 % of the kids will improve the condition and go into complete remission before the puberty [18, 19, 115, 127–132]. However, this has been questioned

more recently in a large cross-sectional and cohort study which suggests that mild to moderate forms of atopic dermatitis may persist well into the second decade and even longer, strongly suggesting that atopic dermatitis should be considered as a lifelong condition [133].

5.3.3 Semiology of the Skin Lesions

Although atopic dermatitis is usually characterized by more or less sharply demarcated, erythematous, and scaly lesions mainly localized on typical body sites such as the head, neck, flexures, and hands, this archetypical kind of morphology may not be applied to all patients suffering from this disease (Fig. 5.3) [117]. Indeed, besides clear evidences of dry skin (xerosis), the semiology of the skin lesions can also be very diverse including, e.g., isolated retroauricular fissures or mainly highly infiltrated and lichenified lesions on other places, sometimes isolated or combined with a strong pruritus (the so-called lichen Vidal). Finally, the so-called nummular eczema is also considered as a possible variant of atopic dermatitis for which, besides the possible role of the microbiome and especially *Staphylococcus aureus* [134], no real pathophysiological explanation has been found so far.

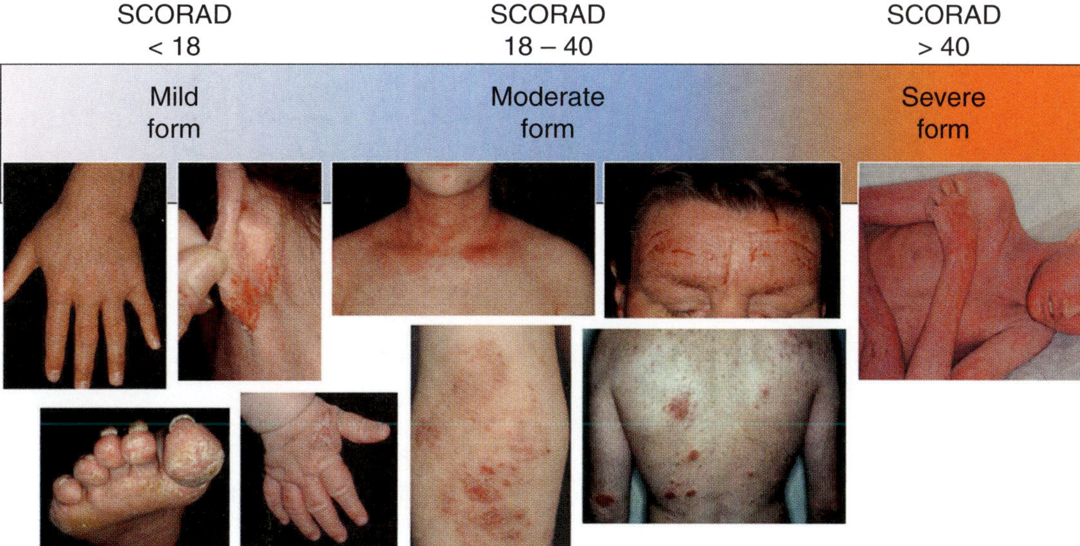

Fig. 5.3 The heterogeneity of the clinical phenotype of atopic dermatitis in relation to the severity grade

5.3.4 Spectrum of the Severity in Atopic Dermatitis

One of the key features of atopic dermatitis remains its wide spectrum of severity, which can be evaluated by different tools. Among the validated tools currently in use in clinical practice as well as in the context of clinical trials are the scoring systems SCORAD [135–139] and EASI [140–142]. Moreover, due to the increased importance of patient-related outcomes under socioeconomic and pharmaco-economic aspects, tools to evaluate the severity from the patients point of view (PO-SCORAD and POEMS) [136, 141, 143–147] as well as questionnaires for the evaluation of the quality of life specifically designed for patients with skin conditions (e.g., DLQI or the Skindex) have been developed [148–156].

Three main severity categories have been defined: mild (including xerosis), moderate, and severe. It has been shown that most of the patients are switching from one category to the other depending on the disease activity, usually dictated by the flares. As expected, disease severity is strongly associated to the frequency of flares. However, in the absence of adequate therapeutic management, the disease keeps a level of severity of its own. Except for the case of the infantile and childhood onsets of the disease where a gradual increase in the affected body regions and body surface area is usually observed during the chronic course of the disease, only few data are available for the natural history in terms of severity with the adult onsets of atopic dermatitis. Among the population of patients suffering from atopic dermatitis, the severity is not evenly distributed, but it is estimated that severe patients represent 10–15 % of the overall AD populations. However, the moderate-to-severe and severe population (SCORAD >30) have the biggest medical unmet need.

5.4 The Quest for Biomarkers Leading to a New Taxonomy of Atopic Dermatitis

The spectrum of possible biomarkers useful in any kind of disease is quite large and much dependent on the kind of disease and the approach selected. Progress in our understanding of the genetic background and the epidemiology and pathophysiology of atopic dermatitis has led to a series of candidate genes and molecules which could be used as biomarkers in the context of personalized medicine. With regard to the particular natural history of atopic dermatitis, a number of

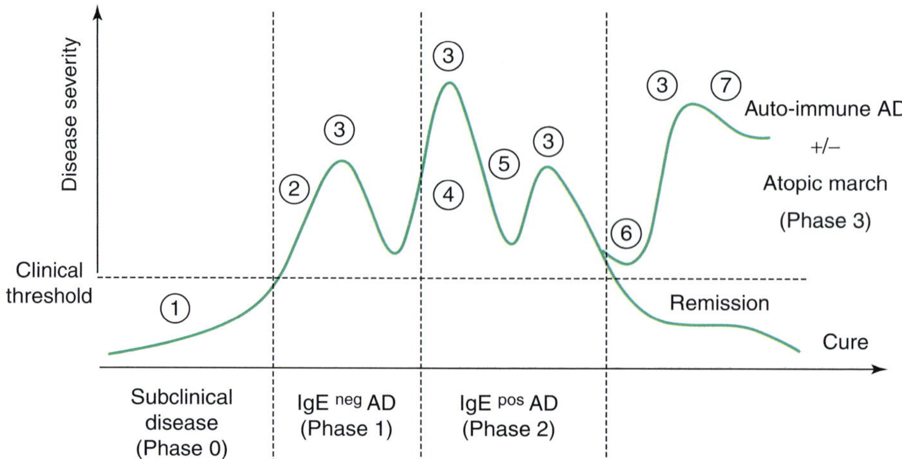

Fig. 5.4 Schematic profile of the natural history of atopic dermatitis with the different time points where a biomarker could be applied (Adapted from [178]). *1* Screening biomarkers for detection of patients at risk for atopic dermatitis. *2* Diagnostic biomarkers. *3* Severity biomarkers. *4* Biomarkers for individualized diagnostics of the sensitization profile. *5* Pharmacogenomic biomarkers predicting the therapeutic response. *6* Prognostic biomarkers predicting the course (complete remission or relapse) of the disease. *7* Diagnostic biomarkers for auto-immunity in atopic dermatitis

different kinds of biomarkers are expected to be discovered. Figure 5.4 shows the typical scenarios of a natural history of atopic dermatitis with early onset and the different time points at which biomarkers could be useful for the management of the disease. Thereby, the following types of biomarkers can be considered:

1. Screening biomarkers which are unable to identify those patients at high risk of developing atopic dermatitis even before the first clinical signs of the disease.
2. Diagnostic biomarkers which could be used at a very early time point in case of differential diagnostic problems.
3. Severity biomarkers typically useful in the setting of clinical trials for the evaluation of therapeutic success or even as surrogate biomarkers for clinical trials and long-lasting control.
4. Biomarkers for individualized diagnostics of the sensitization profile. A determination of specific IgE belongs to this kind of biomarkers already available.
5. Biomarkers predicting the therapeutic response and the risk of side effects for a specific drug (pharmacogenomics).
6. Prognostic biomarkers which may predict the occurrence of remission before puberty or adulthood or a successful disease-modifying strategy.
7. Diagnostic biomarkers for atopic march and/or autoimmunity in atopic dermatitis enabling to identify those patients who would not have benefit from any kind of avoidance strategy with respect to allergens or other environmental factors.

Overall, it is assumed that most of the diseases will not be stratified according to one single biomarker [157–159]. Thus, as our understanding in the genetics and pathophysiology of atopic dermatitis will progress, an increasing number of different biomarkers will be available, and depending on the goal of the stratification, a more or less complex combination of several biomarkers will be considered: they built the so-called endophenotypes. As for other complex diseases, the endophenotype will ultimately lead to a stratification of atopic dermatitis according to a new kind of molecular taxonomy [160]. This stratification will be the basis of future developments in personalized prevention and therapy.

5.5 The Long Way to Personalized Management of Atopic Dermatitis

With regard to the abovementioned complexity of the pathophysiology and clinical phenotype of atopic dermatitis, a number of opportunities can be defined for which a personalized approach could substantially be of benefit for an endophenotype-defined subgroup of patients suffering from this disease.

In the following, a few ideas and speculations are drawn in order to address some key opportunities and goals.

5.5.1 Personalized Prevention to Avoid the Atopic March

The analysis of different kinds of natural history of this disease has strongly suggested that there is one particular subpopulation of patients starting with an early onset which has the highest risk to develop a long life severe form of atopic dermatitis associated with strong sensitization and a high risk to develop allergic asthma, i.e., the atopic march. Preliminary evidence from genetic studies suggests that filaggrin mutations are strongly associated with this particular natural history of the disease [70–73, 161]. However, we will certainly need some other biomarkers related to the immunological sets of genes associated with the regulation of IgE synthesis in order to have a more complete picture of the possible endophenotype associated with individuals at high risk to develop this particular course of the disease. Based on this information provided by a combination of appropriate biomarkers, it could be possible to identify the newborns and children at high risk at a very early time point (Phase 0) and to stratify these populations starting in a way that would allow to provide a more differentiated information to the parents as well as the very early use of particularly adapted prevention measures [162]. This kind of primary prevention could potentially hamper the appearance of the disease or lead to the delay of the first symptoms. Appropriate prevention measures with regard to the exposition to foodstuff and other potential allergens could be designed in order to induce tolerance instead of sensitization. Even if these primary prevention measures would not be effective, and the disease has already started (Phase 1), the knowledge about the risk of atopic march would be very helpful in order to convince the parents about the importance of a good compliance to a therapeutic management plan proposed by the physicians. In this context, a targeted implementation of a long-term proactive management would be of particular benefit and could potentially hamper the emergence of sensitization, i.e., the Phase 2 of the disease.

5.5.2 A Personalized Management to Control a Disease on the Long Run

While the prevention of the atopic march is a strategy which is applicable in infancy and childhood, it would be important to design new approaches for a better control of the flares in patients suffering from a chronic and moderate-to-severe form of atopic dermatitis. Indeed, although it is now well accepted that the control of the flares is mainly reached by a better control of the subclinical information, it is still not clear how long the proactive management has to be provided in order to reach the goal of a complete remission of the disease. Thus, appropriate biomarkers would give us important information about the subclinical inflammation and the time point which should be reached in order to stop the long-term anti-inflammatory treatment.

5.5.3 A Personalized Diagnostic Approach to Identify the Provocation Factors in Atopic Dermatitis

Most of the patients affected by atopic dermatitis display a very wide spectrum of sensitization as detected by either prick test or specific IgE. However, it is well accepted that only a few of these allergens may be relevant for this particular patient [163]. This issue is not specific to atopic dermatitis but remains a challenge for most allergic diseases when allergen-specific immunotherapy is envisaged. Therefore, a refinement of the allergic diagnostic based on new molecular approaches could be very useful in order to detect those allergens which are relevant for each individual patient in order to provide him an appropriate avoidance strategy and thereby to reduce the number of provocations and flares due to contacts with allergens. Most importantly, the hotly debated causative therapy with allergen-specific immunotherapy for atopic dermatitis would have a greater chance of success under these conditions [164–171].

5.5.4 Personalized Approach in the Context of Drug Development

Patients affected by moderate-to-severe atopic dermatitis usually cannot be controlled efficiently on long term using the few approved systemic drugs for these conditions such as cyclosporine. Therefore, a number of patients have to be treated with off-label regimens [172–176]. However, all these treatments which have not been developed specifically for this disease may expose the patients to unwanted, more or less severe side effects. Therefore, the risk-to-benefit ratio for most of the patients treated by systemic immunosuppressive drugs is not satisfactory. A better understanding of the complex pathophysiology of atopic dermatitis and more specifically the role of individual cytokines in the regulation of IgE and in the generation of the skin inflammation in patients with the more severe forms will have a tremendous impact on the discovery of new biomarkers and potentially on the development of new targets for this particular population. Among the biologics which are currently in development, the anti-IL4 strategy seems to be the most promising [177], while it is not clear whether this particular approach will be beneficial only for a subpopulation of patients with AD.

Conclusion

Due to its pathophysiological and clinical complexity, atopic dermatitis is a candidate disease for personalized medicine. Although atopic dermatitis is not life-threatening, it is well accepted that it kills the quality of life of the patients and their relatives. Unfortunately, more than other kinds of disease, atopic dermatitis has so far only been treated with some few standard regimens including emollients and topical anti-inflammatory drugs such as steroids and calcineurin inhibitors. For the most severe forms, depending on the countries, there is no approved systemic drug for the management of this disease. On the other hand, the heterogeneity of the clinical phenotype and our knowledge about the natural history strongly suggest that the management of these patients should be considered in a more differentiated way. While about half of the children affected by atopic dermatitis will experience a remission until adulthood, the other half will have to suffer more or less from this disease for their whole life. Moreover, within this population, a substantial proportion of patients will develop other atopic diseases like rhinitis and allergic asthma, and there is an urgent need and opportunity for early intervention strategies in order to limit the emergence of the atopic march. Thus, one of the primary goals of personalized medicine in the context of atopic dermatitis is to develop new disease-modifying strategies aimed to better control the inflammation in the skin and ideally to hamper the occurrence of IgE sensitization in those patients with high risk to develop an atopic career.

References

1. Bieber T. Atopic dermatitis. N Engl J Med. 2008;358(14):1483–94.
2. Flohr C, Mann J. New insights into the epidemiology of childhood atopic dermatitis. Allergy. 2014;69(1): 3–16. Epub 2014/01/15.
3. Beikert FC, Langenbruch AK, Radtke MA, Kornek T, Purwins S, Augustin M. Willingness to pay and quality of life in patients with atopic dermatitis. Arch Dermatol Res. 2014;306(3):279–86. Epub 2013/08/29.

4. Beattie PE, Lewis-Jones MS. An audit of the impact of a consultation with a paediatric dermatology team on quality of life in infants with atopic eczema and their families: further validation of the Infants' Dermatitis Quality of Life Index and Dermatitis Family Impact score. Br J Dermatol. 2006;155(6):1249–55.

5. Zuberbier T, Orlow SJ, Paller AS, Taieb A, Allen R, Hernanz-Hermosa JM, et al. Patient perspectives on the management of atopic dermatitis. J Allergy Clin Immunol. 2006;118(1):226–32.

6. Healy E, Bentley A, Fidler C, Chambers C. Cost-effectiveness of tacrolimus ointment in adults and children with moderate and severe atopic dermatitis: twice-weekly maintenance treatment vs. standard twice-daily reactive treatment of exacerbations from a third party payer (U.K. National Health Service) perspective. Br J Dermatol. 2011;164(2):387–95. Epub 2010/11/19.

7. Mancini AJ, Kaulback K, Chamlin SL. The socioeconomic impact of atopic dermatitis in the United States: a systematic review. Pediatr Dermatol. 2008;25(1):1–6.

8. Jenner N, Campbell J, Marks R. Morbidity and cost of atopic eczema in Australia. Australas J Dermatol. 2004;45(1):16–22.

9. Lamb SR, Rademaker M. Pharmacoeconomics of drug therapy for atopic dermatitis. Expert Opin Pharmacother. 2002;3(3):249–55.

10. Herd RM. The financial impact on families of children with atopic dermatitis. Arch Dermatol. 2002;138(6):819–20.

11. Ellis CN, Drake LA, Prendergast MM, Abramovits W, Boguniewicz M, Daniel CR, et al. Cost of atopic dermatitis and eczema in the United States. J Am Acad Dermatol. 2002;46(3):361–70.

12. Curtiss FR. Prevalence and costs of atopic dermatitis. J Manag Care Pharm. 2002;8(5):404.

13. Emerson RM, Williams HC, Allen BR. What is the cost of atopic dermatitis in preschool children? Br J Dermatol. 2001;144(3):514–22.

14. Kemp AS. Atopic eczema: its social and financial costs. J Paediatr Child Health. 1999;35(3):229–31.

15. Su JC, Kemp AS, Varigos GA, Nolan TM. Atopic eczema: its impact on the family and financial cost. Arch Dis Child. 1997;76(2):159–62.

16. Herd RM, Tidman MJ, Prescott RJ, Hunter JA. The cost of atopic eczema. Br J Dermatol. 1996;135(1):20–3.

17. Lapidus CS, Schwarz DF, Honig PJ. Atopic dermatitis in children: who cares? Who pays? J Am Acad Dermatol. 1993;28(5 Pt 1):699–703.

18. Williams HC. Clinical practice. Atopic dermatitis. N Engl J Med. 2005;352(22):2314–24.

19. Bieber T, Bussmann C. Atopic dermatitis. In: Bolognia JL, Jorizzo JL, Schaffer JV, editors. Dermatology. 3rd ed. Oxford: Elsevier; 2012.

20. Eichenfield LF, Tom WL, Chamlin SL, Feldman SR, Hanifin JM, Simpson EL, et al. Guidelines of care for the management of atopic dermatitis: section 1. Diagnosis and assessment of atopic dermatitis. J Am Acad Dermatol. 2014;70(2):338–51. Epub 2013/12/03.

21. Rubel D, Thirumoorthy T, Soebaryo RW, Weng SC, Gabriel TM, Villafuerte LL, et al. Consensus guidelines for the management of atopic dermatitis: an Asia-Pacific perspective. J Dermatol. 2013;40(3):160–71. Epub 2013/01/08.

22. Devillers AC, Oranje AP. Wet-wrap treatment in children with atopic dermatitis: a practical guideline. Pediatr Dermatol. 2012;29(1):24–7. Epub 2012/01/20.

23. Katayama I, Kohno Y, Akiyama K, Ikezawa Z, Kondo N, Tamaki K, et al. Japanese guideline for atopic dermatitis. Allergol Int. 2011;60(2):205–20. Epub 2011/06/04.

24. Saeki H, Furue M, Furukawa F, Hide M, Ohtsuki M, Katayama I, et al. Guidelines for management of atopic dermatitis. J Dermatol. 2009;36(10):563–77.

25. Baumer JH. Guideline review: atopic eczema in children, NICE. Arch Dis Child Educ Pract Ed 2008;93(3):93–97.

26. Hanifin JM, Cooper KD, Ho VC, Kang S, Krafchik BR, Margolis DJ, et al. Guidelines of care for atopic dermatitis, developed in accordance with the American Academy of Dermatology (AAD)/ American Academy of Dermatology Association "Administrative Regulations for Evidence-Based Clinical Practice Guidelines". J Am Acad Dermatol. 2004;50(3):391–404.

27. Eichenfield LF. Consensus guidelines in diagnosis and treatment of atopic dermatitis. Allergy. 2004;59 Suppl 78:86–92.

28. Guillet MH, Guillet G. Management of atopic dermatitis: practical guidelines suggested by the conclusion of systematic assessment in 500 children. Allerg Immunol (Paris). 2000;32(8):305–8. La prise en charge allergologique de l'atopique eczemateux: conclusions pratiques de l'exploration systematique de 500 enfants.

29. McNally NJ, Williams HC, Phillips DR, Smallman-Raynor M, Lewis S, Venn A, et al. Atopic eczema and domestic water hardness. Lancet. 1998;352(9127):527–31.

30. Thomas KS, Sach TH. A multicentre randomized controlled trial of ion-exchange water softeners for the treatment of eczema in children: protocol for the Softened Water Eczema Trial (SWET) (ISRCTN: 71423189). Br J Dermatol. 2008;159(3):561–6.

31. Thomas KS, Dean T, O'Leary C, Sach TH, Koller K, Frost A, et al. A randomised controlled trial of ion-exchange water softeners for the treatment of eczema in children. PLoS Med. 2011;8(2):e1000395. Epub 2011/03/02.

32. Chaumont A, Voisin C, Sardella A, Bernard A. Interactions between domestic water hardness, infant swimming and atopy in the development of childhood eczema. Environ Res. 2012;116:52–7. Epub 2012/05/18.

33. Parazzini F, Cipriani S, Zinetti C, Chatenoud L, Frigerio L, Amuso G, et al. Perinatal factors and the

risk of atopic dermatitis: a cohort study. Pediatr Allergy Immunol. 2014;25(1):43–50. Epub 2013/12/10.

34. Kim JH, Jeong KS, Ha EH, Park H, Ha M, Hong YC, et al. Relationship between prenatal and postnatal exposures to folate and risks of allergic and respiratory diseases in early childhood. Pediatr Pulmonol. 2014. Epub 2014/03/13.

35. Illi S, Weber J, Zutavern A, Genuneit J, Schierl R, Strunz-Lehner C, et al. Perinatal influences on the development of asthma and atopy in childhood. Ann Allergy Asthma Immunol. 2014;112(2):132–9 e1. Epub 2014/01/29.

36. Bunyavanich S, Rifas-Shiman SL, Platts-Mills TA, Workman L, Sordillo JE, Camargo Jr CA, et al. Peanut, milk, and wheat intake during pregnancy is associated with reduced allergy and asthma in children. J Allergy Clin Immunol. 2014;133(5): 1373–82.

37. Chen CM, Sausenthaler S, Bischof W, Herbarth O, Borte M, Behrendt H, et al. Perinatal exposure to endotoxin and the development of eczema during the first 6 years of life. Clin Exp Dermatol. 2010;35(3):238–244.

38. Dharmage SC, Lowe AJ, Matheson MC, Burgess JA, Allen KJ, Abramson MJ. Atopic dermatitis and the atopic march revisited. Allergy. 2014;69(1):17–27. Epub 2013/10/15.

39. Illi S, von Mutius E, Lau S, Nickel R, Gruber C, Niggemann B, et al. The natural course of atopic dermatitis from birth to age 7 years and the association with asthma. J Allergy Clin Immunol. 2004;113(5): 925–31.

40. Lack G. Update on risk factors for food allergy. J Allergy Clin Immunol. 2012;129(5):1187–97. Epub 2012/04/03.

41. Roduit C, Frei R, Depner M, Schaub B, Loss G, Genuneit J, et al. Increased food diversity in the first year of life is inversely associated with allergic diseases. J Allergy Clin Immunol. 2014;133(4):1056–64 e7. Epub 2014/02/11.

42. Roduit C, Frei R, Loss G, Buchele G, Weber J, Depner M, et al. Development of atopic dermatitis according to age of onset and association with early-life exposures. J Allergy Clin Immunol. 2012;130(1):130–6 e135.

43. Brauweiler AM, Goleva E, Leung DY. Th2 cytokines increase staphylococcus aureus alpha toxin-induced keratinocyte death through the signal transducer and activator of transcription 6 (STAT6). J Invest Dermatol. 2014;134(8):2114–21.

44. Reginald K, Westritschnig K, Werfel T, Heratizadeh A, Novak N, Focke-Tejkl M, et al. Immunoglobulin E antibody reactivity to bacterial antigens in atopic dermatitis patients. Clin Exp Allergy. 2011;41(3):357–69. Epub 2010/12/16.

45. Leung AD, Schiltz AM, Hall CF, Liu AH. Severe atopic dermatitis is associated with a high burden of environmental Staphylococcus aureus. Clin Exp Allergy. 2008;38(5):789–93.

46. Cardona ID, Cho SH, Leung DY. Role of bacterial superantigens in atopic dermatitis: implications for future therapeutic strategies. Am J Clin Dermatol. 2006;7(5):273–9.

47. Travers JB, Kozman A, Yao Y, Ming W, Yao W, Turner MJ, et al. Treatment outcomes of secondarily impetiginized pediatric atopic dermatitis lesions and the role of oral antibiotics. Pediatr Dermatol. 2012;29(3):289–96. Epub 2011/12/14.

48. Ong PY, Leung DY. The infectious aspects of atopic dermatitis. Immunol Allergy Clin North Am. 2010;30(3):309–21. Epub 2010/07/31.

49. Boguniewicz M, Leung DY. Recent insights into atopic dermatitis and implications for management of infectious complications. J Allergy Clin Immunol. 2010;125(1):4–13; quiz 4–5. Epub 2010/01/30.

50. Kong HH, Segre JA. Skin microbiome: looking back to move forward. J Invest Dermatol. 2012;132(3 Pt 2):933–9. Epub 2011/12/23.

51. Abrahamsson TR, Jakobsson HE, Andersson AF, Bjorksten B, Engstrand L, Jenmalm MC. Low diversity of the gut microbiota in infants with atopic eczema. J Allergy Clin Immunol. 2012;129(2):434–40, 40 e1–2. Epub 2011/12/14.

52. Costello EK, Lauber CL, Hamady M, Fierer N, Gordon JI, Knight R. Bacterial community variation in human body habitats across space and time. Science. 2009;326(5960):1694–7. Epub 2009/11/07.

53. Grice EA, Kong HH, Conlan S, Deming CB, Davis J, Young AC, et al. Topographical and temporal diversity of the human skin microbiome. Science. 2009;324(5931):1190–2. Epub 2009/05/30.

54. Zhou Y, Gao H, Mihindukulasuriya KA, La Rosa PS, Wylie KM, Vishnivetskaya T, et al. Biogeography of the ecosystems of the healthy human body. Genome Biol. 2013;14(1):R1. Epub 2013/01/16.

55. Kong HH, Oh J, Deming C, Conlan S, Grice EA, Beatson MA, et al. Temporal shifts in the skin microbiome associated with disease flares and treatment in children with atopic dermatitis. Genome Res. 2012;22(5):850–9. Epub 2012/02/09.

56. Castelino M, Eyre S, Upton M, Ho P, Barton A. The bacterial skin microbiome in psoriatic arthritis, an unexplored link in pathogenesis: challenges and opportunities offered by recent technological advances. Rheumatology. 2014;53(5):777–84.

57. Chen YE, Tsao H. The skin microbiome: current perspectives and future challenges. J Am Acad Dermatol. 2013;69(1):143–55. Epub 2013/03/16.

58. Zeeuwen PL, Kleerebezem M, Timmerman HM, Schalkwijk J. Microbiome and skin diseases. Curr Opin Allergy Clin Immunol. 2013;13(5):514–20. Epub 2013/08/27.

59. Benjamin K, Waterston K, Russell M, Schofield O, Diffey B, Rees JL. The development of an objective method for measuring scratch in children with atopic dermatitis suitable for clinical use. J Am Acad Dermatol. 2004;50(1):33–40.

60. Kinaciyan T, Natter S, Kraft D, Stingl G, Valenta R. IgE autoantibodies monitored in a patient with

atopic dermatitis under cyclosporin A treatment reflect tissue damage. J Allergy Clin Immunol. 2002;109(4):717–9.

61. Tang TS, Bieber T, Williams HC. Does "autoreactivity" play a role in atopic dermatitis? J Allergy Clin Immunol. 2012;129(5):1209–15 e2. Epub 2012/03/14.

62. Altrichter S, Kriehuber E, Moser J, Valenta R, Kopp T, Stingl G. Serum IgE autoantibodies target keratinocytes in patients with atopic dermatitis. J Invest Dermatol. 2008;128(9):2232–9.

63. Valenta R, Seiberler S, Natter S, Mahler V, Mossabeb R, Ring J, et al. Autoallergy: a pathogenetic factor in atopic dermatitis? J Allergy Clin Immunol. 2000;105(3):432–7.

64. Valenta R, Natter S, Seiberler S, Wichlas S, Maurer D, Hess M, et al. Molecular characterization of an autoallergen, Hom s 1, identified by serum IgE from atopic dermatitis patients. J Invest Dermatol. 1998;111(6):1178–83.

65. Valenta R, Maurer D, Steiner R, Seiberler S, Sperr WR, Valent P, et al. Immunoglobulin E response to human proteins in atopic patients. J Invest Dermatol. 1996;107(2):203–8.

66. Mothes N, Niggemann B, Jenneck C, Hagemann T, Weidinger S, Bieber T, et al. The cradle of IgE autoreactivity in atopic eczema lies in early infancy. J Allergy Clin Immunol. 2005;116(3):706–9.

67. Smith FJ, Irvine AD, Terron-Kwiatkowski A, Sandilands A, Campbell LE, Zhao Y, et al. Loss-of-function mutations in the gene encoding filaggrin cause ichthyosis vulgaris. Nat Genet. 2006;38(3):337–42.

68. Palmer CN, Irvine AD, Terron-Kwiatkowski A, Zhao Y, Liao H, Lee SP, et al. Common loss-of-function variants of the epidermal barrier protein filaggrin are a major predisposing factor for atopic dermatitis. Nat Genet. 2006;38(4):441–6.

69. Kezic S, O'Regan GM, Yau N, Sandilands A, Chen H, Campbell LE, et al. Levels of filaggrin degradation products are influenced by both filaggrin genotype and atopic dermatitis severity. Allergy. 2011;66(7):934–40. Epub 2011/01/26.

70. Marenholz I, Nickel R, Ruschendorf F, Schulz F, Esparza-Gordillo J, Kerscher T, et al. Filaggrin loss-of-function mutations predispose to phenotypes involved in the atopic march. J Allergy Clin Immunol. 2006;118(4):866–71.

71. Schuttelaar ML, Kerkhof M, Jonkman MF, Koppelman GH, Brunekreef B, de Jongste JC, et al. Filaggrin mutations in the onset of eczema, sensitization, asthma, hay fever and the interaction with cat exposure. Allergy. 2009;64(12):1758–65.

72. Spergel JM. From atopic dermatitis to asthma: the atopic march. Ann Allergy Asthma Immunol. 2010;105(2):99–106; quiz 7–9, 17. Epub 2010/08/03.

73. Heimall J, Spergel JM. Filaggrin mutations and atopy: consequences for future therapeutics. Expert Rev Clin Immunol. 2012;8(2):189–97. Epub 2012/02/01.

74. Burgess JA, Lowe AJ, Matheson MC, Varigos G, Abramson MJ, Dharmage SC. Does eczema lead to asthma? J Asthma. 2009;46(5):429–36.

75. Williams H, Flohr C. How epidemiology has challenged 3 prevailing concepts about atopic dermatitis. J Allergy Clin Immunol. 2006;118(1):209–13.

76. Spergel JM. Atopic march: link to upper airways. Curr Opin Allergy Clin Immunol. 2005;5(1):17–21.

77. Walley AJ, Chavanas S, Moffatt MF, Esnouf RM, Ubhi B, Lawrence R, et al. Gene polymorphism in Netherton and common atopic disease. Nat Genet. 2001;29(2):175–8.

78. Sprecher E, Chavanas S, DiGiovanna JJ, Amin S, Nielsen K, Prendiville JS, et al. The spectrum of pathogenic mutations in SPINK5 in 19 families with Netherton syndrome: implications for mutation detection and first case of prenatal diagnosis. J Invest Dermatol. 2001;117(2):179–87.

79. Briot A, Deraison C, Lacroix M, Bonnart C, Robin A, Besson C, et al. Kallikrein 5 induces atopic dermatitis-like lesions through PAR2-mediated thymic stromal lymphopoietin expression in Netherton syndrome. J Exp Med. 2009;206(5):1135–47.

80. Di WL, Hennekam RC, Callard RE, Harper JI. A heterozygous null mutation combined with the G1258A polymorphism of SPINK5 causes impaired LEKTI function and abnormal expression of skin barrier proteins. Br J Dermatol. 2009;161(2):404–12.

81. Meyer-Hoffert U, Wu Z, Schroder JM. Identification of lympho-epithelial Kazal-type inhibitor 2 in human skin as a kallikrein-related peptidase 5-specific protease inhibitor. PLoS One. 2009;4(2):e4372.

82. Briot A, Lacroix M, Robin A, Steinhoff M, Deraison C, Hovnanian A. Par2 inactivation inhibits early production of TSLP, but not cutaneous inflammation, in Netherton syndrome adult mouse model. J Invest Dermatol. 2010;130(12):2736–42. Epub 2010/08/13.

83. Hovnanian A. Netherton syndrome: skin inflammation and allergy by loss of protease inhibition. Cell Tissue Res. 2013;351(2):289–300. Epub 2013/01/25.

84. Weidinger S, Willis-Owen SA, Kamatani Y, Baurecht H, Morar N, Liang L, et al. A genome-wide association study of atopic dermatitis identifies loci with overlapping effects on asthma and psoriasis. Hum Mol Genet. 2013;22(23):4841–56. Epub 2013/07/28.

85. Ellinghaus D, Baurecht H, Esparza-Gordillo J, Rodriguez E, Matanovic A, Marenholz I, et al. High-density genotyping study identifies four new susceptibility loci for atopic dermatitis. Nat Genet. 2013;45(7):808–12. Epub 2013/06/04.

86. Bonnelykke K, Matheson MC, Pers TH, Granell R, Strachan DP, Alves AC, et al. Meta-analysis of genome-wide association studies identifies ten loci influencing allergic sensitization. Nat Genet. 2013;45(8):902–6. Epub 2013/07/03.

87. Sun LD, Xiao FL, Li Y, Zhou WM, Tang HY, Tang XF, et al. Genome-wide association study identifies two new susceptibility loci for atopic dermatitis in the Chinese Han population. Nat Genet. 2011;43(7):690–4. Epub 2011/06/15.

88. Paternoster L, Standl M, Chen CM, Ramasamy A, Bonnelykke K, Duijts L, et al. Meta-analysis of genome-wide association studies identifies three new risk loci for atopic dermatitis. Nat Genet. 2012;44(2):187–92. Epub 2011/12/27.

89. Beyer K, Nickel R, Freidhoff L, Bjorksten B, Huang SK, Barnes KC, et al. Association and linkage of atopic dermatitis with chromosome 13q12-14 and 5q31-33 markers. J Invest Dermatol. 2000;115(5):906–8.

90. Soderhall C, Bradley M, Kockum I, Wahlgren CF, Luthman H, Nordenskjold M. Linkage and association to candidate regions in Swedish atopic dermatitis families. Hum Genet. 2001;109(2):129–35.

91. Tsunemi Y, Saeki H, Nakamura K, Sekiya T, Hirai K, Fujita H, et al. Interleukin-12 p40 gene (IL12B) 3′-untranslated region polymorphism is associated with susceptibility to atopic dermatitis and psoriasis vulgaris. J Dermatol Sci. 2002;30(2):161–6. Epub 2002/11/05.

92. Hershey GK, Friedrich MF, Esswein LA, Thomas ML, Chatila TA. The association of atopy with a gain-of-function mutation in the alpha subunit of the interleukin-4 receptor. N Engl J Med. 1997;337(24):1720–5.

93. Biagini Myers JM, Wang N, Lemasters GK, Bernstein DI, Epstein TG, Lindsey MA, et al. Genetic and environmental risk factors for childhood eczema development and allergic sensitization in the CCAAPS Cohort. J Invest Dermatol. 2010; 130(2):430–437.

94. Turner MJ, Zhou B. A new itch to scratch for TSLP. Trends Immunol. 2014;35(2):49–50. Epub 2014/01/15.

95. Margolis DJ, Kim B, Apter AJ, Gupta J, Hoffstad O, Papadopoulos M, et al. Thymic stromal lymphopoietin variation, filaggrin loss of function, and the persistence of atopic dermatitis. JAMA Dermatol. 2014;150(3):254–9. Epub 2014/01/10.

96. Leyva-Castillo JM, Hener P, Jiang H, Li M. TSLP produced by keratinocytes promotes allergen sensitization through skin and thereby triggers atopic march in mice. J Invest Dermatol. 2013;133(1):154–63. Epub 2012/07/27.

97. Ziegler SF, Artis D. Sensing the outside world: TSLP regulates barrier immunity. Nat Immunol. 2010;11(4):289–93. Epub 2010/03/20.

98. Eyerich K, Novak N. Immunology of atopic eczema: overcoming the Th1/Th2 paradigm. Allergy. 2013;68(8):974–82. Epub 2013/07/31.

99. Eyerich S, Eyerich K, Pennino D, Carbone T, Nasorri F, Pallotta S, et al. Th22 cells represent a distinct human T cell subset involved in epidermal immunity and remodeling. J Clin Invest. 2009;119(12):3573–85. Epub 2009/11/19.

100. Nograles KE, Zaba LC, Shemer A, Fuentes-Duculan J, Cardinale I, Kikuchi T, et al. IL-22-producing "T22" T cells account for upregulated IL-22 in atopic dermatitis despite reduced IL-17-producing TH17 T cells. J Allergy Clin Immunol. 2009;123(6):1244–52 e2.

101. Niebuhr M, Scharonow H, Gathmann M, Mamerow D, Werfel T. Staphylococcal exotoxins are strong inducers of IL-22: a potential role in atopic dermatitis. J Allergy Clin Immunol. 2010;126(6):1176–83 e4. Epub 2010/09/25.

102. Souwer Y, Szegedi K, Kapsenberg ML, de Jong EC. IL-17 and IL-22 in atopic allergic disease. Curr Opin Immunol. 2010;22(6):821–6. Epub 2010/11/23.

103. Auriemma M, Vianale G, Amerio P, Reale M. Cytokines and T cells in atopic dermatitis. Eur Cytokine Netw. 2013;24(1):37–44. Epub 2013/04/24.

104. Yao W, Zhang Y, Jabeen R, Nguyen ET, Wilkes DS, Tepper RS, et al. Interleukin-9 is required for allergic airway inflammation mediated by the cytokine TSLP. Immunity. 2013;38(2):360–72. Epub 2013/02/05.

105. Ma L, Xue HB, Guan XH, Shu CM, Zhang JH, Yu J. Possible pathogenic role of T helper type 9 cells and interleukin (IL)-9 in atopic dermatitis. Clin Exp Immunol. 2014;175(1):25–31. Epub 2013/09/17.

106. Wang YH, Angkasekwinai P, Lu N, Voo KS, Arima K, Hanabuchi S, et al. IL-25 augments type 2 immune responses by enhancing the expansion and functions of TSLP-DC activated Th2 memory cells. J Exp Med. 2007;204(8):1837–47.

107. Hvid M, Vestergaard C, Kemp K, Christensen GB, Deleuran B, Deleuran M. IL-25 in atopic dermatitis: a possible link between inflammation and skin barrier dysfunction? J Invest Dermatol. 2010;130(2):430–437.

108. Hvid M, Vestergaard C, Kemp K, Christensen GB, Deleuran B, Deleuran M. IL-25 in atopic dermatitis: a possible link between inflammation and skin barrier dysfunction? J Invest Dermatol. 2011;131(1):150–7. Epub 2010/09/24.

109. Deleuran M, Hvid M, Kemp K, Christensen GB, Deleuran B, Vestergaard C. IL-25 induces both inflammation and skin barrier dysfunction in atopic dermatitis. Chem Immunol Allergy. 2012;96:45–9. Epub 2012/03/22.

110. Luo Y, Zhou B, Zhao M, Tang J, Lu Q. Promoter demethylation contributes to TSLP overexpression in skin lesions of patients with atopic dermatitis. Clin Exp Dermatol. 2014;39(1):48–53. Epub 2013/12/18.

111. Wang IJ, Chen SL, Lu TP, Chuang EY, Chen PC. Prenatal smoke exposure, DNA methylation, and childhood atopic dermatitis. Clin Exp Allergy. 2013;43(5):535–43. Epub 2013/04/23.

112. van Panhuys N, Le Gros G, McConnell MJ. Epigenetic regulation of Th2 cytokine expression in atopic diseases. Tissue Antigens. 2008;72(2):91–7. Epub 2008/06/17.

113. Han J, Park SG, Bae JB, Choi J, Lyu JM, Park SH, et al. The characteristics of genome-wide DNA methylation in naive CD4+ T cells of patients with psoriasis or atopic dermatitis. Biochem Biophys Res Commun. 2012;422(1):157–63. Epub 2012/05/09.

114. Liang Y, Wang P, Zhao M, Liang G, Yin H, Zhang G, et al. Demethylation of the FCER1G promoter leads to FcepsilonRI overexpression on monocytes of patients with atopic dermatitis. Allergy. 2012;67(3):424–30. Epub 2011/12/14.

115. Garmhausen D, Hagemann T, Bieber T, Dimitriou I, Fimmers R, Diepgen T, et al. Characterization of different courses of atopic dermatitis in adolescent and adult patients. Allergy. 2013;68(4):498–506. Epub 2013/03/05.
116. Roguedas-Contios AM, Misery L. What is intrinsic atopic dermatitis? Clin Rev Allergy Immunol. 2011;41(3):233–6. Epub 2011/05/25.
117. Pugliarello S, Cozzi A, Gisondi P, Girolomoni G. Phenotypes of atopic dermatitis. J Dtsch Dermatol Ges. 2011;9(1):12–20. Epub 2010/11/09.
118. Katsarou A, Armenaka M. Atopic dermatitis in older patients: particular points. J Eur Acad Dermatol Venereol. 2011;25(1):12–8. Epub 2010/06/24.
119. Tokura Y. Extrinsic and intrinsic types of atopic dermatitis. J Dermatol Sci. 2010;58(1):1–7. Epub 2010/03/09.
120. Ott H, Stanzel S, Ocklenburg C, Merk HF, Baron JM, Lehmann S. Total serum IgE as a parameter to differentiate between intrinsic and extrinsic atopic dermatitis in children. Acta Derm Venereol. 2009;89(3):257–61.
121. Novak N, Bieber T. Allergic and nonallergic forms of atopic diseases. J Allergy Clin Immunol. 2003;112(2):252–62.
122. Ozkaya E. Adult-onset atopic dermatitis. J Am Acad Dermatol. 2005;52(4):579–82.
123. Asai T, Horiuchi Y. Senile erythroderma with serum hyper IgE. Int J Dermatol. 1989;28(4):255–8.
124. Tanei R, Katsuoka K. Clinical analyses of atopic dermatitis in the aged. J Dermatol. 2008;35(9):562–9.
125. Tanei R. Atopic dermatitis in the elderly. Inflamm Allergy Drug Targets. 2009;8(5):398–404.
126. Lancrajan C, Bumbacea R, Giurcaneanu C. Erythrodermic atopic dermatitis with late onset – case presentation. J Med Life. 2010;3(1):80–3. Epub 2010/03/23.
127. Roth HL, Kierland RR. The natural history of atopic dermatitis. A 20-year follow-up study. Arch Dermatol. 1964;89:209–14.
128. Williams HC, Strachan DP. The natural history of childhood eczema: observations from the British 1958 birth cohort study. Br J Dermatol. 1998;139(5):834–9.
129. Taieb A. The natural history of atopic dermatitis. J Am Acad Dermatol. 2001;45(1 Suppl):S4–5; discussion S-6.
130. Kadyk DL, McCarter K, Achen F, Belsito DV. Quality of life in patients with allergic contact dermatitis. J Am Acad Dermatol. 2003;49(6):1037–48.
131. Stone KD. Atopic diseases of childhood. Curr Opin Pediatr. 2003;15(5):495–511.
132. Perkin MR, Strachan DP, Williams HC, Kennedy CT, Golding J. Natural history of atopic dermatitis and its relationship to serum total immunoglobulin E in a population-based birth cohort study. Pediatr Allergy Immunol. 2004;15(3):221–9.
133. Margolis JS, Abuabara K, Bilker W, Hoffstad O, Margolis DJ. Persistence of mild to moderate atopic dermatitis. JAMA Dermatol. 2014;150(6):593–600. Epub 2014/04/04.
134. Kim WJ, Ko HC, Kim MB, Kim DW, Kim JM, Kim BS. Features of Staphylococcus aureus colonization in patients with nummular eczema. Br J Dermatol. 2013;168(3):658–60. Epub 2012/05/29.
135. Severity scoring of atopic dermatitis: the SCORAD index. Consensus report of the European Task Force on Atopic Dermatitis. Dermatology. 1993;186(1):23–31.
136. Schram ME, Spuls PI, Leeflang MM, Lindeboom R, Bos JD, Schmitt J. EASI, (objective) SCORAD and POEM for atopic eczema: responsiveness and minimal clinically important difference. Allergy. 2012;67(1):99–106. Epub 2011/09/29.
137. Hon KL, Wang SS, Leung TF. What happens to the severity grading by objective SCORAD if we over- or underestimate disease extent or intensity in patients with atopic dermatitis? Int J Dermatol. 2012;51(3):295–9. Epub 2012/02/22.
138. Oranje AP, Stalder JF, Taieb A, Tasset C, de Longueville M. Scoring of atopic dermatitis by SCORAD using a training atlas by investigators from different disciplines. ETAC Study Group. Early Treatment of the Atopic Child. Pediatr Allergy Immunol. 1997;8(1):28–34.
139. Gelmetti C, Colonna C. The value of SCORAD and beyond. Towards a standardized evaluation of severity? Allergy. 2004;59 Suppl 78:61–5.
140. Tremp M, Knafla I, Burg G, Wuthrich B, Schmid-Grendelmeier P. 'EASIdig' – a digital tool to document disease activity in atopic dermatitis. Dermatology. 2011;223(1):68–73. Epub 2011/08/26.
141. Schmitt J, Langan S, Williams HC. What are the best outcome measurements for atopic eczema? A systematic review. J Allergy Clin Immunol. 2007;120(6):1389–98.
142. Holm EA, Wulf HC, Thomassen L, Jemec GB. Assessment of atopic eczema: clinical scoring and noninvasive measurements. Br J Dermatol. 2007;157(4):674–80.
143. Vourc'h-Jourdain M, Barbarot S, Taieb A, Diepgen T, Ambonati M, Durosier V, et al. Patient-oriented SCORAD: a self-assessment score in atopic dermatitis. A preliminary feasibility study. Dermatology. 2011;66(8):1114–21.
144. Ricci G, Dondi A, Patrizi A. Useful tools for the management of atopic dermatitis. Am J Clin Dermatol. 2009;10(5):287–300.
145. Armstrong AW, Kim RH, Idriss NZ, Larsen LN, Lio PA. Online video improves clinical outcomes in adults with atopic dermatitis: a randomized controlled trial. J Am Acad Dermatol. 2011;64(3):502–7. Epub 2011/01/18.
146. Stalder JF, Barbarot S, Wollenberg A, Holm EA, De Raeve L, Seidenari S, et al. Patient-oriented SCORAD (PO-SCORAD): a new self-assessment scale in atopic dermatitis validated in Europe. Allergy. 2011;66(8):1114–21. Epub 2011/03/19.
147. Meni C, Bodemer C, Toulon A, Merhand S, Perez-Cullell N, Branchoux S, et al. Atopic dermatitis burden scale: creation of a specific burden questionnaire for families. J Eur Acad Dermatol Venereol. 2013;27(11):1426–32. Epub 2013/05/17.
148. Nijsten T. Dermatology life quality index: time to move forward. J Invest Dermatol. 2012;132(1):11–3. Epub 2011/12/14.

149. Maksimovic N, Jankovic S, Marinkovic J, Sekulovic LK, Zivkovic Z, Spiric VT. Health-related quality of life in patients with atopic dermatitis. J Dermatol. 2012;39(1):42–7. Epub 2011/11/03.

150. Rehal B, Armstrong AW. Health outcome measures in atopic dermatitis: a systematic review of trends in disease severity and quality-of-life instruments 1985–2010. PLoS One. 2011;6(4):e17520. Epub 2011/05/03.

151. Misery L, Finlay AY, Martin N, Boussetta S, Nguyen C, Myon E, et al. Atopic dermatitis: impact on the quality of life of patients and their partners. Dermatology. 2007;215(2):123–9.

152. Ganemo A, Svensson A, Lindberg M, Wahlgren CF. Quality of life in Swedish children with eczema. Acta Derm Venereol. 2007;87(4):345–9.

153. Hon KL, Kam WY, Lam MC, Leung TF, Ng PC. CDLQI, Scorad and Ness: are they correlated? Qual Life Res. 2006;15(10):1551–8.

154. Holm EA, Wulf HC, Stegmann H, Jemec GB. Life quality assessment among patients with atopic eczema. Br J Dermatol. 2006;154(4):719–25.

155. Brenninkmeijer EE, Legierse CM, Sillevis Smitt JH, Last BF, Grootenhuis MA, Bos JD. The course of life of patients with childhood atopic dermatitis. Pediatr Dermatol. 2009;26(1):14–22.

156. Augustin M, Wenninger K, Amon U, Schroth MJ, Kuster W, Chren M, et al. German adaptation of the Skindex-29 questionnaire on quality of life in dermatology: validation and clinical results. Dermatology. 2004;209(1):14–20.

157. Vieths S, Bieber T. Personalised medicine for the diagnosis and treatment of allergic diseases. Bundesgesundheitsblatt Gesundheitsforschung Gesundheitsschutz. 2013;56(11):1531–7. Epub 2013/10/31. Personalisierte Ansatze zur Diagnostik und Therapie von Allergien.

158. Broich K, Bieber T. Personalised medicine. Bundesgesundheitsblatt Gesundheitsforschung Gesundheitsschutz. 2013;56(11):1465–7. Epub 2013/10/31. Personalisierte Medizin.

159. Bieber T, Broich K. Personalised medicine. Aims and challenges. Bundesgesundheitsblatt Gesundheitsforschung Gesundheitsschutz. 2013;56(11):1468–72. Epub 2013/10/31. Personalisierte Medizin. Zielsetzungen und Herausforderungen.

160. Bieber T. Atopic dermatitis 2.0: from the clinical phenotype to the molecular taxonomy and stratified medicine. Allergy. 2012;67(12):1475–82. Epub 2012/10/31.

161. Suzuki Y, Kodama M, Asano K. Skin barrier-related molecules and pathophysiology of asthma. Allergol Int. 2011;60(1):11–5. Epub 2011/01/22.

162. Bieber T, Cork M, Reitamo S. Atopic dermatitis: a candidate for disease-modifying strategy. Allergy. 2012;67(8):969–75. Epub 2012/06/08.

163. Wu LC, Zarrin AA. The production and regulation of IgE by the immune system. Nat Rev Immunol. 2014;14(4):247–59. Epub 2014/03/15.

164. Bae JM, Choi YY, Park CO, Chung KY, Lee KH. Efficacy of allergen-specific immunotherapy for atopic dermatitis: a systematic review and meta-analysis of randomized controlled trials. J Allergy Clin Immunol. 2013;132(1):110–7. Epub 2013/05/08.

165. Nahm DH, Kim ME. Treatment of severe atopic dermatitis with a combination of subcutaneous allergen immunotherapy and cyclosporin. Yonsei Med J. 2012;53(1):158–63. Epub 2011/12/22.

166. Novak N, Thaci D, Hoffmann M, Folster-Holst R, Biedermann T, Homey B, et al. Subcutaneous immunotherapy with a depigmented polymerized birch pollen extract–a new therapeutic option for patients with atopic dermatitis. Int Arch Allergy Immunol. 2011;155(3):252–6. Epub 2011/02/05.

167. Darsow U, Forer I, Ring J. Allergen-specific immunotherapy in atopic eczema. Curr Allergy Asthma Rep. 2011;11(4):277–83. Epub 2011/04/05.

168. BuBmann C, Bieber T, Novak N. Systemic therapeutic options for severe atopic dermatitis. J Dtsch Dermatol Ges. 2009;7(3):205–19.

169. Niebuhr M, Kapp A, Werfel T. Specific immunotherapy (SIT) in atopic dermatitis and food allergy. Hautarzt. 2008;59(7):544–50.

170. Novak N. Allergen specific immunotherapy for atopic dermatitis. Curr Opin Allergy Clin Immunol. 2007;7(6):542–56.

171. Werfel T, Breuer K, Rueff F, Przybilla B, Worm M, Grewe M, et al. Usefulness of specific immunotherapy in patients with atopic dermatitis and allergic sensitization to house dust mites: a multi-centre, randomized, dose-response study. Allergy. 2006;61(2):202–5.

172. Bieber T. Off-label prescription in atopic dermatitis. Allergy. 2015;70(1):6–11.

173. Roekevisch E, Spuls PI, Kuester D, Limpens J, Schmitt J. Efficacy and safety of systemic treatments for moderate-to-severe atopic dermatitis: a systematic review. J Allergy Clin Immunol. 2014;133(2):429–38. Epub 2013/11/26.

174. Schram ME, Roekevisch E, Leeflang MM, Bos JD, Schmitt J, Spuls PI. Response to a randomized trial of methotrexate vs. azathioprine for severe atopic eczema: a critical appraisal. Br J Dermatol. 2012;166(4):704. Epub 2012/03/29.

175. Schram ME, Roekevisch E, Leeflang MM, Bos JD, Schmitt J, Spuls PI. A randomized trial of methotrexate versus azathioprine for severe atopic eczema. J Allergy Clin Immunol. 2011;128(2):353–9. Epub 2011/04/26.

176. Schmitt J, Schakel K, Schmitt N, Meurer M. Systemic treatment of severe atopic eczema: a systematic review. Acta Derm Venereol. 2007;87(2):100–11.

177. Beck LA, Thaçi D, Hamilton JD, Graham NM, Bieber T, Rocklin R, et al. Dupilumab treatment of adults with moderate-to-severe atopic dermatitis. N Engl J Med. 2014;371(7):130–9.

178. Bieber T. Stratified medicine: a new challenge for academia, industry, regulators and patients. London: Future Science; 2013. Available from: http://www.futuremedicine.com/doi/book/10.2217/9781780843186.

Targeted Therapies and Biomarkers for Personalized Treatment of Psoriasis

Federica Villanova, Paola Di Meglio, and Frank O. Nestle

6

Contents

Federica Villanova and Paola Di Meglio contributed equally

F. Villanova, PhD • F.O. Nestle, MD (✉)
St John's Institute of Dermatology,
King's College London,
London SE1 9RT, UK
e-mail: federica.villanova@kcl.ac.uk;
frank.nestle@kcl.ac.uk

P. Di Meglio, MPharm, PhD
Molecular Immunology, MRC NIMR,
London NW7 1AA, UK
e-mail: pdmegl@nimr.mrc.ac.uk

6.1 Introduction

Psoriasis is a complex disease, resulting from the interaction of genetic, immunological, and environmental factors [1, 2]. The complex nature of the disease is mirrored by a spectrum of clinical phenotypes, which often associates with comorbidities (e.g., psoriatic arthritis (PsA), cardiovascular diseases (CVD), and metabolic disease) that are also multifactorial. Moreover, psoriasis is always accompanied by a psychosocial disability with patients struggling to adapt to the chronic yet variable and unpredictable nature of the disease and to cope with the anticipated negative reactions of shame or stigmatization of others. Thus, clinicians are presented with the challenging task of managing a multifaceted and lifelong disease which, although not lethal, severely affects patients' quality of life.

The current therapeutic portfolio for psoriasis is wide, spanning from local to systemic therapies, from old-fashioned drugs discovered by serendipitous circumstances to innovative targeted therapies.

T. Bieber, F. Nestle (eds.), *Personalized Treatment Options in Dermatology*,
DOI 10.1007/978-3-662-45840-2_6, © Springer-Verlag Berlin Heidelberg 2015

In the presence of such clinical heterogeneity and given the availability of multiple treatment options to which patients unfortunately do not respond in the same manner, the successful control of the disease is usually achieved after various therapeutic attempts until the best-matched treatment for that specific patient, at that disease stage, is identified.

Thus, personalized medicine approaches are highly needed in the context of psoriasis, in order to maximize therapeutic efficacy, shift risk-benefit balance, and reduce costs. Biomarkers predicting therapy response (so-called theranostic biomarkers [3]) or disease prognosis would be extremely helpful to stratify patients and apply personalized medicine in an effective and quick manner, but unfortunately there are no such biomarkers available yet. Nonetheless, continuous advances in elucidating psoriasis immunopathogenesis and developing more and more powerful technologies have led to the identification of several potential biomarkers which could meet this clinical need in the near future. Here, we review the current knowledge about psoriasis pathogenesis, including the latest genetic and immunological findings, and discuss current and future therapeutic options, as well as innovative tools and strategies currently in place to realize the promise of personalized medicine approaches in the treatment of psoriasis.

6.2 Epidemiology, Clinical Phenotypes, and Etiopathogenesis of Psoriasis

Psoriasis is a common disease, affecting 2–4 % of the population in western countries, with prevalence rates influenced by age, geographic location, and genetic background [4]. Prevalence is higher in adults (from 0.91 to 8.5 %) as compared to children (from 0 to 2.1 %), and two peaks of onset have been observed: an early onset, before the age of 40, which is often associated with familiar disease history and showing high association with the human leukocyte antigen

(HLA)-Cw0602 allele (type I psoriasis), and a late onset, after the age of 40 (type II psoriasis) [5]. Geographical patterns of prevalence suggest lower prevalence in those closer to the equator, in keeping with the beneficial effects of UV radiation exposure [6]. Prevalence is higher in individuals of European descent (from 0.73 to 2.9 %) as compared to those of African and Asiatic background (from 0 to <0.5 %).

The term psoriasis encompasses a number of distinct clinical phenotypes. According to the International Psoriasis Council, there are four main forms of psoriasis: plaque type (Fig. 6.1), guttate, generalized pustular psoriasis (GPP), erythroderma, plus several further sub-phenotypes defined based on different parameters, i.e., the distribution, anatomical localization, size and thickness of plaques, onset, and disease activity [7]. It is becoming increasingly clear that this phenotypic heterogeneity is likely to reflect not only a dynamic, anatomical, or qualitative spectrum of the same disease, but also to pin down the existence of different disease entities, such as GPP. Plaque-type psoriasis, occurring in 85–90 % of affected patients, is the most common form of psoriasis and is characterized by oval- or irregularly shaped, red, sharply demarcated, raised plaques, covered by silvery scales [1]. Epidermal thickening (acanthosis), incomplete keratinocyte terminal differentiation with retention of the nucleus by corneocytes (parakeratosis), and elongation of the rete ridges extending downward between dermal papillae (papillomatosis) are the key histological features of psoriasis, together with blood vessel dilation and immune cell infiltration into the skin. In the epidermis, neutrophils accumulate into the parakeratotic scales in the *stratum corneum*, while lymphocytes, mainly CD8+T cells, are interspersed between keratinocytes. The dermis is heavily infiltrated by T cells (mainly CD4+) and dendritic cells (DC).

Guttate psoriasis is characterized by multiple small scaly plaques with often sudden onset, usually within few weeks after a bacterial infection of the upper airways, notably streptococcal pharyngitis in children and young adults [8].

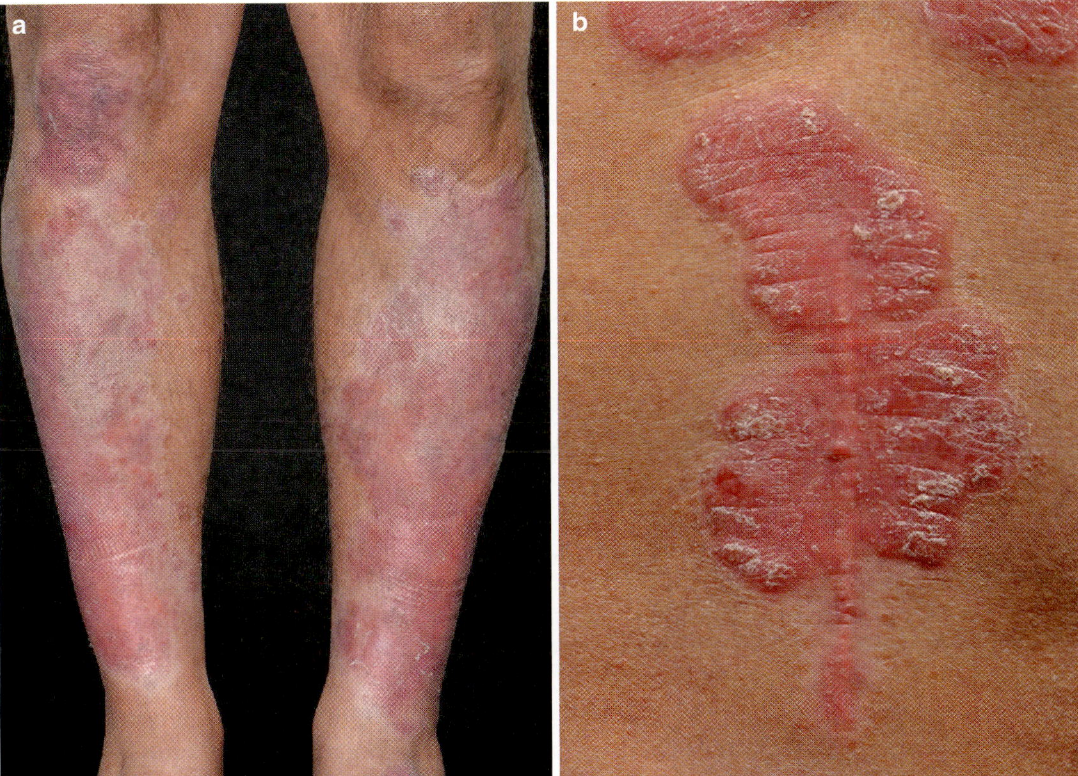

Fig. 6.1 (**a**) Clinical features of chronic plaque-type psoriasis. Clinical pictures of chronic plaque-type psoriasis characterized by scaly, red, extended skin lesions. In (**b**), note psoriatic lesion surrounding a scar

GPP is a rare but potentially life-threatening disease characterized by episodic, widespread skin and systemic inflammation including high fever, fatigue, and neutrophil leukocytosis. Recent genetic data support the hypothesis that GPP is a disease of distinct etiology, being inherited as an autosomal recessive due with mutations in the *IL36RN* gene encoding the anti-inflammatory IL-36-receptor antagonist, IL-36Ra [9, 10].

Erythrodermic psoriasis is characterized by diffuse erythema, with or without scaling, and represents the most severe, albeit rare, phenotype.

About 20–30 % of psoriasis patients develop psoriatic arthritis (PsA), a seronegative, chronic, inflammatory musculoskeletal disorder with a wide spectrum of clinical disease presentation, expression, and clinical course [11, 12]. Since about 80 % of the patients develop PsA following psoriasis [13], PsA is sometimes considered as a disease within a disease, with the skin manifestation being the parent disease [14].

Psoriasis etiopathogenesis is that of a complex disease with disease initiation taking place in genetically predisposed individuals, in which a dysregulated immune response occurs following exposure to certain environmental triggers.

Genetic predisposition to psoriasis is supported by population and family studies as well as higher concordance rates in monozygotic twins, compared with dizygotic twins (up to 73 vs 20 %, depending on the population studied) [15–18]. Large efforts have been made in the past two decades to understand the genetic architecture of psoriasis. The psoriasis genetic landscape emerging from recent genome-wide association studies (GWAS) (See also Sect. 6.7) and their meta-analysis [19–28] includes 36 independent psoriasis-associated genetic regions in individuals of European ancestry, plus five more uniquely associated in the Chinese population [29]. Psoriasis susceptibility genes encompass skin-specific genes and immune-related genes, with the latter belonging to either the innate or the adaptive immunity, as well as bridging the two arms of the immune system. Psoriasis susceptibility region 1 (PSORS1) within the major histocompatibility complex is the strongest susceptibility locus [30, 31], and the HLA-Cw*0602 allele of the MHC class I molecule HLA-C is considered to be the primary associated allele, as confirmed by early sequence and haplotype analysis [32], genome-wide association studies (GWASs) [21, 22, 27], and analysis of high-density SNP data [33]. Among immune genes, the overrepresentation of four fundamental immunological processes and pathways strongly points towards their critical contribution to disease susceptibility: antigen presentation (HLA-C and ERAP1), NF-κb signaling (e.g., TNFAIP3, TNIP1, TRAF3IP2, CARD14), IL-23/IL-17 axis (e.g., IL-23, IL12B, and IL23R), and type I INF pathway (e.g., IL28RA and RNF114) [34]. The critical involvement in disease pathogenesis of the IL-23/IL17 pathway has been particularly well documented by a wealth of clinical and experimental studies showing a pivotal role for IL-23-induced and IL-17-mediated responses in psoriasis [35]. Moreover, the genetic association with IL23R is one of the very few supported by functional evidence with reduced IL-17 responses in carriers of the protective Arg381Gln IL23R allele [36, 37].

In contrast to the fast-growing list of psoriasis susceptibility genes, the environmental factors initiating the disease are still ill defined. Among known environmental triggers of psoriasis are drugs (the antiviral and antiproliferative agent imiquimod, lithium, beta-blockers, the cytokine INF-α, and anti-cytokine therapies such as anti-TNF agents), infections (streptococcal, HIV), physical trauma (tattoos, scars), smoking, alcohol, and stress [8].

The contribution of the immune system to psoriasis is not less complex than the overall disease pathogenesis, with a variety of innate and adaptive immune cells and proinflammatory mediators involved, possibly at different stages of the disease. The current view of psoriasis pathogenesis implies that the aberrant immune and epidermal response seen in psoriasis is sustained by a pathogenic cross talk between epithelial and immune cells [38, 39]. This interplay is primarily driven by the critical proinflammatory molecules, TNF, IL-23, and IL-17, whose direct therapeutic targeting has proven to be clinically effective, with other mediators, such as IFN-α, IFN-γ, and IL-22 also contributing to the initiation, amplification, and maintenance of the disease (Fig. 6.2).

In the initiation phase, LL-37 released by KCs, following physical trauma (Koebner phenomenon) or infection, binds to self-DNA/RNA fragments [40, 41], released by stressed or dying keratinocytes. LL-37/self-DNA complexes activate pDCs to produce IFNα [40], while self-RNA-LL-37 complexes, keratinocyte-derived IL-1β, IL-6, TNF, and pDC-derived IFNα activate DC. DC migrate to the skin-draining lymph nodes to present as yet unknown antigen (either of self or of microbial origin) to naive T cells. DDC activation and their interaction with T cells are central to plaque progression as it creates an IL-23/IL-17 inflammatory environment in which DC and macrophage-derived IL-23 promote an IL-17-rich proinflammatory environment sustained by Th17 cells [42, 43], Tc17 [44–47], γδ-T cells [48, 49], NCR$^+$ group 3 innate lymphocytes (ILC3) [50–52], and possibly neutrophils and mast cells [53], producing IL-17A and IL-17 F, as well as IL-22 and IFN-γ. IL-17A and IL-17 F, sharing high structural and functional homology, activate keratinocytes to produce an array of molecules with chemoattractant properties, including neutrophil (CXCL1, CXCL2, CXCL5, CXCL8)- and T-cell (CCL20)-recruiting chemokines and AMP (LL37, S100A7/8/9/15) [54, 55]. Moreover, IL-22 produced by Th, Tc, and NCR$^+$ ILC3 mediates most of the epidermal hyperplasia by impairing KC differentiation [56, 57]. Finally, a recent study has identified IL-9-producing Th cells in psoriatic lesions although their pathogenic relevance has not been established to date [58].

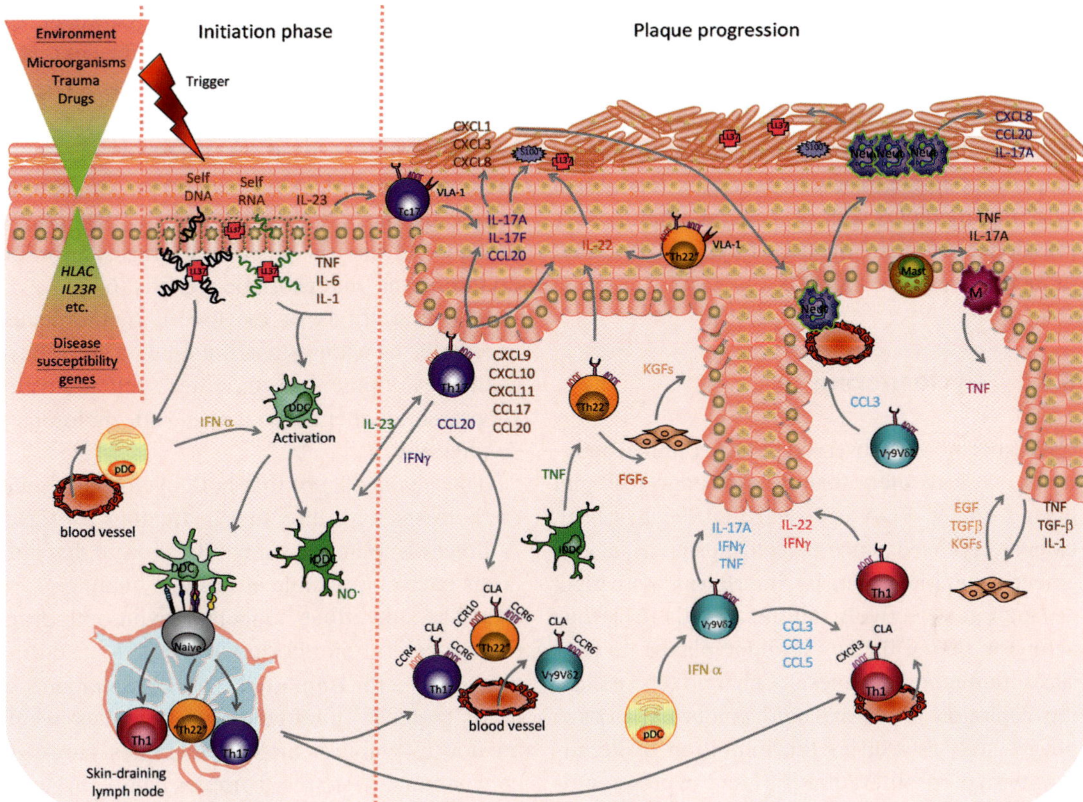

Fig. 6.2 Psoriasis etiopathogenesis. The combination of environmental factors with psoriasis susceptibility genes triggers a cascade of pathogenic events leading to disease initiation and plaque formation. In the initiation phase, proinflammatory cross talk between injured or stressed keratinocytes (*KCs*), releasing self-nucleic acids and LL-37, recruited plasmacytoid dendritic cells (*pDCs*), activated dermal DC (*DDCs*), and inflammatory DDC (*iDDCs*), producing IL-23, TNF, and nitric oxide radicals (*NO·*), promote the activation of skin-resident and newly recruited T cells that lead to plaque formation. IL-23 stimulates T helper 17 (*Th17*) and T cytotoxic 17 (*Tc17*) cells, expressing cutaneous leukocyte antigen (*CLA*), CCR6, and CCR4, plus very late antigen (*VLA*)-1 in the epidermis, to release IL-17A, IL-17 F, IL-22, and IFN-γ. IFN-γ further activates DDC. IL-17A and IL-17 F act on KCs promoting production of T cells and neutrophil-attracting chemokines (CXCL1,3,8-11;CCL17-20) and antimicrobial peptides (*AMPs*): S100 proteins and LL-37. CCL-20 favors the recruitment of more Th17 cells. IL-22, also produced by Th1 cells, expressing CXCR3 and skin-homing marker CLA, and "Th22"/"Tc22" cells, expressing CCR6, CCR10, and CLA, induces epidermal hyperplasia by impairing KC terminal differentiation. Recruited unconventional Vγ9vδ2 T cells, expressing CLA and CCR6, are activated by pDC-derived IFN-α and release further proinflammatory cytokines (IL-17A, IFNγ, TNF) as well as neutrophils (*Neut*) and Th-1-attracting chemokines (CCL3-5). Infiltrating Neut, mast cells, and macrophages (*M*) contribute to the proinflammatory environment producing cytokines (IL-17A, TNF), AMPs (S100 proteins, LL-37), and chemokines. Cross talk between keratinocytes producing IL-1, TNF and transforming growth factor beta (*TGFβ*), and fibroblasts, which in turn release keratinocyte growth factor (*KGF*), epidermal growth factor (*EGF*), and TGFβ, and possibly Th22 cells releasing fibroblast growth factor (*FGF*), contributes to tissue reorganization (Reproduced with permission from Di Meglio et al. [38])

6.3 Immunosuppressant Therapy

At present, there is no definitive cure for psoriasis, and all the available treatments aim at inducing disease remission for the longest period of time. Treatments are chosen according to disease severity; however, all patients should be counseled for their psychosocial disability [59].

Most psoriasis patients (65 %) present with a mild form of disease which is usually treated with topical agents, with local anti-inflammatory and/or antiproliferative action.

However, moderate (25 %) and severe disease (8 %) cases require systemic treatment. Systemic treatment usually comes after unsuccessful topical strategies, in a two-tiered approach where systemic therapy is used as a second-line treatment of moderate to severe psoriasis. Traditional systemic therapies aim at general immunosuppression and include the use of cyclosporine and/or methotrexate (MTX).

6.3.1 Cyclosporine

Cyclosporine was observed to have clinical activity in psoriasis more than 30 years ago [60] and having gained FDA approval in 1997 has been extensively used since. Cyclosporine is a calcineurin inhibitor that, by interfering with IL-2 production, selectively inhibits T cells [61], thus acting on one of the key immune players in psoriasis immunopathogenesis. Other effects include the depletion of dermal and epidermal macrophages [62] as well as the inhibition of keratinocyte hyperproliferation [63] and expression of adhesion molecules [64]. The benefits of treatment with cyclosporine are rapidly seen, and the efficacy is dose dependent. However, improved efficacy obtained by using high doses (higher than 5 mg/kg/day) is counteracted by increased side effects. Although generally well tolerated, safety concerns are related to nephrotoxicity and neurotoxicity [65]. To minimize toxicity, a reduced dose of cyclosporine can be combined with topical and systemic treatments [66].

6.3.2 Methotrexate

Methotrexate is an effective first-line oral therapy, and it is considered the gold-standard comparator for new drugs such as biologics. Its efficacy in psoriasis was discovered in the 1950s, and it was officially approved for this indication in the early 1970s [67]. Methotrexate is an antifolate prodrug which is converted in its active form within the cells where it inhibits the enzymes involved in DNA synthesis. Such interference with DNA replication is most effective at high doses, and it is the basis of its antiproliferative effect, widely applied in the anticancer therapy. However, the mechanism of action of this drug in the context of psoriasis accounts for both antiproliferative and anti-inflammatory effects, which are seen at the low drug doses used in psoriasis treatment. Methotrexate (MTX) is effective in chronic plaque psoriasis not responding to conventional therapy but also in pustular psoriasis, psoriatic erythroderma, and psoriatic arthritis [68].

The limitations of the use of methotrexate, especially as a long-term treatment, are related to the development of toxicities such as myelosuppression, hepatotoxicity, and pulmonary damage [69].

There is no doubt that both cyclosporine and methotrexate are effective in treating psoriasis. A direct comparative study [70] showed that both drugs have comparable efficacy in treating psoriasis. The side effects associated with both drugs require careful monitoring of the patients during treatment and supported the development of more targeted immunological therapies which are now available as biologic therapies. However, conventional systemic therapies can be up to 20 times cheaper than biologics [71].

6.4 Biologic Therapy

In the last decade, the advancements in understanding psoriasis immunopathogenesis have been translated into better therapies. In particular, antibody- or fusion protein-based drugs, known as biologics, have been developed to target a specific immune receptor or cytokine. Biologics have proven to be an effective third-line therapy in moderate-to-severe psoriasis patients, unresponsive to non-biologic systemic agents. There are currently five biologics approved for the treatment of psoriasis, targeting either T cells or cytokines such as TNF or IL-12/IL-23 [8] (Table 6.1).

6.4.1 Anti-T-Cell Therapy

The first biologics to be approved for psoriasis treatment were anti-T-cell therapies (alefacept and efalizumab), targeting T-cell adhesion or activation.

Table 6.1 Biologics approved for the treatment of psoriasis

Mechanism of action	Name	Molecular target	Phase	Biologic	Administration route	Company	References
Anti-T cells	Alefacept	CD2	Approved 2003 (US)	Human LFA-3/IgG1 fusion protein	IM or IV	Biogen	[72, 73]
Anti-cytokine	Etanercept	TNF	Approved 2004 (US and EU)	Human TNF-R(p75)-lgG1 fusion protein	SC	Amgen	[74–77]
	Infliximab	TNF	Approved 2006 (US and EU)	Mouse-human IgG1 chimeric monoclonal antibody	IV	Janssen Biotech	[78–80]
	Adalimumab	TNF	Approved 2007 (EU) 2008 (US)	Human IgG1 monoclonal antibody	SC	Abbott	[81, 82]
	Ustekinumab	IL12p40 (IL-12, IL-23)	Approved 2009 (US and EU)	Human IgG1 monoclonal antibody	SC	Janssen Biotech	[83, 84]

Alefacept, approved in 2003, is an LFA-3/IgG1 fusion protein which binds CD2 on T cells, thus blocking the interaction with antigen-presenting cells (APC) and inducing antibody-dependent cytotoxicity. The approval of this first biologic drug for treating psoriasis followed the successful completion of phase 3 clinical trials [72, 73] showing that 40 % of patients achieved a PASI 75 (75 % reduction of the PASI) response.

Efalizumab is a humanized monoclonal antibody targeting CD11a (alpha chain of LFA-1) therefore blocking the interaction of T cells with both APC and the blood vessels, inhibiting cutaneous infiltration. Efalizumab showed good efficacy in phase 3 clinical trials [85–91], but three cases of progressive multifocal leukoencephalopathy [92] caused the withdrawal from the market in 2009, highlighting the importance of carefully monitoring the long-term safety of immunomodulatory therapies.

Overall, notwithstanding good efficacy, anti-T-cell-targeted agents associate with general immunosuppression, and there are now available alternative biologic drugs with more targeted effects and therefore a better safety profile.

6.4.2 Anti-cytokine Therapies

The importance of a cytokine network mediating the cross talk between immune cells and keratinocytes to sustain the inflammatory loop in psoriasis has been further confirmed by the clinical success of targeting key cytokine pathways with specific biologic therapies. The first cytokine whose blockade showed therapeutic benefit in psoriasis was TNF. This was a serendipitous discovery made during the treatment with the anti-TNF drug infliximab of a patient affected by inflammatory bowel disease with concomitant psoriasis [74]. Currently there are three anti-TNF biologics approved for psoriasis each of them blocking TNF in a slightly different manner: infliximab and adalimumab are monoclonal antibodies against TNF, while etanercept is a human p75 TNF receptor fusion protein. TNF inhibitor efficacy has been shown in phase III clinical trials with up to 80 % of patients under treatment achieving PASI75 within 10–12 weeks of treatment [75–82]. Disease resolution is accompanied by normalization of KC differentiation and proliferation, downregulation of DC activation markers and downstream effector molecules, as well as reduction of Th17 responses [93, 94]. Interestingly downregulation of IL-17 pathway genes correlates with successful therapy response to etanercept [94, 95].

The second category of anti-cytokine biologics approved for psoriasis includes an antibody blocking the p40 subunit shared by IL-12 and IL-23 (ustekinumab) thus simultaneously blocking IL-12 and IL-23. Its efficacy is high, with 67 % of patients achieving PASI75 at 12 weeks of treatment [83]. A direct comparison of etanercept and ustekinumab showed that, despite both drugs achieved a PASI75 response in most patients, ustekinumab was clinically superior to etanercept as evaluated by the Physician Global Assessment with similar safety over a 12-week period [84]. Moreover, among patients who did not respond to etanercept, half of them achieved PASI75 after crossing over ustekinumab for 12 weeks.

The downside of the high efficacy rates of biologics is the potential of some serious adverse events, such as opportunistic infections and reactivation of latent tuberculosis [96]. However etanercept and ustekinumab have shown a good long-term safety profile in studies assessing safety up to 4- and 5-year treatment [75–77, 97, 98].

6.4.3 Emerging Biologics

New biologics have been developed so to specifically target either IL-17 or IL-23, and these molecules are currently tested for their safety and efficacy in clinical trials (Table 6.2).

Blockage of IL-17 is presently investigated using monoclonal antibodies targeting either IL-17A (ixekizumab and secukinumab) or IL-17RA (brodalumab). In the latter case, the inhibition is not limited to IL-17A but covers also IL-17 F, IL17A/F, IL-25, and potentially IL-17C. All anti-IL17 biologics have shown striking efficacy in phase 2 clinical trials with more than 70 % of patients achieving PASI 75

Table 6.2 Emerging biologics and small molecules for the treatment of psoriasis

Type	Mechanism of action	Name	Molecular target	Phase	Biologic/Compound	Administration route	Company	References
Biologics	Anti-cytokine	Tildrakizumab (MK-3222)	IL-23p19	Phase III	Humanized IgG1 monoclonal antibody	SC	Merck	[99, 100]
		Guselkumab (CNTO 1959)	IL-23p19	Phase II	Human IgG1 monoclonal antibody	SC	Janssen Biotech	[101, 102]
		BI655066	IL-23p19	Phase II	Humanized IgG1 monoclonal antibody	SC	Boehringer Ingelheim	[103]
		Brodalumab (AMG 827)	IL-17R	Phase III	Human IgG2 monoclonal antibody	SC	Amgen	[104]
		Ixekizumab (LY2439821)	IL-17	Phase III	Humanized IgG4 monoclonal antibody	SC	Eli Lilly	[105]
		Secukinumab (AIN457)	IL-17	Phase III	Human IgG1 monoclonal antibody	SC or IV	Novartis	[106]
Small molecule	PDE4 inhibitor	Apremilast (CC-10004)	PDE4	Phase III	N/A	Oral	Celgene	[107, 108]
	JAK inhibitor	Tofacitinib (CP-690,550)	JAK1 and JAK3	Phase II	N/A	Oral	Pfizer	[109, 110]
		Tofacitinib (CP-690,550)	JAK1 and JAK3	Phase II	N/A	Topical	Pfizer	[111]

and more than half achieving a notable PASI 90 [104–106].

Phase III clinical trials are ongoing to further confirm the safety and efficacy of these drugs while comparing them with approved biologics such as ustekinumab and etanercept. At the molecular level, IL-17 blockade showed a greater magnitude in regulating the expression of genes synergistically regulated by IL-17 and TNF-α as compared to TNF blockade [112].

There are three antibodies (BI655066, tildrakizumab, and guselkumab) specifically targeting the IL-23p19 subunit which are currently being tested in phase II [103], III [99], or have recently completed phase II [101] clinical trials, respectively. Preliminary data for guselkumab and tildrakizumab, presented at the American Academy of Dermatology meeting in 2013 and 2014, are very encouraging. Phase IIb data for guselkumab showed up to 81 % of patients receiving the highest dose achieving PASI75 response [102], while phase 3 data for tildrakizumab showed PASI75 response rates of 64–74 %, [100].

6.5 Emerging Small Molecules

The therapy revolution introduced by biologics in psoriasis is challenged by the high cost of about £10 k per patient/per year [113] by about 20–30 % of nonresponder patients and by the loss of response of some patients due to the development of antidrug antibodies which can decrease the drug bioavailability or induce side effects [114, 115]. Moreover, clinicians prefer to go for a safer option, at least for milder forms of disease. This has encouraged the exploration of small molecules as an alternative therapeutic option. Small molecules are low molecular weight compounds which target specific intracellular molecules involved in pivotal cellular signaling pathways [116]. Based on the importance of the cytokine-driven inflammatory pathways in psoriasis, the most promising small molecules currently under testing (Table 6.2) are targeting key cellular components in cytokine signaling such as Janus kinases (JAK) as well as enzymes involved in cytokine production. Among the JAK inhibitors

tofacitinib, which specifically inhibits JAK1 and 3 and is approved for RA treatment, showed good efficacy in phase II trials of both oral and topical formulation of the drug [109, 111]. 66.7 % of patients treated with the highest dose of oral tofacitinib reached the end point PASI 75 at 12 weeks as compared to 2 % in the placebo-controlled group in a phase 2b study [110]. The other small molecule showing good results in phase II trials is apremilast, a phosphodiesterase 4 inhibitor that by inhibiting an enzyme involved in the breakdown of cAMP, suppresses the production of proinflammatory cytokines. Phase IIb clinical trials [107, 108] showed that the drug is safe and well tolerated. Efficacy as compared to placebo was significant with 41 % of patients achieving PASI75 at week 16 at the highest drug dose, advocating for additional clinical studies to test this small molecule.

Despite the potentially lower efficacy of small molecules as compared to biologics, the advantages are in the cheaper manufacturing process, the route of administration (oral or topical vs injectable), and a good safety profile in some cases. Thus, their use in mild to moderate form of psoriasis is foreseeable, although long-term safety data are required.

6.6 Concepts and Principles of Personalized Medicine: Patient Stratification and Biomarkers

The aspiration of tailoring medicine to the individual characteristics of each patient has long been a central vision of medicine. Pioneering studies resulting in the genetic diagnosis of Mendelian diseases and in the understanding that individual genetic variation affects how drugs are absorbed and metabolized laid the foundation of personalized medicine in the twentieth century.

In 1902, the first genetic disorder, alkaptonuria, was identified by Sir Archibald Garrod, who linked for the first time disease occurrence with genetic inheritance [117], laying the foundation of genetic diagnosis. In 1956, the genetic basis for selective drug toxicity was first postulated in the case of the antimalarial drug primaquine [118] and further strengthened later on by the discovery of the drug-metabolizing activity of the cytochrome P450 family enzymes [119] and the subsequent understanding of how their variation can affect the effective dose of a drug, launching the science of genetic variation in drug response or pharmacogenomics [120].

It is in the twenty-first century, however, that personalized medicine has begun in earnest, building upon the tremendous advances in the understanding of human diseases that have been enabled by the technological developments discussed in Sect. 6.7.

Genetics has taken the lead with a number of initiatives that have revolutionized our knowledge. The completion of the first draft of the human genome in 2001 [121, 122], complemented by the release and periodic update (1998–ongoing) of the Single Nucleotide Polymorphism Database (dbSNP, currently dbSNP 138) [123], provided the foundation for the advanced study of human genetics. Next, the launch and completion (2002–2009) of the International HapMap Project [124], listing allele frequencies and the correlation patterns between nearby gene variants, a phenomenon known as linkage disequilibrium (LD), across several populations for several million SNPs has made possible the discovery of disease susceptibility gene by means of genome-wide association studies (GWAS). Finally, the 1,000 Genome project (2008–ongoing) [125], aimed at sequencing the genome of 2,500 individuals from about 25 populations around the world, is poised to produce an extensive public catalog of human genetic variation to further support medical research studies, including personalized medicine approaches.

A number of objectives aimed at improving patient care are within the scope of personalized medicine: to predict individual susceptibility to disease, based on genetic or environmental factors; to detect the onset of disease at the very earliest stages; to predict and preempt disease progression; to develop novel targeted therapies; and to prescribe safe and effective medicines to each patient. The implementation of such objectives is also expected to increase the efficiency of the health-care system by improving quality, accessibility, and affordability.

In order to achieve such ambitious goals, personalized medicine is fast moving beyond the genome to encompass the entire spectrum of molecular medicine, including the proteome, metabolome, and epigenome, again fueled by improved knowledge and technology.

At the heart of personalized medicine is patient stratification, or the classification of individuals into subpopulations that differ in their susceptibility to a particular disease, or the natural history of their disease or their response to a specific treatment. Genetic and epigenetic testing, together with more conventional types of analysis (blood, urine, etc.), as well as with the careful consideration of lifestyle and other environmental factors, can effectively guide patient stratification, overcoming heterogeneity and aiding in disease diagnosis, prognosis, and therapy (Fig. 6.3).

Critical to the implementation of stratified and personalized medicine approaches are biomarkers or biological characteristics that are measured and evaluated objectively as an indicator of normal biological processes, pathogenic responses, or to pharmacological responses to therapeutic intervention.

Biomarkers can be classified in diagnostic biomarkers, indicating the existence of disease; prognostic biomarkers, able to forecast disease progression, with or without treatment; and predictive or theranostic biomarkers, able to predict the probable response to a particular treatment.

Thus, biomarkers can be distinguished in *disease-related* (diagnostic and prognostic) and *drug-related biomarkers* (pharmacokinetic and pharmacodynamic biomarker), the latter indicating how the patient's body will process it and whether or not the drug will be effective.

An alternative classification, according to the NIH Biomarkers Definitions Working Group, distinguishes biomarkers in three categories: type 0 biomarkers, correlating longitudinally with the severity of disease; type 1 biomarkers, reflecting the effect of an intervention according to the mechanism of action of therapy itself (drug endotype); and type 2 biomarkers which are surrogate end points for a therapy [126].

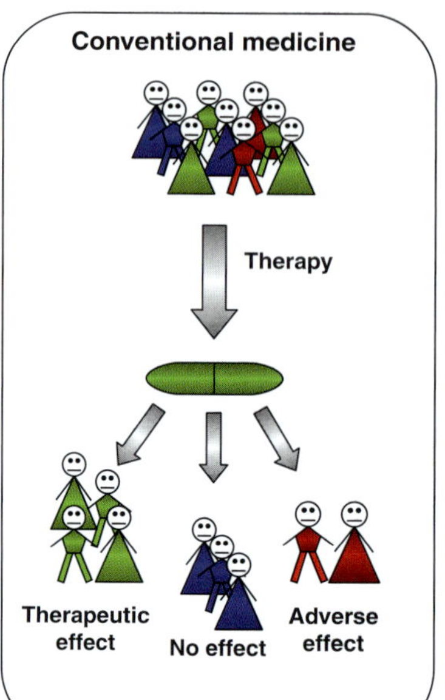
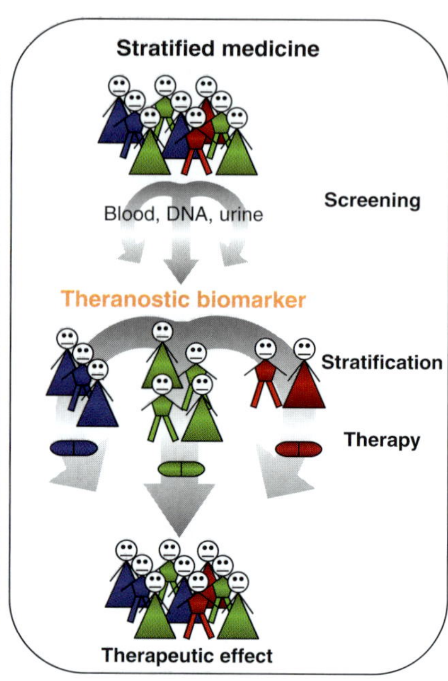

Fig. 6.3 Conventional versus stratified medicine. In conventional medicine approaches (*left*), patients receive the same drug which will have a therapeutic effect on the majority of them but will be ineffective in some and cause adverse events in others. In personalized medicine approaches, patients undergo screening using biological materials (DNA, urine, blood) to identify theranostic biomarkers allowing their stratification to receive the most appropriate and effective drug for each individual

Finally, biomarkers can be classified according to their ontogeny in genetic, epigenetics, transcriptional, soluble, and cellular biomarkers.

The classical biomarker discovery pipeline is a three-step process, from discovery to validation and clinical adoption [127]. A key element in translating biomarkers into clinical practice is the validation process. Tests used in the clinic to measure biomarkers must be reliable, with an acceptably low rate of false-positive and/or false-negative results. Sensitivity, specificity, positive predictive value (PPV), and negative predictive value (NPV) are key parameters to take in account when evaluating the performance of such tests [128]. Only biomarkers with high sensitivity and specificity can enter to the clinical practice, explaining why only a small fraction of potential biomarkers translate into clinical use.

Personalized medicine approaches are already established in modern clinical oncology, where a number of reliable biomarkers aiding in patients stratification have been identified and implemented in clinical practice. One of the first examples is the overexpression of the human epidermal growth factor receptor (Her2) in breast cancer tissue of certain patients. Her2 is a twofold biomarker, being a prognostic marker of more aggressive disease, but also a theranostic marker supporting the use of trastuzumab, a monoclonal antibody binding to Her2 used in the treatment of Her2-positive metastatic breast cancer [129].

6.7 Novel Technologies for Stratified Medicine in Psoriasis

The identification of biomarkers for patient stratification purposes can be done by using either a hypothesis- or a non-hypothesis-driven approach. While the former was the most common approach in the past, the latter has become a popular method in recent years thanks to the tremendous advancements in technologies in multiple areas of medical research. Overall, the recently developed technologies allow deep analysis of biological samples available in limited quantity, in a high-throughput manner permitting almost simultaneous genomics, proteomics, transcriptomics, and metabolomics analysis.

The most striking progresses have been made in the genomic sequencing field, where novel high-throughput technologies and next-generation sequencing (NGS) have enabled the genomics community to comprehensively characterize human DNA sequence variation, quantitating transcript abundance, detecting methylated region of the genome, and characterizing different gene isoforms. While a fully automated application of first-generation sequencing, such as the chain termination method developed by Sanger in 1975 [130], has been the mainstay for the original sequencing of the human genome, this has come with a cost of 3 billion dollars and took almost 10 years to complete [131]. The increasing demand for low-cost and high-throughput sequencing has driven the development of NGS technologies (second- and third-generation sequencing) that parallelize the sequencing process, producing thousands or millions of sequences concurrently, at a fraction of the initial costs. Moreover, the impact of these technologies extends far beyond genomic DNA sequencing. Traditional methods for studying DNA modification and its interactions with other cellular components or gene expression are being redesigned to take advantage of these powerful technologies, e.g., ChIP-Seq, to interrogate whole-genome histone modifications, whole-genome bisulfite sequencing of the DNA methylome, or deep-RNA sequencing [132, 133]. In psoriasis, high-throughput genotyping has enabled the identification of 36 psoriasis susceptibility genes by means of GWAS in which common genetic variations such as SNPs are examined in patients and control individuals to identify association with the disease [27]. Moreover, NSG have enabled the refining of the psoriasis transcriptome [134, 135] via RNA sequencing, building upon array-based analysis [136, 137].

Array-based technologies have also been used for DNA methylation profiling resulting in the identification of detection of different methylation profiles between lesional and nonlesional psoriatic skin [138].

Genetic, transcriptional, and epigenetic analysis can be complemented by the multiparameter analysis of samples at cellular level. Multidimensional analysis at single-cell level classically performed via flow cytometry has greatly improved in terms of number (up to 20 parameters) and types of markers (surface, intracellular, and phospho proteins) which can

be measured thanks to advances in both instrumentations and reagents. Efforts have also been made to standardize the technology to be more applicable in clinical trials, for example, with the use of lyoplates, which are preformatted plates containing lyophilized cocktails of antibodies. Sample staining and acquisition for flow cytometry analysis using lypolates increase reproducibility, standardization, and medium throughput processing of the samples [139]. Intrinsic flow cytometry limitations in marker detection due to the spectral overlap of fluorochromes have been recently overcome by a novel technology for multiparameter cellular analysis named mass cytometry. By replacing the detection of fluorochromes with that of metal stable isotopes allows the investigation of up to 100 markers at the same time [140]. Studies using human samples have demonstrated the power of mass cytometry to identify highly diverse cell subsets [141, 142], resulting in a fine and detailed mapping of immune cells and their response. Moreover, mass cytometry-based analysis has recently elucidated a previously unappreciated role for CD8+ and $\gamma\delta$ T cells in celiac disease following short-term gluten challenge, suggesting that immunological changes after short-term gluten exposure could be used to develop a novel diagnostic tool much faster than those currently in use requiring a longer exposure to the antigen [143].

Another powerful flow-based technology is phospho-flow cytometry, which quantifies the amount of phosphorylated intracellular signaling proteins before and after relevant cell stimulation, thus characterizing the functional state of complex immune cell populations in single individuals. Phospho-flow-based studies in immune-mediated disease such as SLE and RA have indicated signaling heterogeneity of different cell populations and different signaling profiles in different disease states [144], while similar studies are awaited in psoriasis.

Another area of recent investigation is metabolomics, which consists in the quantification of the metabolites in a biological system, by using complex technologies such as nuclear magnetic resonance and mass spectrometry. Both the quantification of specific metabolites and an untargeted and comprehensive metabolic profile associated to disease status can be obtained by metabolomics analysis [145]. This type of analysis has been proved successful in distinguishing different clinical phenotypes in complex disease such as CVD, cancer, and asthma [146]. Clinically relevant metabolite present in easily accessible samples such as urine could lead to the identification of metabolic biomarkers in psoriasis.

All the aforementioned technologies each generate a vast amount of data. Moreover, they are often used in combination to analyze the same biological sample, thus resulting in an escalating amount of data which require powerful bioinformatics tools not only to analyze, but also to integrate, handle, manage, and store these "omics" data [147]. Computational analysis approaches applied to the analysis of large data in psoriasis has already proven successful in a number of studies, especially taking advantage of the large amount of publicly available gene expression data from psoriasis skin. A meta-analytic approach has recently been used to combine the results of five microarray datasets obtaining the Meta-Analysis Derived (MAD) psoriasis transcriptome [134]. The overrepresentation of atherosclerosis signaling and fatty acid metabolism pathways in lesional skin support the close relationship between psoriasis and systemic manifestations [134]. A set of 20 "classifier" genes clearly separating lesional from nonlesional psoriasis skin has also been identified [134], to contain many genes that were part of the residual disease genomic profile, or "molecular scar', still present in psoriasis skin after successful treatment [148] or genes with differential methylation status [138].

From skin gene expression data, ensembles of decision tree predictors were used to cluster psoriatic samples, and the analysis revealed distinct molecular subgroups within the clinical phenotype of plaque psoriasis [149]. In another study, cytokines and cell-type specific signatures were identified according to differentially expressed genes in the lesions, uncovering a range of inflammatory- and cytokine-associated gene expression patterns able to differentiate between etanercept responders and nonresponders [137].

Data from human samples can also be integrated with data from in vivo models to overcome the translational gap in the development of new targeted therapies. For example, the role of IL-22 in psoriasis has been recently evaluated by comparing the publicly available psoriasis transcriptome with the transcriptome derived from humanized mouse models of disease (i.e., IL-22 injection into xenografts of normal human skin) or inhibition of disease (i.e., antibody-mediated blockade of IL-22 into xenografts of psoriasis human skin). Mapping the in vivo experimental data over the psoriasis transcriptome led to the identification of the serine/threonine kinase PIM1, subsequently validated as a critical checkpoint for human skin inflammation and potential future therapeutic target in psoriasis [150]. Finally, a systems biology approach has been used to model and quantify immune cell interactions contributing to skin inflammation via cytokine signaling [151].

These new technologies provide high-throughput data platforms, shifting the analysis from discrete markers to the analysis of several interconnected systems. Such integrative approach is likely to result in the identification of novel biomarkers in the form of combination of markers or patterns instead of a single measurement.

6.8 Biomarkers in Stratified Medicine Approaches for Psoriasis

Large efforts aimed at the identification of psoriasis biomarkers are ongoing in order to implement stratified medicine approaches in disease management [127].

Psoriasis is diagnosed by clinical assessment by a dermatologist, with rare cases of histological confirmation of the disease. Thus, there is no urgent need for diagnostic biomarkers neither for disease monitoring during treatment as successful therapies are clinically evaluated by plaque resolution. On the contrary, prognostic biomarkers indicating disease severity progression or the onset of cardiovascular or other comorbidities

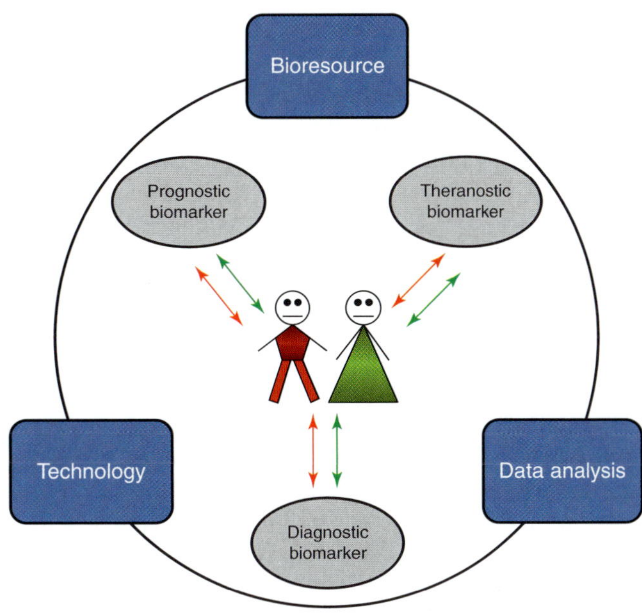

Fig. 6.4 Psoriasis biomarkers in translational research. Psoriasis patients would benefit from the clinical use of diagnostic, prognostic, and theranostic biomarkers. Translational research, involving the integrated use of bioresources, high-throughput technologies, and data analysis, aims to discover biomarkers for stratified medicine approaches in psoriasis

would be extremely useful for better patient management. Moreover, biomarkers for early diagnosis are an unmet need in psoriasis arthritis, where the large disease heterogeneity often hampers proper diagnosis and the progressive course of the disease also calls prognostic biomarkers. Finally, despite the growing number of therapeutic alternatives to treat psoriasis, not all patients respond to the same treatment, and a recent survey has indicated that more than 50 % of patients polled are dissatisfied by the management of their disease [152]. The current therapeutic approach to treat psoriasis, especially in its moderate-to-severe forms, contemplates the use of different treatments, in an empirical attempt to find the most effective one. Patients are therefore likely to experience one or more ineffective therapies with relative associated side effects. Moreover, this approach also results in increased public health costs which are especially relevant in the case of expensive biologic drugs. Thus, biomarkers for better disease management are both a clinical and public health need which would benefit both patients and the health-care system. Despite large efforts in the quest for psoriasis biomarkers, none of those identified so far have entered into clinical use for disease diagnosis, prognosis, or for predicting therapy response

[127]. Here, we describe them according to the type 0, 1, and 2 classification and discuss their potential use in stratified medicine approaches in psoriasis (Fig. 6.4).

6.8.1 Type 0 Psoriasis Biomarkers: Markers of Disease Severity

Type 0 biomarkers, correlating with the severity of psoriasis, include genetic as well as tissue and systemic biomarkers.

HLA-Cw*0602- positive patients have more severe disease and early onset (Type I Psoriasis) compared to HLA-Cw*0602- negative patients [5]. On the contrary, HLA-Cw*0602- positive PsA patients have a less severe clinical course [153].

The altered skin architecture found in psoriatic plaques is reflected by the altered expression of tissue-specific molecules, such as keratins, as well as proinflammatory molecules in the tissue. Keratins associated with cell proliferation such as K6 and K16 are upregulated in psoriatic skin as compared to normal, while those indicating keratinocyte terminal differentiation such as K1 and K10 [154] are decreased. Antiapoptotic proteins are overexpressed in psoriatic skin, and their expression correlates with pathology improvements after successful therapy with anthralin [155] and anti-TNF [156].

However, psoriasis being "more than skin deep," it is not surprising that systemic markers are also altered. Alteration of inflammatory mediators both at tissue and peripheral levels correlates with disease status. Proinflammatory cytokines such as TNF, IFN, IL-6, IL-8, and IL-12 [157, 158] are increased in both psoriatic skin and circulation of psoriatic patients as compared to healthy volunteers. Inflammatory gene expression rapidly reduces after successful anti-TNF treatment [93]. Interesting work by Suarez-Farinas and colleagues [159] showed that inflammatory cytokines increased in psoriatic serum were also increased in the skin, suggesting that peripheral blood can mirror the skin. The study of circulating markers has been extensively investigated due to the easy access to patients' peripheral blood samples, with the view to develop a minimally invasive biomarker test. IL-22 serum levels are increased in psoriasis patients, and they show a positive correlation with PASI [160, 161]. Cellular and molecular components of the key IL-23/Th17 axis are associated with psoriasis severity. IL23, IL23R, and Th17 cytokines are increased in lesional psoriatic skin [162], and IL23R is overexpressed in circulating T cells [163]. However, it is not clear yet whether IL-17A serum levels are altered in psoriatic disease as compared to healthy status as inconsistent results have been found in different studies, possibly due to low levels and sensitivity issues of the detection assays [158–161, 164]. Nevertheless, high IL17-A serum levels, together with high IL1RA, correlate with the eruptive inflammatory form of the disease and not with chronic and stable psoriasis [165]. Investigating at the cells producing these cytokines, results indicate an increased frequency of T-cell subsets such as Th1, Th17, and Th22 cells in the circulation of psoriasis patients as well as in the tissue [43, 166, 167]. Interestingly, also innate cells involved in the production of IL-17 and IL-22 such as ILC3 are increased in the skin and blood of psoriasis patients and decrease in the circulation after successful anti-TNF treatment [50–52]. Besides the alteration of markers related to the specific immunopathogenesis of the disease, psoriasis patients present high level of generic inflammation markers shared with other inflammatory conditions (e.g., CRP, haptoglobin, and platelet P-selectin) [168] as well as lipids and oxidative status alterations [169, 170] shared with metabolic diseases. The heterogeneity of the type 0 psoriasis biomarkers further highlights the complex nature of psoriasis and the difficulty to find psoriasis-specific biomarkers.

6.8.2 Type 1 Psoriasis Biomarkers: Drug Endotype

Type 1 biomarkers, reflecting the effect of an intervention according to the mechanism of action of therapy itself are being identified as results of targeted therapies involving the use of biologic drugs targeting specific immune circuits which are dysregulated in psoriasis. In particular, anti-IL12/23 and anti-IL17 biologics act on the central IL23/IL17 axis in psoriasis. The molecules directly targeted by these drugs have the potential to be used as prognostic or theranostic biomarkers to monitor the actual suppression of the targeted pathway and the associated clinical improvements.

Blockade of IL-17 with ixekizumab leads to decrease of IL-17 and other inflammatory mediators (IFN, IL-22) in the tissue as well as of IL-17-regulated molecules in epidermal keratinocytes (LL37, beta-defensin 2, S100A7, S100A8) already after 2 weeks of treatment. This in turn leads to the decrease of lymphocytic and dendritic cell infiltration as well as normalization of keratinocyte structural and activation markers within 6 weeks of treatment. This correlates with the rapid clinical improvements suggesting that IL-17 is a key marker whose regulation is sufficient to normalize many other circuits that deregulate in psoriatic skin [112]. Downregulation of IL17 and its immediate regulated genes is also necessary for positive response to the anti-TNF biologic etanercept [94, 95], suggesting that the efficacy of TNF blockade is ultimately down to the inhibition of IL17 signaling.

Interestingly, the beneficial effects of non-targeted immunosuppressant therapies, such as cyclosporine [171] and UVB therapy [172], have also been associated to the inhibition of the IL-17 axis. As the mechanism of action of these drugs in psoriasis has not fully been elucidated, a better understanding of such mechanisms could help to develop type 2 biomarkers for psoriasis.

6.8.3 Type 2 Biomarkers: Predictive or Theranostic Biomarkers

Type 2 biomarkers, which are surrogate end points for therapy, have predictive value and theranostic use.

As already highlighted earlier, the identification, validation, and implementation of this type of biomarker is most urgently needed in psoriasis. Soluble, circulatory, or genetic markers associated to therapy response would be ideal theranostic biomarkers in psoriasis, being not or minimally invasive.

In a small study, a disease response classifier including 23 genes using gene expression of PBMCs has been obtained to accurately predict response to alefacept [173]. Among circulating markers, the relative frequency of some peripheral immune cell populations within the first few weeks of treatment has been shown to correlate with more long-term therapy response. T regulatory cells that increase within 8 weeks of anti-TNF therapy predict good therapeutic response [174], while the expression of cutaneous lymphocyte-associated antigen (CLA) on lymphocytes negatively correlates with PASI at 6 weeks [175]. A number of genetic biomarkers have also been shown or have the potential to play a theranostic role and guide patient stratification. Conventional pharmacogenetic studies focused on genes involved in drug transport and metabolism such as ABCC1 and ABCG2 have identified SNPs in these genes associated with good response to methotrexate [176]. Another approach focuses on psoriasis susceptibility genes identified by GWASs which represent a potential gold mine for the identification of theranostic biomarkers. SNPs in TNAFAIP3, encoding for a zinc finger protein (A20) that is a negative regulator of TNF-induced pathways, are associated with improved response to anti-TNF agents [177]. Moreover, a small cohort of HLA-Cw06+ patients have been shown to respond better and faster to ustekinumab [178]. An obvious potential candidate to probe is the *IL23R* R381Q SNP in IL-23R, given its functional role in downregulating IL-23 responses in psoriasis patients [37].

The perceived need to identify theranostic biomarkers has resulted in the establishment of a number of UK-wide initiatives with the aim of identifying biomarkers predicting therapy response (BSTOP study – Biomarkers of Systemic Treatment Outcomes in Psoriasis) [179] and developing an algorithm to guide psoriasis management (PSORT – Psoriasis Stratification to Optimise Relevant Therapy) [180]. The PSORT consortium is formed by world-leading psoriasis experts from both academia and industry which are working together to effectively deliver personalized medicine to psoriasis patients.

Conclusion

The complex pathogenesis of psoriasis has been untangled in the last 40 years, yet specific genetic factors, environmental triggers, and immune dysregulation which predict disease progression therapeutic response at a single patient level are unknown. However, tremendous advances in technologies and data analysis are providing researchers with powerful discovery tools at the bench, while clinicians are evaluating the results of novel targeted therapies at the bedside. The integration of such basic and clinical activities results in a lively translation of research process, whose aim is to identify ways to stratify the patient population to predict therapy response and to achieve efficient disease management, thus benefiting both patients and the healthcare system. The concept of personalized medicine is therefore central in the multifaceted reality of psoriasis disease, and prognostic and theranostic biomarker discovery, validation, and implementation in the clinical practice are eagerly awaited. Personalized medicine lessons learned in psoriasis could also be of interest to other immune-mediated inflammatory diseases, with which psoriasis shares inflammatory mechanisms, genetic traits, and therapeutic options.

Acknowledgments We are in debt to psoriasis patients and healthy volunteers for their courage, trust, and generosity in donating clinical specimens to make psoriasis research possible. We thank FON laboratory members for their contribution over the years to the work cited in this chapter. We thank Hemawtee Sreeneebus and Thomas Walters for their help with Fig. 6.1. We acknowledge support by the following grant bodies: Wellcome Trust Programme GR078173MA (FON) and National Institute for Health Research (NIHR) Biomedical Research Centre based at Guy's and St Thomas' NHS Foundation Trust and King's College London. The views expressed are those of the authors and not necessarily those of the NHS, the NIHR, or the Department of Health. FON has been a consultant for companies producing targeted therapies for treatment of patients with psoriasis. The other authors state no conflict of interest.

References

1. Nestle FO, Kaplan DH, Barker J. Psoriasis. N Engl J Med. 2009;361(5):496–509.
2. Lowes MA, Suarez-Farinas M, Krueger JG. Immunology of psoriasis. Annu Rev Immunol. 2014;32:227–55.
3. Kelkar SS, Reineke TM. Theranostics: combining imaging and therapy. Bioconjug Chem. 2011;22(10):1879–903.
4. Parisi R, Symmons DP, Griffiths CE, Ashcroft DM. Global epidemiology of psoriasis: a systematic review of incidence and prevalence. J Invest Dermatol. 2013;133(2):377–85.
5. Henseler T, Christophers E. Psoriasis of early and late onset: characterization of two types of psoriasis vulgaris. J Am Acad Dermatol. 1985;13(3):450–6.
6. Hart PH, Gorman S, Finlay-Jones JJ. Modulation of the immune system by UV radiation: more than just the effects of vitamin D? Nat Rev Immunol. 2011;11(9):584–96.
7. Griffiths CE, Christophers E, Barker JN, Chalmers RJ, Chimenti S, Krueger GG, et al. A classification of psoriasis vulgaris according to phenotype. Br J Dermatol. 2007;156(2):258–62.
8. Perera GK, Di Meglio P, Nestle FO. Psoriasis. Annu Rev Pathol. 2012;7:385–422.
9. Marrakchi S, Guigue P, Renshaw BR, Puel A, Pei XY, Fraitag S, et al. Interleukin-36-receptor antagonist deficiency and generalized pustular psoriasis. N Engl J Med. 2011;365(7):620–8.
10. Onoufriadis A, Simpson MA, Pink AE, Di Meglio P, Smith CH, Pullabhatla V, et al. Mutations in IL36RN/IL1F5 are associated with the severe episodic inflammatory skin disease known as generalized pustular psoriasis. Am J Hum Genet. 2011;89(3):432–7.
11. Anandarajah AP, Ritchlin CT. The diagnosis and treatment of early psoriatic arthritis. Nat Rev Rheumatol. 2009;5(11):634–41.
12. Gladman DD, Antoni C, Mease P, Clegg DO, Nash P. Psoriatic arthritis: epidemiology, clinical features, course, and outcome. Ann Rheum Dis. 2005;64 Suppl 2:ii14–7.
13. Ellinghaus E, Stuart PE, Ellinghaus D, Nair RP, Debrus S, Raelson JV, et al. Genome-wide meta-analysis of psoriatic arthritis identifies susceptibility locus at REL. J Invest Dermatol. 2012;132(4):1133–40.
14. Eder L, Chandran V, Pellett F, Pollock R, Shanmugarajah S, Rosen CF, et al. IL13 gene polymorphism is a marker for psoriatic arthritis among psoriasis patients. Ann Rheum Dis. 2011;70(9):1594–8.
15. Brandrup F, Hauge M, Henningsen K, Eriksen B. Psoriasis in an unselected series of twins. Arch Dermatol. 1978;114(6):874–8.
16. Duffy DL, Spelman LS, Martin NG. Psoriasis in Australian twins. J Am Acad Dermatol. 1993;29(3):428–34.
17. Farber EM, Nall ML, Watson W. Natural history of psoriasis in 61 twin pairs. Arch Dermatol. 1974;109(2):207–11.
18. Lonnberg AS, Skov L, Skytthe A, Kyvik KO, Pedersen OB, Thomsen SF. Heritability of psoriasis in a large twin sample. Br J Dermatol. 2013;169:412–6.
19. Capon F, Bijlmakers MJ, Wolf N, Quaranta M, Huffmeier U, Allen M, et al. Identification of ZNF313/RNF114 as a novel psoriasis susceptibility gene. Hum Mol Genet. 2008;17(13):1938–45.
20. Ellinghaus E, Ellinghaus D, Stuart PE, Nair RP, Debrus S, Raelson JV, et al. Genome-wide association study identifies a psoriasis susceptibility locus at TRAF3IP2. Nat Genet. 2010;42(11):991–5.
21. Nair RP, Duffin KC, Helms C, Ding J, Stuart PE, Goldgar D, et al. Genome-wide scan reveals association of psoriasis with IL-23 and NF-kappaB pathways. Nat Genet. 2009;41(2):199–204.
22. Strange A, Capon F, Spencer CC, Knight J, Weale ME, Allen MH, et al. A genome-wide association study identifies new psoriasis susceptibility loci and an interaction between HLA-C and ERAP1. Nat Genet. 2010;42(11):985–90.
23. Stuart PE, Nair RP, Ellinghaus E, Ding J, Tejasvi T, Gudjonsson JE, et al. Genome-wide association analysis identifies three psoriasis susceptibility loci. Nat Genet. 2010;42(11):1000–4.
24. Zhang XJ, Huang W, Yang S, Sun LD, Zhang FY, Zhu QX, et al. Psoriasis genome-wide association study identifies susceptibility variants within LCE gene cluster at 1q21. Nat Genet. 2009;41(2):205–10.
25. de Cid R, Riveira-Munoz E, Zeeuwen PL, Robarge J, Liao W, Dannhauser EN, et al. Deletion of the late cornified envelope LCE3B and LCE3C genes as a susceptibility factor for psoriasis. Nat Genet. 2009;41(2):211–5.

26. Huffmeier U, Uebe S, Ekici AB, Bowes J, Giardina E, Korendowych E, et al. Common variants at TRAF3IP2 are associated with susceptibility to psoriatic arthritis and psoriasis. Nat Genet. 2010;42(11):996–9.

27. Tsoi LC, Spain SL, Knight J, Ellinghaus E, Stuart PE, Capon F, et al. Identification of 15 new psoriasis susceptibility loci highlights the role of innate immunity. Nat Genet. 2012;44(12):1341–8.

28. Ellinghaus D, Ellinghaus E, Nair RP, Stuart PE, Esko T, Metspalu A, et al. Combined analysis of genome-wide association studies for Crohn disease and psoriasis identifies seven shared susceptibility loci. Am J Hum Genet. 2012;90(4):636–47.

29. Sun LD, Cheng H, Wang ZX, Zhang AP, Wang PG, Xu JH, et al. Association analyses identify six new psoriasis susceptibility loci in the Chinese population. Nat Genet. 2010;42(11):1005–9.

30. Nair RP, Stuart P, Henseler T, Jenisch S, Chia NV, Westphal E, et al. Localization of psoriasis-susceptibility locus PSORS1 to a 60-kb interval telomeric to HLA-C. Am J Hum Genet. 2000;66(6):1833–44.

31. Trembath RC, Clough RL, Rosbotham JL, Jones AB, Camp RD, Frodsham A, et al. Identification of a major susceptibility locus on chromosome 6p and evidence for further disease loci revealed by a two stage genome-wide search in psoriasis. Hum Mol Genet. 1997;6(5):813–20.

32. Nair RP, Stuart PE, Nistor I, Hiremagalore R, Chia NV, Jenisch S, et al. Sequence and haplotype analysis supports HLA-C as the psoriasis susceptibility 1 gene. Am J Hum Genet. 2006;78(5):827–51.

33. Clop A, Bertoni A, Spain SL, Simpson MA, Pullabhatla V, Tonda R, et al. An in-depth characterization of the major psoriasis susceptibility locus identifies candidate susceptibility alleles within an HLA-C enhancer element. PLoS One. 2013;8(8):e71690.

34. Capon F, Burden AD, Trembath RC, Barker JN. Psoriasis and other complex trait dermatoses: from Loci to functional pathways. J Invest Dermatol. 2012;132(3 Pt 2):915–22.

35. Di Cesare A, Di Meglio P, Nestle FO. The IL-23/Th17 axis in the immunopathogenesis of psoriasis. J Invest Dermatol. 2009;129(6):1339–50.

36. Di Meglio P, Di Cesare A, Laggner U, Chu CC, Napolitano L, Villanova F, et al. The IL23R R381Q gene variant protects against immune-mediated diseases by impairing IL-23-induced Th17 effector response in humans. PLoS One. 2011;6(2):e17160.

37. Di Meglio P, Villanova F, Napolitano L, Tosi I, Terranova Barberio M, Mak RK, et al. The IL23R A/Gln381 allele promotes IL-23 unresponsiveness in human memory T-helper 17 cells and impairs Th17 responses in psoriasis patients. J Invest Dermatol. 2013;133(10):2381–9.

38. Di Meglio P, Perera GK, Nestle FO. The multitasking organ: recent insights into skin immune function. Immunity. 2011;35(6):857–69.

39. Lowes MA, Russell CB, Martin DA, Towne JE, Krueger JG. The IL-23/T17 pathogenic axis in psoriasis is amplified by keratinocyte responses. Trends Immunol. 2013;34(4):174–81.

40. Lande R, Gregorio J, Facchinetti V, Chatterjee B, Wang YH, Homey B, et al. Plasmacytoid dendritic cells sense self-DNA coupled with antimicrobial peptide. Nature. 2007;449(7162):564–9.

41. Ganguly D, Chamilos G, Lande R, Gregorio J, Meller S, Facchinetti V, et al. Self-RNA-antimicrobial peptide complexes activate human dendritic cells through TLR7 and TLR8. J Exp Med. 2009;206(9):1983–94.

42. Lowes MA, Kikuchi T, Fuentes-Duculan J, Cardinale I, Zaba LC, Haider AS, et al. Psoriasis vulgaris lesions contain discrete populations of Th1 and Th17 T cells. J Invest Dermatol. 2008;128(5):1207–11.

43. Kagami S, Rizzo HL, Lee JJ, Koguchi Y, Blauvelt A. Circulating Th17, Th22, and Th1 cells are increased in psoriasis. J Invest Dermatol. 2010;130(5):1373–83.

44. Austin LM, Ozawa M, Kikuchi T, Walters IB, Krueger JG. The majority of epidermal T cells in Psoriasis vulgaris lesions can produce type 1 cytokines, interferon-gamma, interleukin-2, and tumor necrosis factor-alpha, defining TC1 (cytotoxic T lymphocyte) and TH1 effector populations: a type 1 differentiation bias is also measured in circulating blood T cells in psoriatic patients. J Invest Dermatol. 1999;113(5):752–9.

45. Kryczek I, Bruce AT, Gudjonsson JE, Johnston A, Aphale A, Vatan L, et al. Induction of IL-17+ T cell trafficking and development by IFN-gamma: mechanism and pathological relevance in psoriasis. J Immunol. 2008;181(7):4733–41.

46. Ortega C, Fernandez AS, Carrillo JM, Romero P, Molina IJ, Moreno JC, et al. IL-17-producing CD8+ T lymphocytes from psoriasis skin plaques are cytotoxic effector cells that secrete Th17-related cytokines. J Leukoc Biol. 2009;86(2):435–43.

47. Hijnen D, Knol EF, Gent YY, Giovannone B, Beijn SJ, Kupper TS, et al. CD8(+) T cells in the lesional skin of atopic dermatitis and psoriasis patients are an important source of IFN-gamma, IL-13, IL-17, and IL-22. J Invest Dermatol. 2013;133(4):973–9.

48. Cai Y, Shen X, Ding C, Qi C, Li K, Li X, et al. Pivotal role of dermal IL-17-producing gammadelta T cells in skin inflammation. Immunity. 2011;35(4):596–610.

49. Laggner U, Di Meglio P, Perera GK, Hundhausen C, Lacy KE, Ali N, et al. Identification of a novel proinflammatory human skin-homing Vgamma9Vdelta2 T cell subset with a potential role in psoriasis. J Immunol. 2011;187(5):2783–93.

50. Villanova F, Flutter B, Tosi I, Grys K, Sreeneebus H, Perera GK, et al. Characterization of innate lymphoid cells in human skin and blood demonstrates increase of NKp44+ ILC3 in psoriasis. J Invest Dermatol. 2014;134(4):984–91.

51. Dyring-Andersen B, Geisler C, Agerbeck C, Lauritsen JP, Gudjonsdottir SD, Skov L, et al. Increased number and frequency of group 3 innate lymphoid cells in nonlesional psoriatic skin. Br J Dermatol. 2014;170(3):609–16.

52. Teunissen MB, Munneke JM, Bernink JH, Spuls PI, Res PC, Te Velde A, et al. Composition of Innate Lymphoid Cell (ILC) Subsets in the human skin: Enrichment of NCR ILC3 in lesional skin and blood of psoriasis patients. J Invest Dermatol. 2014;134:2351–60.

53. Lin AM, Rubin CJ, Khandpur R, Wang JY, Riblett M, Yalavarthi S, et al. Mast cells and neutrophils release IL-17 through extracellular trap formation in psoriasis. J Immunol. 2011;187(1):490–500.

54. Wilson NJ, Boniface K, Chan JR, McKenzie BS, Blumenschein WM, Mattson JD, et al. Development, cytokine profile and function of human interleukin 17-producing helper T cells. Nat Immunol. 2007; 8(9):950–7.

55. Wolf R, Mascia F, Dharamsi A, Howard OM, Cataisson C, Bliskovski V, et al. Gene from a psoriasis susceptibility locus primes the skin for inflammation. Sci Transl Med. 2010;2(61):61ra90.

56. Zheng Y, Danilenko DM, Valdez P, Kasman I, Eastham-Anderson J, Wu J, et al. Interleukin-22, a T(H)17 cytokine, mediates IL-23-induced dermal inflammation and acanthosis. Nature. 2007;445(7128):648–51.

57. Ma HL, Liang S, Li J, Napierata L, Brown T, Benoit S, et al. IL-22 is required for Th17 cell-mediated pathology in a mouse model of psoriasis-like skin inflammation. J Clin Invest. 2008;118(2):597–607.

58. Schlapbach C, Gehad A, Yang C, Watanabe R, Guenova E, Teague JE, et al. Human TH9 cells are skin-tropic and have autocrine and paracrine proinflammatory capacity. Sci Transl Med. 2014;6(219):219ra8.

59. Griffiths CE, Clark CM, Chalmers RJ, Li Wan Po A, Williams HC. A systematic review of treatments for severe psoriasis. Health Technol Assess. 2000;4(40):1–125.

60. Mueller W, Herrmann B. Cyclosporin A for psoriasis. N Engl J Med. 1979;301(10):555.

61. Amor KT, Ryan C, Menter A. The use of cyclosporine in dermatology: part I. J Am Acad Dermatol. 2010;63(6):925–46; quiz 47–8.

62. Gupta AK, Baadsgaard O, Ellis CN, Voorhees JJ, Cooper KD. Lymphocytes and macrophages of the epidermis and dermis in lesional psoriatic skin, but not epidermal Langerhans cells, are depleted by treatment with cyclosporin A. Arch Dermatol Res. 1989;281(4):219–26.

63. Gottlieb SL, Heftler NS, Gilleaudeau P, Johnson R, Vallat VP, Wolfe J, et al. Short-contact anthralin treatment augments therapeutic efficacy of cyclosporine in psoriasis: a clinical and pathologic study. J Am Acad Dermatol. 1995;33(4):637–45.

64. Edwards BD, Andrew SM, O'Driscoll JB, Chalmers RJ, Ballardie FW, Freemont AJ. Changes in numbers of epidermal cell adhesion molecules caused by oral cyclosporin in psoriasis. J Clin Pathol. 1993;46(8):713–7.

65. Burdmann EA, Andoh TF, Yu L, Bennett WM. Cyclosporine nephrotoxicity. Semin Nephrol. 2003;23(5):465–76.

66. Colombo MD, Cassano N, Bellia G, Vena GA. Cyclosporine regimens in plaque psoriasis: an overview with special emphasis on dose, duration, and old and new treatment approaches. Sci World J. 2013;2013:805705.

67. Weinstein GD. Methotrexate. Ann Intern Med. 1977;86(2):199–204.

68. Prodanovic EM, Korman NJ. Traditional systemic therapy I: methotrexate and cyclosporine. In: Treatment of psoriasis. Basel/Boston: Birkhauser; 2008. p. 103–20.

69. Shen S, O'Brien T, Yap LM, Prince HM, McCormack CJ. The use of methotrexate in dermatology: a review. Australas J Dermatol. 2012;53(1):1–18.

70. Heydendael VM, Spuls PI, Opmeer BC, de Borgie CA, Reitsma JB, Goldschmidt WF, et al. Methotrexate versus cyclosporine in moderate-to-severe chronic plaque psoriasis. N Engl J Med. 2003;349(7):658–65.

71. Ramirez-Fort MK, Levin AA, Au SC, Gottlieb AB. Continuous versus intermittent therapy for moderate-to-severe psoriasis. Clin Exp Rheumatol. 2013;31(4 Suppl 78):S63–70.

72. Krueger GG, Papp KA, Stough DB, Loven KH, Gulliver WP, Ellis CN. A randomized, double-blind, placebo-controlled phase III study evaluating efficacy and tolerability of 2 courses of alefacept in patients with chronic plaque psoriasis. J Am Acad Dermatol. 2002;47(6):821–33.

73. Lebwohl M, Christophers E, Langley R, Ortonne JP, Roberts J, Griffiths CE. An international, randomized, double-blind, placebo-controlled phase 3 trial of intramuscular alefacept in patients with chronic plaque psoriasis. Arch Dermatol. 2003;139(6):719–27.

74. Oh CJ, Das KM, Gottlieb AB. Treatment with anti-tumor necrosis factor alpha (TNF-alpha) monoclonal antibody dramatically decreases the clinical activity of psoriasis lesions. J Am Acad Dermatol. 2000;42(5 Pt 1):829–30.

75. Leonardi CL, Powers JL, Matheson RT, Goffe BS, Zitnik R, Wang A, et al. Etanercept as monotherapy in patients with psoriasis. N Engl J Med. 2003;349(21):2014–22.

76. Papp KA, Tyring S, Lahfa M, Prinz J, Griffiths CE, Nakanishi AM, et al. A global phase III randomized controlled trial of etanercept in psoriasis: safety, efficacy, and effect of dose reduction. Br J Dermatol. 2005;152(6):1304–12.

77. Tyring S, Gottlieb A, Papp K, Gordon K, Leonardi C, Wang A, et al. Etanercept and clinical outcomes, fatigue, and depression in psoriasis: double-blind placebo-controlled randomised phase III trial. Lancet. 2006;367(9504):29–35.

78. Gottlieb AB, Evans R, Li S, Dooley LT, Guzzo CA, Baker D, et al. Infliximab induction therapy for patients with severe plaque-type psoriasis: a randomized, double-blind, placebo-controlled trial. J Am Acad Dermatol. 2004;51(4):534–42.

79. Reich K, Nestle FO, Papp K, Ortonne JP, Evans R, Guzzo C, et al. Infliximab induction and maintenance therapy for moderate-to-severe psoriasis: a phase III, multicentre, double-blind trial. Lancet. 2005;366(9494):1367–74.

80. Menter A, Feldman SR, Weinstein GD, Papp K, Evans R, Guzzo C, et al. A randomized comparison of continuous vs. intermittent infliximab maintenance regimens over 1 year in the treatment of

moderate-to-severe plaque psoriasis. J Am Acad Dermatol. 2007;56(1):31 e1–15.

81. Gordon KB, Langley RG, Leonardi C, Toth D, Menter MA, Kang S, et al. Clinical response to adalimumab treatment in patients with moderate to severe psoriasis: double-blind, randomized controlled trial and open-label extension study. J Am Acad Dermatol. 2006;55(4):598–606.

82. Saurat JH, Stingl G, Dubertret L, Papp K, Langley RG, Ortonne JP, et al. Efficacy and safety results from the randomized controlled comparative study of adalimumab vs. methotrexate vs. placebo in patients with psoriasis (CHAMPION). Br J Dermatol. 2008;158(3):558–66.

83. Leonardi CL, Kimball AB, Papp KA, Yeilding N, Guzzo C, Wang Y, et al. Efficacy and safety of ustekinumab, a human interleukin-12/23 monoclonal antibody, in patients with psoriasis: 76-week results from a randomised, double-blind, placebo-controlled trial (PHOENIX 1). Lancet. 2008;371(9625):1665–74.

84. Griffiths CE, Strober BE, van de Kerkhof P, Ho V, Fidelus-Gort R, Yeilding N, et al. Comparison of ustekinumab and etanercept for moderate-to-severe psoriasis. N Engl J Med. 2010;362(2):118–28.

85. Leonardi C, Menter A, Hamilton T, Caro I, Xing B, Gottlieb AB. Efalizumab: results of a 3-year continuous dosing study for the long-term control of psoriasis. Br J Dermatol. 2008;158(5):1107–16.

86. Lebwohl M, Tyring SK, Hamilton TK, Toth D, Glazer S, Tawfik NH, et al. A novel targeted T-cell modulator, efalizumab, for plaque psoriasis. N Engl J Med. 2003;349(21):2004–13.

87. Gordon KB, Papp KA, Hamilton TK, Walicke PA, Dummer W, Li N, et al. Efalizumab for patients with moderate to severe plaque psoriasis: a randomized controlled trial. JAMA. 2003;290(23):3073–80.

88. Menter A, Gordon K, Carey W, Hamilton T, Glazer S, Caro I, et al. Efficacy and safety observed during 24 weeks of efalizumab therapy in patients with moderate to severe plaque psoriasis. Arch Dermatol. 2005;141(1):31–8.

89. Leonardi CL, Papp KA, Gordon KB, Menter A, Feldman SR, Caro I, et al. Extended efalizumab therapy improves chronic plaque psoriasis: results from a randomized phase III trial. J Am Acad Dermatol. 2005;52(3 Pt 1):425–33.

90. Gottlieb AB, Hamilton T, Caro I, Kwon P, Compton PG, Leonardi CL. Long-term continuous efalizumab therapy in patients with moderate to severe chronic plaque psoriasis: updated results from an ongoing trial. J Am Acad Dermatol. 2006;54(4 Suppl 1):S154–63.

91. Papp KA, Bressinck R, Fretzin S, Goffe B, Kempers S, Gordon KB, et al. Safety of efalizumab in adults with chronic moderate to severe plaque psoriasis: a phase IIIb, randomized, controlled trial. Int J Dermatol. 2006;45(5):605–14.

92. Tan CS, Koralnik IJ. Progressive multifocal leukoencephalopathy and other disorders caused by JC virus: clinical features and pathogenesis. Lancet Neurol. 2010;9(4):425–37.

93. Gottlieb AB, Chamian F, Masud S, Cardinale I, Abello MV, Lowes MA, et al. TNF inhibition rapidly down-regulates multiple proinflammatory pathways in psoriasis plaques. J Immunol. 2005;175(4):2721–9.

94. Zaba LC, Cardinale I, Gilleaudeau P, Sullivan-Whalen M, Suarez-Farinas M, Fuentes-Duculan J, et al. Amelioration of epidermal hyperplasia by TNF inhibition is associated with reduced Th17 responses. J Exp Med. 2007;204(13):3183–94.

95. Zaba LC, Suarez-Farinas M, Fuentes-Duculan J, Nograles KE, Guttman-Yassky E, Cardinale I, et al. Effective treatment of psoriasis with etanercept is linked to suppression of IL-17 signaling, not immediate response TNF genes. J Allergy Clin Immunol. 2009;124(5):1022–10 e1-395.

96. Sivamani RK, Goodarzi H, Garcia MS, Raychaudhuri SP, Wehrli LN, Ono Y, et al. Biologic therapies in the treatment of psoriasis: a comprehensive evidence-based basic science and clinical review and a practical guide to tuberculosis monitoring. Clin Rev Allergy Immunol. 2013;44(2):121–40.

97. Papp KA, Poulin Y, Bissonnette R, Bourcier M, Toth D, Rosoph L, et al. Assessment of the long-term safety and effectiveness of etanercept for the treatment of psoriasis in an adult population. J Am Acad Dermatol. 2012;66(2):e33–45.

98. Papp KA, Griffiths CE, Gordon K, Lebwohl M, Szapary PO, Wasfi Y, et al. Long-term safety of ustekinumab in patients with moderate-to-severe psoriasis: final results from 5 years of follow-up. Br J Dermatol. 2013;168(4):844–54.

99. Merck. A Study to evaluate the efficacy and safety/tolerability of subcutaneous SCH 900222/MK-3222 in participants with moderate-to-severe chronic plaque psoriasis (P07771/MK-3222-011). Available from: http://clinicaltrials.gov/ct2/show/NCT01729754. Accessed 26 Mar 2014.

100. Papp K. Dose-dependent improvement in chronic plaque psoriasis following treatment with anti-IL-23p19 humanized monoclonal antibody (MK-3222). Presented at American Academy of Dermatology conference, Miami, 2013.

101. Jannsenn Inc. A study to evaluate CNTO 1959 in the treatment of patients with moderate to severe plaque-type psoriasis (X-PLORE). Available from: http://clinicaltrials.gov/ct2/show/NCT01483599. Accessed 26 Mar 2014

102. Callis Duffin K. A phase 2 multicenter, randomized, placebo- and active-comparator controlled, dose-ranging trial to evaluate Guselkumab for the treatment of patients with moderate to severe plaque-type psoriasis (X-PLORE). Presented at American Academy of Dermatology conference, Denver, 2014.

103. Boehringer Ingelheim. BI 655066 Dose ranging in psoriasis, active comparator Ustekinumab. Available from: http://clinicaltrials.gov/ct2/show/NCT02054481. Accessed 26 Mar 2014.

104. Papp KA, Leonardi C, Menter A, Ortonne JP, Krueger JG, Kricorian G, et al. Brodalumab, an anti-interleukin-17-receptor antibody for psoriasis. N Engl J Med. 2012;366(13):1181–9.
105. Leonardi C, Matheson R, Zachariae C, Cameron G, Li L, Edson-Heredia E, et al. Anti-interleukin-17 monoclonal antibody ixekizumab in chronic plaque psoriasis. N Engl J Med. 2012;366(13):1190–9.
106. Papp KA, Langley RG, Sigurgeirsson B, Abe M, Baker DR, Konno P, et al. Efficacy and safety of secukinumab in the treatment of moderate-to-severe plaque psoriasis: a randomized, double-blind, placebo-controlled phase II dose-ranging study. Br J Dermatol. 2013;168(2):412–21.
107. Papp KA, Kaufmann R, Thaci D, Hu C, Sutherland D, Rohane P. Efficacy and safety of apremilast in subjects with moderate to severe plaque psoriasis: results from a phase II, multicenter, randomized, double-blind, placebo-controlled, parallel-group, dose-comparison study. J Eur Acad Dermatol Venereol. 2013;27(3):e376–83.
108. Papp K, Cather JC, Rosoph L, Sofen H, Langley RG, Matheson RT, et al. Efficacy of apremilast in the treatment of moderate to severe psoriasis: a randomised controlled trial. Lancet. 2012; 380(9843):738–46.
109. Boy MG, Wang C, Wilkinson BE, Chow VF, Clucas AT, Krueger JG, et al. Double-blind, placebo-controlled, dose-escalation study to evaluate the pharmacologic effect of CP-690,550 in patients with psoriasis. J Invest Dermatol. 2009;129(9):2299–302.
110. Papp KA, Menter A, Strober B, Langley RG, Buonanno M, Wolk R, et al. Efficacy and safety of tofacitinib, an oral Janus kinase inhibitor, in the treatment of psoriasis: a Phase 2b randomized placebo-controlled dose-ranging study. Br J Dermatol. 2012;167(3):668–77.
111. Ports WC, Khan S, Lan S, Lamba M, Bolduc C, Bissonnette R, et al. A randomized phase 2a efficacy and safety trial of the topical Janus kinase inhibitor tofacitinib in the treatment of chronic plaque psoriasis. Br J Dermatol. 2013;169(1):137–45.
112. Krueger JG, Fretzin S, Suarez-Farinas M, Haslett PA, Phipps KM, Cameron GS, et al. IL-17A is essential for cell activation and inflammatory gene circuits in subjects with psoriasis. J Allergy Clin Immunol. 2012;130(1):145–54 e9.
113. National Institute for Health and Care Excellence. Costing statement: Ustekinumab for the treatment of adults with moderate to severe psoriasis. 2009. Available from: http://www.nice.org.uk/guidance/ta180/resources/ta180-psoriasis-ustekinumab-costing-statement2
114. Vincent FB, Morand EF, Murphy K, Mackay F, Mariette X, Marcelli C. Antidrug antibodies (ADAb) to tumour necrosis factor (TNF)-specific neutralising agents in chronic inflammatory diseases: a real issue, a clinical perspective. Ann Rheum Dis. 2013;72(2):165–78.
115. Sathish JG, Sethu S, Bielsky MC, de Haan L, French NS, Govindappa K, et al. Challenges and approaches for the development of safer immunomodulatory biologics. Nat Rev Drug Discov. 2013;12(4):306–24.
116. Garcia-Perez ME, Stevanovic T, Poubelle PE. New therapies under development for psoriasis treatment. Curr Opin Pediatr. 2013;25(4):480–7.
117. Garrod AE. About Alkaptonuria. Med Chir Trans. 1902;85:69–78.
118. Alving AS, Carson PE, Flanagan CL, Ickes CE. Enzymatic deficiency in primaquine-sensitive erythrocytes. Science. 1956;124(3220):484–5.
119. Cooper DY, Levin S, Narasimhulu S, Rosenthal O. Photochemical action spectrum of the terminal oxidase of mixed function oxidase systems. Science. 1965;147(3656):400–2.
120. Vogel F. Moderne problem der humangenetik. Ergeb Inn Med U Kinderheilk. 1959;12:52–125.
121. Venter JC, Adams MD, Myers EW, Li PW, Mural RJ, Sutton GG, et al. The sequence of the human genome. Science. 2001;291(5507):1304–51.
122. Lander ES, Linton LM, Birren B, Nusbaum C, Zody MC, Baldwin J, et al. Initial sequencing and analysis of the human genome. Nature. 2001;409(6822):860–921.
123. Sherry ST, Ward MH, Kholodov M, Baker J, Phan L, Smigielski EM, et al. dbSNP: the NCBI database of genetic variation. Nucleic Acids Res. 2001;29(1):308–11.
124. Altshuler DM, Gibbs RA, Peltonen L, Dermitzakis E, Schaffner SF, Yu F, et al. Integrating common and rare genetic variation in diverse human populations. Nature. 2010;467(7311):52–8.
125. Abecasis GR, Auton A, Brooks LD, DePristo MA, Durbin RM, Handsaker RE, et al. An integrated map of genetic variation from 1,092 human genomes. Nature. 2012;491(7422):56–65.
126. Biomarkers Definitions Working Group. Biomarkers and surrogate endpoints: preferred definitions and conceptual framework. Clin Pharmacol Ther. 2001;69(3):89–95.
127. Villanova F, Di Meglio P, Nestle FO. Biomarkers in psoriasis and psoriatic arthritis. Ann Rheum Dis. 2013;72 Suppl 2:ii104–10.
128. Soreide K. Receiver-operating characteristic curve analysis in diagnostic, prognostic and predictive biomarker research. J Clin Pathol. 2009;62(1):1–5.
129. Hudis CA. Trastuzumab–mechanism of action and use in clinical practice. N Engl J Med. 2007;357(1):39–51.
130. Sanger F, Coulson AR. A rapid method for determining sequences in DNA by primed synthesis with DNA polymerase. J Mol Biol. 1975;94(3):441–8.
131. Schadt EE, Turner S, Kasarskis A. A window into third-generation sequencing. Hum Mol Genet. 2010;19(R2):R227–40.
132. Ku CS, Naidoo N, Wu M, Soong R. Studying the epigenome using next generation sequencing. J Med Genet. 2011;48(11):721–30.

133. Wang Z, Gerstein M, Snyder M. RNA-Seq: a revolutionary tool for transcriptomics. Nat Rev Genet. 2009;10(1):57–63.

134. Tian S, Krueger JG, Li K, Jabbari A, Brodmerkel C, Lowes MA, et al. Meta-analysis derived (MAD) transcriptome of psoriasis defines the "core" pathogenesis of disease. PLoS One. 2012;7(9):e44274.

135. Jabbari A, Suarez-Farinas M, Dewell S, Krueger JG. Transcriptional profiling of psoriasis using RNA-seq reveals previously unidentified differentially expressed genes. J Invest Dermatol. 2012;132(1):246–9.

136. Suarez-Farinas M, Lowes MA, Zaba LC, Krueger JG. Evaluation of the psoriasis transcriptome across different studies by gene set enrichment analysis (GSEA). PLoS One. 2010;5(4):e10247.

137. Swindell WR, Johnston A, Voorhees JJ, Elder JT, Gudjonsson JE. Dissecting the psoriasis transcriptome: inflammatory- and cytokine-driven gene expression in lesions from 163 patients. BMC Genomics. 2013;14:527.

138. Roberson ED, Liu Y, Ryan C, Joyce CE, Duan S, Cao L, et al. A subset of methylated CpG sites differentiate psoriatic from normal skin. J Invest Dermatol. 2012;132(3 Pt 1):583–92.

139. Villanova F, Di Meglio P, Inokuma M, Aghaeepour N, Perucha E, Mollon J, et al. Integration of lyoplate based flow cytometry and computational analysis for standardized immunological biomarker discovery. PLoS One. 2013;8(7):e65485.

140. Bendall SC, Nolan GP, Roederer M, Chattopadhyay PK. A deep profiler's guide to cytometry. Trends Immunol. 2012;33(7):323–32.

141. Bendall SC, Simonds EF, Qiu P, el Amir AD, Krutzik PO, Finck R, et al. Single-cell mass cytometry of differential immune and drug responses across a human hematopoietic continuum. Science. 2011;332(6030):687–96.

142. Newell EW, Sigal N, Bendall SC, Nolan GP, Davis MM. Cytometry by time-of-flight shows combinatorial cytokine expression and virus-specific cell niches within a continuum of CD8+ T cell phenotypes. Immunity. 2012;36(1):142–52.

143. Han A, Newell EW, Glanville J, Fernandez-Becker N, Khosla C, Chien YH, et al. Dietary gluten triggers concomitant activation of CD4+ and CD8+ alphabeta T cells and gammadelta T cells in celiac disease. Proc Natl Acad Sci U S A. 2013;110(32):13073–8.

144. Covey TM, Cesano A, Parkinson DR. Single-cell network profiling (SCNP) by flow cytometry in autoimmune disease. Autoimmunity. 2010;43(7):550–9.

145. Putri SP, Yamamoto S, Tsugawa H, Fukusaki E. Current metabolomics: technological advances. J Biosci Bioeng. 2013;116(1):9–16.

146. Reisdorph N, Wechsler ME. Utilizing metabolomics to distinguish asthma phenotypes: strategies and clinical implications. Allergy. 2013;68(8):959–62.

147. Berger B, Peng J, Singh M. Computational solutions for omics data. Nat Rev Genet. 2013;14(5):333–46.

148. Suarez-Farinas M, Fuentes-Duculan J, Lowes MA, Krueger JG. Resolved psoriasis lesions retain expression of a subset of disease-related genes. J Invest Dermatol. 2011;131(2):391–400.

149. Ainali C, Valeyev N, Perera G, Williams A, Gudjonsson JE, Ouzounis CA, et al. Transcriptome classification reveals molecular subtypes in psoriasis. BMC Genomics. 2012;13:472.

150. Perera GK, Ainali C, Semenova E, Hundhausen C, Barinaga G, Kassen D, et al. Integrative biology approach identifies cytokine targeting strategies for psoriasis. Sci Transl Med. 2014;6(223):223ra22.

151. Valeyev NV, Hundhausen C, Umezawa Y, Kotov NV, Williams G, Clop A, et al. A systems model for immune cell interactions unravels the mechanism of inflammation in human skin. PLoS Comput Biol. 2010;6(12):e1001024.

152. Armstrong AW, Robertson AD, Wu J, Schupp C, Lebwohl MG. Undertreatment, treatment trends, and treatment dissatisfaction among patients with psoriasis and psoriatic arthritis in the United States: findings from the National Psoriasis Foundation surveys, 2003–2011. JAMA Dermatol. 2013;149(10):1180–5.

153. Ho PY, Barton A, Worthington J, Plant D, Griffiths CE, Young HS, et al. Investigating the role of the HLA-Cw*06 and HLA-DRB1 genes in susceptibility to psoriatic arthritis: comparison with psoriasis and undifferentiated inflammatory arthritis. Ann Rheum Dis. 2008;67(5):677–82.

154. Piruzian E, Bruskin S, Ishkin A, Abdeev R, Moshkovskii S, Melnik S, et al. Integrated network analysis of transcriptomic and proteomic data in psoriasis. BMC Syst Biol. 2010;4:41.

155. Yamamoto T, Nishioka K. Alteration of the expression of Bcl-2, Bcl-x, Bax, Fas, and Fas ligand in the involved skin of psoriasis vulgaris following topical anthralin therapy. Skin Pharmacol Appl Skin Physiol. 2003;16(1):50–8.

156. Kokolakis G, Giannikaki E, Stathopoulos E, Avramidis G, Tosca AD, Kruger-Krasagakis S. Infliximab restores the balance between pro- and anti-apoptotic proteins in regressing psoriatic lesions. Br J Dermatol. 2012;166(3):491–7.

157. Rashmi R, Rao KS, Basavaraj KH. A comprehensive review of biomarkers in psoriasis. Clin Exp Dermatol. 2009;34(6):658–63.

158. Arican O, Aral M, Sasmaz S, Ciragil P. Serum levels of TNF-alpha, IFN-gamma, IL-6, IL-8, IL-12, IL-17, and IL-18 in patients with active psoriasis and correlation with disease severity. Mediators Inflamm. 2005;2005(5):273–9.

159. Suarez-Farinas M, Li K, Fuentes-Duculan J, Hayden K, Brodmerkel C, Krueger JG. Expanding the psoriasis disease profile: interrogation of the skin and serum of patients with moderate-to-severe psoriasis. J Invest Dermatol. 2012;132(11):2552–64.

160. Meephansan J, Ruchusatsawat K, Sindhupak W, Thorner PS, Wongpiyabovorn J. Effect of metho-

trexate on serum levels of IL-22 in patients with psoriasis. Eur J Dermatol. 2011;21(4):501–4.

161. Michalak-Stoma A, Bartosinska J, Kowal M, Juszkiewicz-Borowiec M, Gerkowicz A, Chodorowska G. Serum levels of selected Th17 and Th22 cytokines in psoriatic patients. Dis Markers. 2013;35(6):625–31.

162. Di Meglio P, Nestle FO. The role of IL-23 in the immunopathogenesis of psoriasis. F1000 Biol Rep. 2010;2:40.

163. Tonel G, Conrad C, Laggner U, Di Meglio P, Grys K, McClanahan TK, et al. Cutting edge: A critical functional role for IL-23 in psoriasis. J Immunol. 2010;185(10):5688–91.

164. El-Moaty Zaher HA, El-Komy MH, Hegazy RA, Mohamed E, Khashab HA, Ahmed HH. Assessment of interleukin-17 and vitamin D serum levels in psoriatic patients. J Am Acad Dermatol. 2013; 69(5):840–2.

165. Choe YB, Hwang YJ, Hahn HJ, Jung JW, Jung HJ, Lee YW, et al. A comparison of serum inflammatory cytokines according to phenotype in patients with psoriasis. Br J Dermatol. 2012;167(4):762–7.

166. Cheuk S, Wiken M, Blomqvist L, Nylen S, Talme T, Stahle M, et al. Epidermal Th22 and Tc17 cells form a localized disease memory in clinically healed psoriasis. J Immunol. 2014;192:3111–20.

167. Benham H, Norris P, Goodall J, Wechalekar MD, FitzGerald O, Szentpetery A, et al. Th17 and Th22 cells in psoriatic arthritis and psoriasis. Arthritis Res Ther. 2013;15(5):R136.

168. Rocha-Pereira P, Santos-Silva A, Rebelo I, Figueiredo A, Quintanilha A, Teixeira F. The inflammatory response in mild and in severe psoriasis. Br J Dermatol. 2004;150(5):917–28.

169. Gupta M, Chari S, Borkar M, Chandankhede M. Dyslipidemia and oxidative stress in patients of psoriasis. Biomed Res. 2011;22(2):221–4.

170. Tekin NS, Tekin IO, Barut F, Sipahi EY. Accumulation of oxidized low-density lipoprotein in psoriatic skin and changes of plasma lipid levels in psoriatic patients. Mediators Inflamm. 2007;2007:78454.

171. Haider AS, Lowes MA, Suarez-Farinas M, Zaba LC, Cardinale I, Khatcherian A, et al. Identification of cellular pathways of "type 1," Th17 T cells, and TNF- and inducible nitric oxide synthase-producing dendritic cells in autoimmune inflammation through pharmacogenomic study of cyclosporine A in psoriasis. J Immunol. 2008;180(3):1913–20.

172. Johnson-Huang LM, Suarez-Farinas M, Sullivan-Whalen M, Gilleaudeau P, Krueger JG, Lowes MA. Effective narrow-band UVB radiation therapy suppresses the IL-23/IL-17 axis in normalized psoriasis plaques. J Invest Dermatol. 2010;130(11):2654–63.

173. Suarez-Farinas M, Shah KR, Haider AS, Krueger JG, Lowes MA. Personalized medicine in psoriasis: developing a genomic classifier to predict histological response to Alefacept. BMC Dermatol. 2010;10:1.

174. Richetta AG, Mattozzi C, Salvi M, Giancristoforo S, Cantisani C, D'Epiro S, et al. Downregulation of circulating CD4+ CD25(bright) Foxp3+ T cells by cyclosporine therapy and correlation with clinical response in psoriasis patients: report of three cases. Int J Dermatol. 2013;52(11):1437–9.

175. Jokai H, Szakonyi J, Kontar O, Barna G, Inotai D, Karpati S, et al. Cutaneous lymphocyte-associated antigen as a novel predictive marker of TNF-alpha inhibitor biological therapy in psoriasis. Exp Dermatol. 2013;22(3):221–3.

176. Warren RB, Smith RL, Campalani E, Eyre S, Smith CH, Barker JN, et al. Genetic variation in efflux transporters influences outcome to methotrexate therapy in patients with psoriasis. J Invest Dermatol. 2008;128(8):1925–9.

177. Tejasvi T, Stuart PE, Chandran V, Voorhees JJ, Gladman DD, Rahman P, et al. TNFAIP3 gene polymorphisms are associated with response to TNF blockade in psoriasis. J Invest Dermatol. 2012;132(3 Pt 1):593–600.

178. Talamonti M, Botti E, Galluzzo M, Teoli M, Spallone G, Bavetta M, et al. Pharmacogenetics of psoriasis: HLA-Cw6 but not LCE3B/3C deletion nor TNFAIP3 polymorphism predisposes to clinical response to interleukin 12/23 blocker ustekinumab. Br J Dermatol. 2013;169(2):458–63.

179. BSTOP. Biomarkers of Systemic Treatment Outcomes in Psoriasis (BSTOP) study. Available from: http://www.kcl.ac.uk/medicine/research/divisions/gmm/departments/dermatology/Research/stru/groups/bstop/index.aspx. Accessed 26 Mar 2014.

180. PSORT. Psoriasis Stratification to Optimise Relevant Therapy. Available from: www.psort.org.uk. Accessed 26 Mar 2014.

Autoinflammatory Syndromes: Relevance to Inflammatory Skin Diseases and Personalized Medicine

Dan Lipsker

Contents

D. Lipsker, MD, PhD
Department of Dermatology, Faculté de Médecine,
Université de Strasbourg et Clinique Dermatologique,
Hôpitaux Universitaires, Strasbourg 67000, France
e-mail: dan.lipsker@chru-strasbourg.fr

7.1   Introduction

The comprehension of the pathogenetic mechanisms of the autoinflammatory disorders has profoundly changed the nosology of inflammatory disorders [1]. It has opened the path to a *sign-based*, personalized approach to the patient with an inflammatory disorder, allowing optimized treatment and avoiding unnecessary overtreatment [2].

The term autoinflammatory syndrome (AIS) refers to a group of monogenic disorders characterized by seemingly unprovoked bouts of recurrent inflammation [3]. Inflammatory flares can occur in many organs, especially in the skin, joints, eyes, and serous membranes. It is an underlying genetic abnormality involving actors of the innate immune system that predisposes the affected individual to an exaggerated inflammatory response to exogenous or endogenous triggering factors. Markers of autoimmunity are absent. However, a few novel conditions present with both autoimmune and autoinflammatory disease presentation, and therefore innate and adaptive immunity should be considered as two extremes of a continuous spectrum. According to Jesus and Goldbach-Mansky, it is probably more accurate to consider the autoinflammatory syndromes as dysregulatory conditions marked by excessive inflammation, mediated predominantly by cells and molecules of the innate immune system and with significant host predisposition [4]. Some sporadic or polygenic disorders are closely

T. Bieber, F. Nestle (eds.), *Personalized Treatment Options in Dermatology*,
DOI 10.1007/978-3-662-45840-2_7, © Springer-Verlag Berlin Heidelberg 2015

related to the AIS and involve similar pathogenic mechanisms. It is therefore important to distinguish between monogenic AIS and complex disorders with underlying AI mechanisms such as gout, adult-onset Still's disease, or Schnitzler's syndrome. Indeed, the comprehension and genetic deciphering of the AIS has allowed a new classification of inflammatory diseases in general [1]. The same or shared mechanisms that underlie those rare disorders also contribute to inflammation in many frequent complex polygenic disorders. Thus, the importance of the comprehension of their pathogenesis reaches far beyond the simple comprehension of this group of diseases. Skin signs can be the presenting sign or one of the main clinical finding in many of these disorders. The relevance of AI mechanisms in much commoner inflammatory dermatoses, such as the neutrophilic dermatoses, will be emphasized.

7.2 Monogenic Mainly IL-1-Mediated AIS

Table 7.1 summarizes the general clinical characteristics of the major AIS. Familial Mediterranean fever (FMF) is a relatively common disorder in some parts of the world, while most other disorders are extremely rare diseases, sometimes reported only in few families. For FMF, the highest prevalence rates are found in the Sephardic Jewish, Turkish, Armenian, and Arab populations; prevalence rates of 1:248 to 1:1,000 and carrier rates of 1:3 to 1–7 are reported [5].

An AIS should be suspected in every patient with otherwise unexplained recurrent flares of inflammation with or without fever. Age of onset, type of involvement, and duration of the attacks will help establishing a correct diagnosis (Table 7.1). In this author's experience, a significant number of patients have however all the characteristics of a typical AIS, but they do not fit into established nosology, as the whole spectrum of these disorders is so far not delineated and new entities are regularly reported and mutations in new genes described.

We shall only briefly describe the cutaneous findings of some of these disorders, especially those that are clearly IL-1 mediated [4]. This will allow us to draw conclusions that we can apply to the much commoner complex polygenic disorders.

7.2.1 Clearly IL-1-Mediated AIS: IL-1 Is the Only or Main Pathogenic Factor

7.2.1.1 Excessive IL-1 Production: Cryopyrinopathies or Cold-Induced Autoinflammatory Syndromes (CAPS)

They include three, partially overlapping autosomal dominant entities related to mutations in the same *NLRP3/CIAS1* gene: familial cold autoinflammatory syndrome (FCAS), Muckle-Wells syndrome (MWS), and chronic infantile neurological and articular (CINCA)/neonatal onset multi-inflammatory disorder (NOMID) [3, 4]. Within the CAPS spectrum, FCAS is the least severe entity, while CINCA is the most severe.

A closely related syndrome to the milder FCAS/MWS variants was described in patients with a *NLRP12* mutation [6].

The three disorders usually start in the newborn or during early infancy with fever, fatigue, a flu-like syndrome, and rash. The flares are triggered by exposure to cold in FCAS – after an interval of 1–2 h – and are accompanied by thirst, transpiration, joint pain, and conjunctivitis. Cold-stimulation tests (ice cube, immersion) can be negative, as ventilated cold is the usual trigger. Cold dependency of flares is less marked in MWS, but this disorder is more severe and patients develop sensorineural hearing loss and they are at risk of AA amyloidosis.

Continuous flares with neutrophilic aseptic meningitis, dysmorphism, mental retardation, sensorineural deafness, and deforming arthropathy characterize CINCA, a very severe disorder. Diagnosis is based on typical clinical and biological findings; evidencing an autosomal dominant mutation in *NLRP3/CIAS1* gene is helpful, but the mutation will not be present in all patients.

Table 7.1 Clinical characteristics and treatment of selected AIS

Disease	Mode of inheritance	Predominant ethnic group	Age at onset	Typical duration of flare	Typical frequency of flares	Typical/distinctive clinical features	Treatment
FMF	AR; rarely AD	Eastern Mediterranean	Childhood to early adulthood	1–3 days	Variable	Colchicine responsiveness Pseudo-appendicular pain Erysipelas-like erythema	Colchicine Anakinra
TRAPS	AD	Northern European; numerous other ethnic groups	Childhood/early adulthood; rarely late onset	>7 days; may be prolonged over many weeks	Variable	Longer duration of attack; migratory myalgia with erythema; periorbital edema	Steroids on demand Etanercept
MVK deficiency/ HIDS	AR	Northern European	Infancy	3–7 days	1–2 monthly	Palpable lymph nodes; diarrhea; triggered by vaccinations	Steroids on demand Anti-TNF Anti-IL-1
FCAS	AD	Northern European	Childhood	24 h	Depends on exposure to cold	Triggered by exposure to cold Neutrophilic urticarial dermatosis Conjunctivitis Thirst and transpiration Spectacular response to anakinra	Cold avoidance Anti-IL-1
MWS	AD	Northern European	Neonatal/infancy	Continuous; worse in the evening	Often daily	Neutrophilic urticarial dermatosis Hearing loss Spectacular response to anakinra	Anti-IL-1
CINCA	Sporadic	Northern European	Neonatal/infancy	Continuous	Continuous	Neutrophilic urticarial dermatosis Dysmorphia Aseptic meningitis Deforming arthropathy Spectacular response to anakinra	Anti-IL-1
PAPA	AD	Northern European	Childhood	Intermittent	Variable	Pathergy Notion of familial pyoderma gangrenosum Migratory arthritis in early childhood	Anti-TNF Anti-IL-1
DIRA	AR	Newfoundland; Brazil; Lebanon; Puerto Rican, Dutch	Neonatal/infancy	Continuous	Continuous	Pustules Osteolytic bone lesions Spectacular response to anakinra	Anti-IL-1
CANDLE	AR	Japan	Infancy	Continuous	Continuous	Exacerbated in winter Plaques with atypical myeloid infiltrate Pernio-like lesions Lipoatrophy Basal ganglia calcification	No efficient treatment known
Blau syndrome	AD	Not known	Childhood	Continuous	Continuous	Granulomatous dermatitis Uveitis	Steroids Anti-TNF

FMF familial Mediterranean fever, *TRAPS* TNF-receptor-associated periodic syndrome, *MVK* mevalonate kinase, *HIDS* hyper-IgD syndrome, *FCAS* familial cold autoinflammatory syndrome, *MWS* Muckle-Wells syndrome, *CINCA* chronic infantile neurological and articular, *PAPA* pyogenic sterile arthritis, pyoderma gangrenosum, and acne, *DIRA* deficiency of interleukin-1 receptor antagonist, *CANDLE* chronic atypical neutrophilic dermatosis with lipodystrophy and elevated temperature

Skin Findings and Histopathology

Neutrophilic urticarial dermatosis (NUD; see also below) is the classic cutaneous manifestations in those children [7, 8]. An urticarial rash with a neutrophilic intravascular, perivascular, perieccrine, and interstitial infiltrate on histopathologic evaluation is typical. In this author's experience, leukocytoclasia is frequent in patients with NUD in the context of Schnitzler's syndrome (see below) but much less so in children with CAPS.

7.2.1.2 Deficient IL-1 Inhibition: Deficiency of Interleukin-1 Receptor Antagonist (DIRA)

DIRA is suspected in every newborn with a pustular dermatitis, multifocal osteomyelitis, and periostitis with marked elevation of acute phase reactants though fever is only low grade or absent. Pustules are aseptic. Chronic lung disease, respiratory distress syndrome, and central nervous system vasculitis were rarely described. Fatal evolution is reported [9, 10]. Diagnosis relies on clinical and radiological findings (widened rips and clavicles, osteolytic lesions of long bones) and is supported by evidencing an autosomal recessive loss-of-function mutation in *IL-1Rn* gene [9].

Skin Findings

Grouped pustules on an erythematous base in the newborn or within the first 3 weeks and evolution toward yellowish crusts [9, 11]. The lesions can be localized or widespread, including face and scalp involvement. Bullae with hypopyon can be present. Evolution toward ichthyosiform lesions with diffuse desquamating scaly and sometimes slightly red skin can occur [12]. Oral mucosa and nail can be affected, with pitting and onychomadesis.

Histopathology

Epidermal spongiosis and acanthosis and most notably a neutrophilic infiltrate of the epidermis, with intracorneal, subcorneal, and intraepidermal microabscesses, as well as a neutrophilic infiltrate in the dermis and the perifollicular and periecccrine areas [9, 11]. Neutrophilic syringotropism could be a distinctive feature [12], and this latter finding is also found in CINCA syndrome [8].

7.2.2 AIS in Which IL-1 Plays an Important Role, but Other Factors Are Involved

7.2.2.1 Familial Mediterranean Fever (FMF)

The disease usually starts before the age of thirty with recurrent flares of fever; abdominal pain, sometimes mimicking an acute abdomen; pleurisy; and large joint arthritis that last between 1 and 3 days. The major risk is the development of inflammatory AA amyloidosis, and this risk can be largely prevented with continuous treatment with colchicine. Diagnosis is supported by evidencing a pathogenic autosomal recessive *MEFV* gene mutation (rare dominant variant exist); diagnosis is based on the Livneh criteria [13].

Typical Skin Findings

The most typical cutaneous finding is the socalled erysipelas-like erythema [14, 15]. It consists of a red edematous, warm, swollen erythema, more often than a circumscribed plaque. The erythema is usually localized on the lower limbs below the knee, typically in the perimalleolar area or the dorsum of the foot.

Histopathology

A sparse neutrophilic infiltrate in the upper dermis is the hallmark of the erysipelas-like erythema [14, 15]. Leukocytoclasia can be present but no significant vasculitis. Histiocytes and eosinophils can also be present.

7.2.2.2 Pyogenic Sterile Arthritis, Pyoderma Gangrenosum, and Acne (PAPA) Syndrome

Early-onset childhood flares of recurrent painful sterile arthritis, sterile abscesses, and pathergy are typical. By puberty, joint symptoms tend to subside, while skin symptoms increase. Diagnosis is established on grounds of clinical history and finding an autosomal dominant mutation in *PSTPIP1* [16].

Skin Findings

Pathergy and aseptic abscesses, as well as ulcerations related to pyoderma gangrenosum, can occur from childhood on. Gingival pustules can also occur from childhood on [16]. By puberty, severe nodulocystic acne develops. PAPA should be considered in every patient with a familial history of pathergy and/or pyoderma gangrenosum.

Hidradenitis suppurativa can also develop and has been reported in a patient with a novel *PSTPIP1* mutation; authors then called this expanded entity PAPASH [17]. A related entity referred to as "PASH syndrome" has been described [18]. These patients lack the sterile arthritis, but they have nodulocystic acne and pyoderma gangrenosum; in addition, they develop hidradenitis suppurativa. The underlying genetic abnormality is so far unknown.

Histopathology
There are no specific histopathological findings reported so far.

7.3 Pathophysiology

CAPS are related to mostly missense mutations in the *NLRP3/CIAS1* gene encoding a death domain protein known as NLRP3 (or cryopyrin). This protein is expressed in the epithelial cells of the skin and the mucosa, the granulocytes, the dendritic cells, and the T and B cells. A variety of danger signals, including "pathogen-associated molecular pattern" (PAMP), induce association of NLRP3 with other members of the death domain superfamily to form a cytosolic protein complex named the "inflammasome." This results in activation of caspase 1 which cleaves biologic inactive pro-IL 1β into biologic active IL-1β [3, 4]. It also upregulates NF-κB expression and thereby increases IL-1 gene expression. IL-1 is a major proinflammatory cytokine and the key mediator of the manifestations of CAPS. This assumption is supported by the observation that IL-1 blockade induces rapid and complete response in patients with CAPS.

DIRA is related to a deficiency of the naturally occurring antagonist of the IL-1 receptor (IL-1Rn) [9, 11]. The result is an excess in IL-1-mediated inflammation, by lack of inhibition of (initially) normally produced IL-1.

The pathophysiology of FMF is less clear. FMF is usually an autosomal recessive disorder related to mutations in the *MEFV* gene, though rare dominant mutations exist [19]. MEFV encodes pyrin, which plays probably an important role in the modulation of caspase 1 and thus the production of IL-1.

Mutations in *PSTPIP1* that alter its interaction with pyrin and the inflammasome and induce overproduction of active IL-1β are found in patients with PAPA syndrome [3, 4].

7.4 Other AIS

There are numerous other AIS which will not be addressed here; excellent review articles have been published during the last years [3, 20]. The key features of some of them like partial mevalonate kinase deficiency (or HIDS, hyper-IgD syndrome), TNF-receptor-associated periodic syndrome (TRAPS), Blau syndrome, or Nakajo-Nishimura syndrome are summarized in Table 7.1.

Some particular variants of psoriasis are AIS, challenging the nosology of this entity. This is the case for recessive familial generalized pustular psoriasis related to a deficiency of interleukin-36 receptor antagonist (DITRA) [21] and for CARD14-mediated psoriasis (CAMPS) [22]. The latter was found to cause plaque psoriasis and generalized pustular psoriasis, as well as familial pityriasis rubra pilaris. It is therefore not surprising that some variants of pustular psoriasis respond to IL-1 inhibition with anakinra [2, 23].

Majeed syndrome is related to autosomal recessive loss-of-function mutations of the *LPIN2* gene and presents with neonatal recurrent multifocal osteomyelitis and congenital dyserythropoietic anemia. Neutrophilic dermatoses are frequent in the rare patients reported to have Majeed's syndrome: no further specified pustular lesions, pustular psoriasis, and Sweet syndrome [24].

7.5 A Synopsis of the Cutaneous Findings in Monogenic AIS and Their Relevance to Sporadic Diseases

A careful analysis of the cutaneous findings reported in the patients with IL-1-mediated AIS shows that they are always neutrophilic aseptic dermatoses. Table 7.2 summarizes the dermatologic findings and provides comparison with related complex/polygenic disorders. It is therefore tempting to speculate that the *pathomechanisms underlying all neutrophilic (aseptic) dermatoses involve autoinflammatory mechanisms.*

Neutrophilic urticarial dermatosis deserves a special mention, as this entity is not only characteristic of CAPS but strongly associated with systemic complex disorders [7]. The rash is peculiar: it consists of rose or red macules or only slightly elevated plaques. Significant edema is rare. Pruritus is usually initially absent. Dermographism can be present. Lesion resolves within some hours. From a histopathological point of view, there is a significant interstitial neutrophilic infiltrate, with leukocytoclasia, sometimes small foci of necrobiosis, but without vasculitis and without significant dermal edema. Especially two diseases,

now considered as polygenic expression of autoinflammation, display this type of rash: adult-onset Still's disease (AOSD) (Fig. 7.1) and Schnitzler's syndrome (Fig. 7.2) [7, 25, 26]. Both disorders are characterized by high fever, joint pain, and rash. Pharyngitis, hepatitis, and very high ferritin levels are suggestive of AOSD, while a monoclonal IgM gammopathy is suggestive of Schnitzler's syndrome (see Table 7.3 for diagnostic criteria of the latter entity). In every patient with NUD, an underlying autoinflammatory

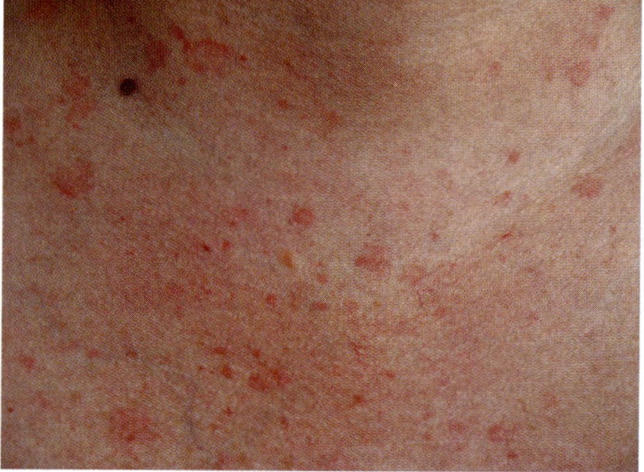

Fig. 7.1 Discrete red macules in a patient with adult-onset Still's disease. Lesions resolve within hours. Biopsy revealed typical findings of neutrophilic urticarial dermatosis

Table 7.2 Examples of neutrophilic dermatoses responsive to IL-1 inhibition occurring in monogenic and complex disorders

Dermatological sign with tissular neutrophilic aseptic infiltration (nosologic entity)	Hereditary autoinflammatory syndrome	Related sporadic or complex disorder
Evanescent maculopapular rash (nosology = *neutrophilic urticarial dermatosis*)	CAPS	Schnitzler's syndrome
		Adult-onset Still's disease
		Systemic-onset juvenile idiopathic arthritis
Ulceration (nosology = *pyoderma gangrenosum*)	PAPA	Pyoderma gangrenosum "idiopathic" or occurring in the setting of a nosologically characterized inflammatory disease
Pustule (aseptic)	DIRA	Generalized pustular psoriasis
	PAPA	Impetigo herpetiformis
		SAPHO syndrome
		Acne fulminans
Edematous plaque (nosology = *Sweet syndrome*)	Majeed syndrome	Sweet syndrome either "idiopathic" or occurring in the setting of a nosologically characterized inflammatory disease

CAPS cryopyrin-associated periodic syndrome, *DIRA* deficiency of interleukin-1 receptor antagonist, *PAPA* pyogenic arthritis, pyoderma gangrenosum, and acne

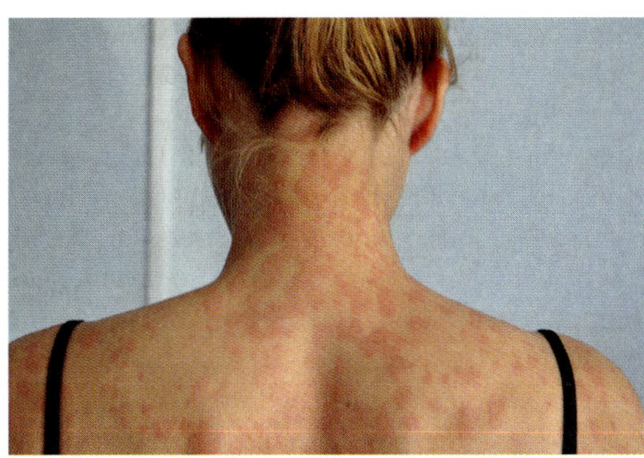

Fig. 7.2 Red macules, papules, and plaques in a patient with Schnitzler's syndrome. Lesions resolve within hours. Biopsy revealed an interstitial neutrophilic infiltrate in the dermis, without vasculitis and without edema, typical of neutrophilic urticarial dermatosis

Table 7.3 Schnitzler's syndrome: Strasbourg diagnostic criteria

Obligate criteria
Chronic urticarial rash +
Monoclonal IgM or IgG
Minor criteria
Recurrent fever[a]
Objective findings of abnormal bone remodeling with or without bone pain[b]
A neutrophilic dermal infiltrate without vasculitis on skin biopsy[c]
Leukocytosis and/or elevated CRP[d]
Definite diagnosis if
2 obligate criteria and at least 2 minor criteria if IgM and 3 minor criteria if IgG
Probable diagnosis if
2 obligate criteria and at least 1 minor criterion if IgM and 2 minor criteria if IgG

[a]A valid criterion if objectively measured. Must be >38 °C and otherwise unexplained. Occurs usually – but not obligatory – together with the skin rash
[b]As assessed by bone scintigraphy, MRI, or elevation of bone alkaline phosphatase
[c]Corresponds usually to the entity described as "neutrophilic urticarial dermatosis" (*Medicine* 2009;88:23–31); absence of fibrinoid vessel wall necrosis and absence of significant dermal edema
[d]Neutrophils >10,000/mm^3 and/or CRP >30 mg/l

mechanism should be suspected, and treatment option should firsthand target neutrophils and/or IL-1 production.

7.6 Treatment of Dermatoses with a Supposed AIS Mechanism

As is shown in Table 7.1, colchicine (in FMF) and IL-1 antagonists are the main treatments for the IL-1-mediated AIS. In particular, the prognosis of CAPS has been completely changed since IL-1 inhibitors are available. Before IL-1 inhibition, there was no efficient treatment for affected children, while a single injection of anakinra controls all clinical signs of the disease within hours. The response is very impressive for both the patient and the physician. The same is true for the complex disorders AOSD and Schnitzler's syndrome that are now commonly included in the spectrum of AIS. The response in patients with Schnitzler's syndrome is as complete and immediate as the one observed in CAPS. This strongly points to the fact that the clinical manifestations of Schnitzler's syndrome are solely IL-1 mediated, though that has not been proven so far. In AOSD, the situation is interesting: the "rheumatologic variants" with much pain and less intense systemic signs are only poorly responsive or unresponsive to IL-1 inhibition, while the "dermatologic variants" with high fever and rash, sometimes complicated by macrophage activation syndrome, usually respond well to IL-1 inhibition [27, 28].

When we now turn to the treatment of the neutrophilic aseptic dermatoses, it is obvious that drugs should target the key tissue effector, the neutrophils. As in FMF, colchicine, an inhibitor of neutrophil migration, is sometimes useful. Dapsone inhibits neutrophil chemotaxis but also the generation of five lipoxygenase products, and it binds and inactivates myeloperoxidase. It is a very useful drug in many of the neutrophilic dermatoses. Though it is not the aim of this chapter to address the treatment of the neutrophilic dermatoses, I will only briefly mention the fact that in some difficult-to-treat patients with neutrophilic dermatoses, either because they are refractory to standard treatment or because of contraindications, the lessons learned from the AIS can apply to this group of diseases. Indeed,

IL-1 inhibition can be a very efficient alternative treatment, and this has already been published in some examples: neutrophilic urticarial dermatosis, Sweet syndrome, neutrophilic panniculitis, pustular psoriasis, and relapsing polychondritis (reviewed in [29]). In this author's experience, however, IL-1 inhibitors will provide significant relief only in those patients with a neutrophilic dermatosis and systemic signs of IL-1 impregnation such as fever, leukocytosis, and elevated CRP levels.

Therefore, dermatologists should become familiar with the handling of the IL-1 inhibitor anakinra [29]. Anakinra has a short half-life of 4–6 h and is rapidly completely eliminated from the body; therefore, daily injections (100 mg, subcutaneous) are required. In the aforementioned situations, it is worth to be tried as response is usually rapid, occurring a couple of hours after the first injection; if there is no response after 3 days of treatment, the dermatosis is usually not responsive and treatment can be interrupted. Injection site reactions are very frequent with anakinra, but otherwise the drug is well tolerated. In case of long-term use (e.g., Schnitzler's syndrome, CAPS), neutrophil count, liver function tests, and triglycerides should be monitored. The usage of the other longer-acting IL-1 antagonists (gevokizumab, canakinumab, rilonacept) should be restricted to physicians with extensive experience, because of longer half-life and exorbitant price for those so far available.

7.7   Non-IL-1-mediated AIS and Their Relevance to Inflammatory Dermatoses

There are more and more reports of non-IL-1-mediated AIS [3, 20, 30–33]. Their description is beyond the scope of this book. It is probable that we will learn a lot from those disorders in the coming years. The Nakajo-Nishimura/CANDLE (chronic atypical neutrophilic dermatosis with lipodystrophy and elevated temperature) syndrome is a serious disorder with prominent dermatologic involvement [30–33]. It is characterized by early onset of recurrent fever, rash,

arthralgia, or arthritis and increase in acute phase reactants. Violaceous pernio-like eyelid and finger swelling is characteristic, as is lipoatrophy, which can be secondary to panniculitis. Enlarged lymph nodes, spleen, and/or liver as well as increased liver function test are frequent. Basal ganglia calcification and muscle atrophy are also reported. Up to 50 % of patients could die before adulthood. The remaining develop muscle atrophy, cardiac arrhythmias, and dilated cardiomyopathy. Diagnostic criteria were published by Japanese authors [31]. Abnormal signaling in the interferon pathways characterizes Nakajo-Nishimura and/or CANDLE syndrome [30, 31]. This syndrome, first reported in Japan, is related to a mutation in the *PMSB8* gene, encoding the ß5i subunit of the (immuno)proteasome, which is highly expressed in hematopoietic cells and is involved in protein degradation [33]. It is probable, from a clinico-biologic perspective, that this syndrome shares many features with a subgroup of patients with dermatomyositis and lupus erythematosus.

7.8   The Concept of Autoimmunity and Autoinflammation in Clinical Practice: A Paradigmatic Case Report Highlighting Bedside Relevance of These Concepts

Case Report A 22-year-old girl developed joint pain with effusion, autoimmune hemolytic Coombs-positive anemia, and abdominal pain with diarrhea. She was found to have high titer of ANA (1:2,048), anti-dsDNA, anti-SSA, and anti-SSB antibodies. Imaging revealed intestinal thickening, abnormal bowel wall enhancement, increased fat attenuation, engorgement of mesenteric vessels with increased number of visible vessels, and features highly suggestive of lupus enteritis. She was treated with steroid pulse therapy and mycophenolate mofetil for lupus enteritis in the context of SLE. After the acute enteric episode had resolved, steroids were tapered.

Hydroxychloroquine was then added. Two years later while still being treated with prednisone 10 mg/day, hydroxychloroquine 400 mg/day, and mycophenolate mofetil 1 g/day, she had daily episodes of joint pain, red eyes related to episcleritis, and an urticarial rash. As all these signs fit perfectly in her known SLE, increasing steroid and mycophenolate mofetil dosages was considered, but a second opinion was required in our institution. A skin biopsy showed the typical findings of neutrophilic urticarial dermatosis. As there were no other signs of active SLE, we therefore stopped mycophenolate mofetil, tapered prednisone at a rate of 1 mg/month, and started dapsone 100 mg/day. Response was immediate and spectacular; within days, rash ceased, joint pain and swelling regressed, and eyes normalized.

This case report highlights the importance of distinguishing between autoimmune and autoinflammatory pathomechanisms. It also underlines that classic autoimmune diseases can have autoinflammation-driven symptoms and that *every sign must be pathogenetically deciphered.*

Indeed, SLE is a paradigm of an autoimmune disorder, and definitely the initial signs of this patient, namely, hemolytic Coombs-positive anemia and enteric vasculitis, were clearly autoantibody mediated. However, 2 years later, she had NUD with joint pain and episcleritis. It was important at that stage to perform biopsy and to distinguish between urticarial vasculitis and NUD, as NUD is almost always a cutaneous expression of an autoinflammatory mechanism [7]; autoinflammation can also occur in a subset of patients with SLE, especially those with neutrophilic cutaneous LE [34]. Recognition is essential as it prevents unnecessary overtreatment with steroids and immunosuppressors, treatments that are more toxic than the drugs targeting autoinflammatory mechanisms and, by the way, much less efficient to treat these symptoms, as highlighted by this case report.

In summary, when dealing with patients with inflammatory disorders, we should be able to classify the disorder rather as having underlying autoimmune pathogenesis (e.g., SLE, pemphigus, etc.) or an autoinflammatory pathogenesis (AOSD, Crohn's diseases, ankylosing spondylitis, etc.). But as the previous case report highlights, though general disease mechanism provides a broad pathogenic approach, actually each sign must be analyzed in terms of pathogenicity; this is bedside personalized medicine with direct therapeutic consequences. In the era of next-generation sequencing, we will certainly learn in the coming years that the shared genetic background of many inflammatory diseases is modulated by sign-specific genetic signatures. So far, a careful clinicopathological analyses can already provide meaningful and therapeutically revealed informations, many of which we have learned from the genetic deciphering of the rare monogenic AIS.

References

1. McGonagle D, McDermott MF. A proposed classification of the immunological diseases. PLoS Med. 2006;3(8):e297.
2. Lutz V, Lipsker D. Acitretin- and tumor necrosis factor inhibitor-resistant acrodermatitis continua of Hallopeau responsive to the interleukin 1 receptor antagonist anakinra. Arch Dermatol. 2012; 148:297–9.
3. Goldbach-Mansky R. Immunology in clinic review series; focus on autoinflammatory diseases: update on monogenic autoinflammatory diseases: the role of interleukin (IL)-1 and an emerging role for cytokines beyond IL-1. Clin Exp Immunol. 2012; 167(3):391–404.
4. Jesus AA, Goldbach-Mansky R. IL-1 blockade in autoinflammatory syndromes. Ann Rev Med. 2014;65:223–44.
5. Stoffman N, Magal N, Shohat T, et al. Higher than expected carrier rates for familial Mediterranean fever in various Jewish ethnic groups. Eur J Hum Genet. 2000;8:307–10.
6. Jéru I, Le Borgne G, Cochet E, et al. Identification and functional consequences of a recurrent NLRP12 missense mutation in periodic fever syndromes. Arthritis Rheum. 2011;63(5):1459–64.
7. Kieffer C, Cribier B, Lipsker D. Neutrophilic urticarial dermatosis: a variant of neutrophilic urticaria strongly associated with systemic disease. Report of 9 new cases and review of the literature. Medicine (Baltimore). 2009;88(1):23–31.
8. Kolivras A, Theunis A, Ferster A, et al. Cryopyrin-associated periodic syndrome: an autoinflammatory disease manifested as neutrophilic urticarial dermatosis with additional perieccrine involvement. J Cutan Pathol. 2011;38(2):202–8.

9. Aksentijevich I, Masters SL, Ferguson PJ, et al. An autoinflammatory disease with deficiency of the interleukin-1-receptor antagonist. N Engl J Med. 2009;360(23):2426–37.

10. Altiok E, Aksoy F, Perk Y, Taylan F, Kim PW, Ilıkkan B, Asal GT, Goldbach-Mansky R, Sanal O. A novel mutation in the interleukin-1 receptor antagonist associated with intrauterine disease onset. Clin Immunol. 2012;145(1):77–81.

11. Reddy S, Jia S, Geoffrey R, Lorier R, et al. An autoinflammatory disease due to homozygous deletion of the IL1RN locus. N Engl J Med. 2009;360(23):2438–44.

12. Minkis K, Aksentijevich I, Goldbach-Mansky R, Magro C, Scott R, Davis JG, Sardana N, Herzog R. Interleukin 1 receptor antagonist deficiency presenting as infantile pustulosis mimicking infantile pustular psoriasis. Arch Dermatol. 2012;148(6):747–52.

13. Livneh A, Langevitz P, Zemer D, et al. Criteria for the diagnosis of familial Mediterranean fever. Arthritis Rheum. 1997;40(10):1879–85.

14. Radakovic S, Holzer G, Tanew A. Erysipelas-like erythema as a cutaneous sign of familial Mediterranean fever: a case report and review of the histopathologic findings. J Am Acad Dermatol. 2013;68(2):e61–3.

15. Barzilai A, Langevitz P, Goldberg I, et al. Erysipelas-like erythema of familial Mediterranean fever: clinicopathologic correlation. J Am Acad Dermatol. 2000;42:791–5.

16. Demidowich AP, Freeman AF, Kuhns DB, et al. Brief report: genotype, phenotype, and clinical course in five patients with PAPA syndrome (pyogenic sterile arthritis, pyoderma gangrenosum, and acne). Arthritis Rheum. 2012;64(6):2022–7.

17. Marzano AV, Trevisan V, Gattorno M, et al. Pyogenic arthritis, pyoderma gangrenosum, acne, and hidradenitis suppurativa (PAPASH): a new autoinflammatory syndrome associated with a novel mutation of the PSTPIP1 gene. JAMA Dermatol. 2013;149:762–4.

18. Braun-Falco M, Kovnerystyy O, Lohse P, Ruzicka T. Pyoderma gangrenosum, acne, and suppurative hidradenitis (PASH)–a new autoinflammatory syndrome distinct from PAPA syndrome. J Am Acad Dermatol. 2012;66(3):409–15.

19. Koné-Paut I, Hentgen V, Guillaume-Czitrom S, et al. The clinical spectrum of 94 patients carrying a single mutated MEFV allele. Rheumatology (Oxford). 2009;48(7):840–2.

20. Masters SL, Simon A, Aksentijevich I, Kastner DL. Horror autoinflammaticus: the molecular pathophysiology of autoinflammatory disease. Annu Rev Immunol. 2009;27:621–68.

21. Marrakchi S, Guigue P, Renshaw BR, et al. Interleukin-36-receptor antagonist deficiency and generalized pustular psoriasis. N Engl J Med. 2011;365(7):620–8.

22. Jordan CT, Cao L, Roberson ED, et al. PSORS2 is due to mutations in CARD14. Am J Hum Genet. 2012;90(5):784–95.

23. Viguier M, Guigue P, Pagès C, Smahi A, Bachelez H. Successful treatment of generalized pustular psoriasis with the interleukin-1-receptor antagonist anakinra: lack of correlation with IL1RN mutations. Ann Intern Med. 2010;153(1):66–7.

24. Herlin T, Fiirgaard B, Bjerre M, et al. Efficacy of anti-IL-1 treatment in Majeed syndrome. Ann Rheum Dis. 2013;72(3):410–3.

25. Lipsker D, Veran Y, Grunenberger F, et al. The Schnitzler syndrome. Four new cases and review of the literature. Medicine (Baltimore). 2001;80(1):37–44.

26. Simon A, Asli B, Braun-Falco M, et al. Schnitzler's syndrome: diagnosis, treatment, and follow-up. Allergy. 2013;68(5):562–8.

27. Quartier P, Allantaz F, Cimaz R, Pillet P, Messiaen C, Bardin C, et al. A multicentre, randomised, double-blind, placebo-controlled trial with the interleukin-1 receptor antagonist anakinra in patients with systemic-onset juvenile idiopathic arthritis (ANAJIS trial). Ann Rheum Dis. 2011;70:747–54.

28. Laskari K, Tzioufas AG, Moutsopoulos HM. Efficacy and long-term follow-up of IL-1R inhibitor anakinra in adults with Still's disease: a case-series study. Arthritis Res Ther. 2011;13:R91.

29. Lipsker D, Lenormand C. Indications et modalities d'utilisation des anti-IL-1 dans les dermatoses inflammatoires. Ann Dermatol Venereol. 2012;139:459–67.

30. Kanazawa N. Nakajo-Nishimura syndrome: an autoinflammatory disorder showing pernio-like rashes and progressive partial lipodystrophy. Allergol Int. 2012;61(2):197–206.

31. Kunimoto K, Kimura A, Uede K, et al. A new infant case of Nakajo-Nishimura syndrome with a genetic mutation in the immunoproteasome subunit: an overlapping entity with JMP and CANDLE syndrome related to PSMB8 mutations. Dermatology. 2013;227:26–30.

32. Torrelo A, Patel S, Colmenero I, et al. Chronic atypical neutrophilic dermatosis with lipodystrophy and elevated temperature (CANDLE) syndrome. J Am Acad Dermatol. 2010;62(3):489–95.

33. Liu Y, Ramot Y, Torrelo A, et al. Mutations in proteasome subunit β type 8 cause chronic atypical neutrophilic dermatosis with lipodystrophy and elevated temperature with evidence of genetic and phenotypic heterogeneity. Arthritis Rheum. 2012;64(3):895–907.

34. Lipsker D, Saurat JH. Neutrophilic cutaneous lupus erythematosus. At the edge between innate and acquired immunity. Dermatology. 2008;216:283–6.

The Personalized Treatment for Urticaria

8

Torsten Zuberbier

Contents

8.1 Introduction

Personalized treatment in urticaria is a very important aspect as many urticaria patients have very special triggering factors and also many have a special need for treatment.

On the other hand, the current international guidelines do provide an excellent standard for diagnosis and management which will be sufficient for the vast majority of patients. Still, if some small amendments are made for those who need it, a more personalized approach is warranted. This personalized approach will be successful if the physician is watchful enough to check for the rarer underlying causes and is able to listen to possibly small individual remarks a patient makes.

This chapter has therefore taken into account the international guidelines that have just been published [1]. It will therefore quote the relevant parts of the existing guidelines and add the personalized approaches which are based not only on the level of evidence in the literature but also on the personal experience of the author. Where personal experience has been taken into account it will be marked explicitly.

8.2 Definition and Classification of Urticaria

Urticaria is a disease characterized by the development of wheals (hives), angioedema, or both. Urticaria needs to be differentiated from other

T. Zuberbier
Department of Dermatology and Allergy,
Charité Universitätsmedizin, Berlin 10117, Germany
e-mail: torsten.zuberbier@charite.de

T. Bieber, F. Nestle (eds.), *Personalized Treatment Options in Dermatology*,
DOI 10.1007/978-3-662-45840-2_8, © Springer-Verlag Berlin Heidelberg 2015

medical conditions where wheals, angioedema, or both can occur as a symptom, e.g., skin prick test, anaphylaxis, autoinflammatory syndromes, or hereditary angioedema (bradykinin-mediated angioedema).

8.2.1 Clinical Appearance

Urticaria is characterized by the sudden appearance of wheals, angioedema, or both.

A. A wheal consists of three typical features:
1. It is characterized by a central swelling of variable size, almost invariably surrounded by a reflex erythema.
2. It is associated with itching or sometimes a burning sensation.
3. It has a fleeting nature, with the skin returning to its normal appearance, usually within 1–24 h. Sometimes wheals resolve even more quickly.

B. Angioedema is characterized by:
1. A sudden, pronounced erythematous or skin-colored swelling of the lower dermis and subcutis with frequent involvement below mucous membranes.
2. Sometimes pain rather than itching and frequent involvement below mucous membranes. Its resolution is slower than that for wheals and can take up to 72 h [1].

Surely the definition of the disease leaves very little room for interpretation in a personalized manner, but it needs to be acknowledged that like in all areas of medicine, sometimes the cutoff is not extremely clear. Thus it is important to monitor the duration of the different wheals in the individual patient. In some patients, it may occur that wheals in some areas are typical short-lasting wheals and in other areas show signs of vasculitis although not fully pronounced. This is an important aspect to note as especially the longer-lasting wheals do respond differently on treatment regimes.

In addition to the definition, also the proposed classification of urticaria should be clearly adhered to as it is important for the communication among specialists to use the same terminology even though it may not be perfect in all instances.

8.3 The Personalized Approach in Assessing Disease Severity

The guidelines clearly state that it is important to monitor the quality of life of patients using standardized questionnaires which are available for both wheals and angioedema. Both instruments and the validated Urticaria Activity Score (UAS) are important tools in the personalized approach to the patient. In the course of time, the activity score helps in the discussion especially with those patients who are very unsatisfied with the treatment options and often show an increasing demand for better treatment despite already improved treatment response. The Quality of Life questionnaire allows a better understanding which of the symptoms of the disease are the most bothersome for the patient, requiring a possible amended therapeutic approach. Thus it is striking that the majority of patients feel embarrassed about the way they look and struggle with the feelings of a social dysfunctionality [2]:

Urticaria interferes with my social relationship	67.11 %
I feel embarrassed by urticaria signs on my body	84.21 %
I'm embarrassed in going to public places understanding the personal impact is thus important for the management	72.37 %

8.4 Diagnosis

The guidelines obviously provide a rational approach for the diagnosis of urticaria based on the typical patient and is also based on a concept of an economic use of resources in medicine. The guidelines however also leave freedom for the decision and emphasize that based on the history of the patient, additional diagnostic procedures may be warranted and are mentioned as an extended diagnostic program in Fig. 8.1 [1]:

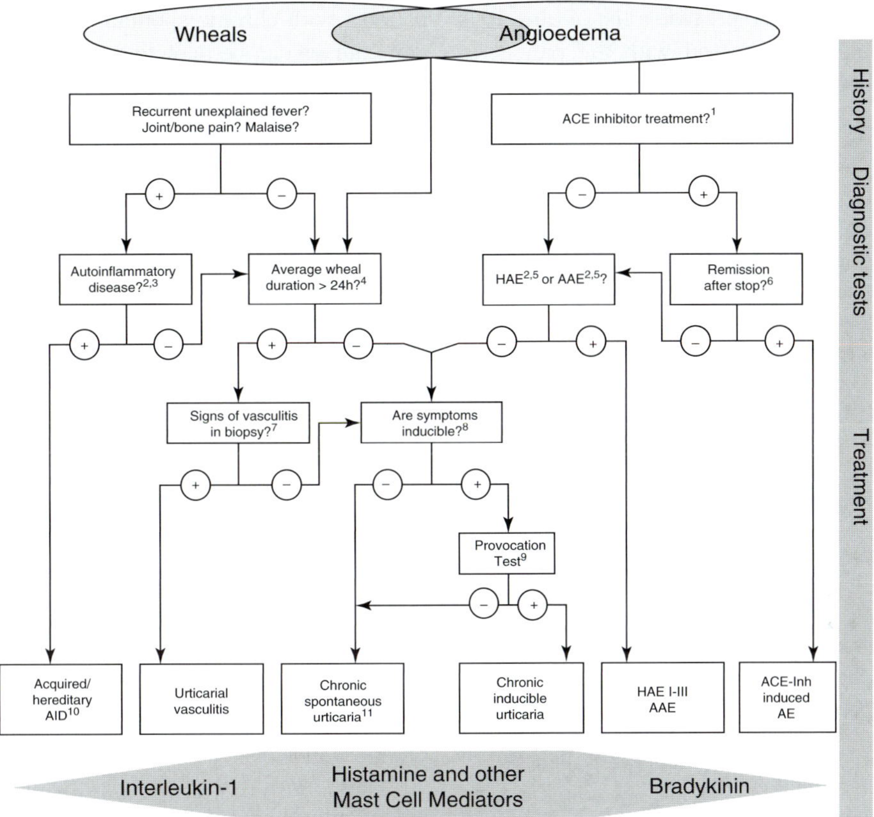

Fig. 8.1 Recommended diagnostic algorithm for patients presenting with wheals, angioedema, or both. *AAE* acquired angioedema due to C1-inhibitor deficiency, *ACE-Inh* angiotensin-converting enzyme inhibitor, *AE* angioedema, *AH* antihistamine, *AID* autoinflammatory disease, *HAE* hereditary angioedema, *IL-1* interleukin-1

1. Other (new) drugs may also induce bradykinin-mediated angioedema.
2. Patients should be asked for a detailed family history and age of disease onset.
3. Test for elevated inflammation markers (C-reactive protein, erythrocyte sedimentation rate), test for paraproteinemia in adults, look for signs of neutrophil-rich infiltrates in skin biopsy; perform gene mutation analysis of hereditary periodic fever syndromes (e.g., cryopyrin-associated periodic syndrome), if strongly suspected.
4. Patients should be asked: "How long do your wheals last?"
5. Test for complement C4 and C1-INH levels and function; in addition, test for C1q and C1-INH antibodies, if AAE is suspected; do gene mutation analysis, if former tests are unremarkable but patient's history suggests hereditary angioedema.
6. Wait for up to 6 months for remission; additional diagnostics to test for C1-inhibitor deficiency should only be performed if the family history suggests hereditary angioedema.
7. Does the biopsy of lesional skin show damage of the small vessels in the papillary and reticular dermis and/or fibrinoid deposits in perivascular and interstitial locations suggestive of UV (urticarial vasculitis)?
8. Patients should be asked: "Can you make your wheals come?"
9. In patients with a history suggestive of inducible urticaria, standardized provocation testing according to international consensus recommendations [3] should be performed.
10. Acquired AIDs (autoinflammatory syndromes) include Schnitzler's syndrome as well as systemic-onset juvenile idiopathic arthritis (sJIA) and adult-onset Still's disease (AOSD); hereditary AIDs include cryopyrin-associated periodic syndromes (CAPS) such as familial cold autoinflammatory syndromes (FCAS), Muckle-Wells syndrome (MWS), and neonatal-onset multisystem inflammatory disease (NOMID), more rarely hyper-IgD syndrome (HIDS) and tumor necrosis factor receptor alpha-associated periodic syndrome (TRAPS).
11. In some rare cases, recurrent angioedema is neither mast cell mediator mediated nor bradykinin mediated, and the underlying pathomechanisms remain unknown. These rare cases are referred to as "idiopathic angioedema" by some authors.

The guidelines also provide a list of questions which should be discussed with the patient to understand possible courses [1]:

1.	Time of onset of disease
2.	Frequency/duration of and provoking factors for wheals
3.	Diurnal variation
4.	Occurrence in relation to weekends, holidays, and foreign travel
5.	Shape, size, and distribution of wheals
6.	Associated angioedema
7.	Associated subjective symptoms of lesions, e.g., itch and pain
8.	Family and personal history regarding urticaria and atopy
9.	Previous or current allergies, infections, internal diseases, or other possible causes
10.	Psychosomatic and psychiatric diseases
11.	Surgical implantations and events during surgery, e.g., after local anesthesia
12.	Gastric/intestinal problems
13.	Induction by physical agents or exercise
14.	Use of drugs (e.g., NSAIDs, injections, immunizations, hormones, laxatives, suppositories, ear and eye drops, and alternative remedies)
15.	Observed correlation to food
16.	Relationship to the menstrual cycle
17.	Smoking habits (esp. use of perfumed tobacco products or cannabis)
18.	Type of work
19.	Hobbies
20.	Stress (eustress and distress)
21.	Quality of life related to urticaria and emotional impact
22.	Previous therapy and response to therapy
23.	Previous diagnostic procedures/results

For the interested physician, it is useful to adapt and possibly extend these questions to a questionnaire which can then be handed out to the patient still in the waiting room. This allows a very quick overview of patient history and also allows the patient a time for reflection saving on the other hand time in the doctor's office. For our urticaria clinic, we have extended the questionnaire to "100 questions on your urticaria." The full questionnaire in English language can be found on the web page www.ecarf.org. In my own experience, taking a very thorough history based on this questionnaire in approximately 20 % of patients with chronic spontaneous urticaria, hidden courses can be detected. Some of them may even be worth to be published such as the use of aspirin as a preservative [4] which I have now discovered is also sometimes used in restaurants especially in Brazil, where salad is sprayed with an aspirin solution to prevent oxidation.

Another aspect which is frequently overlooked but can be discovered by the right questions is subtle underlying inflammatory processes. More severe diseases are certainly noticed by patients, but chronic inflammatory processes, e.g., chronic sinusitis, gastritis, or an inflammation of the bile duct, are often regarded as less noteworthy by patients. However they may be an important causative factor in urticaria. In this instance it is also important to mention that not only the infectious agent, e.g., *Helicobacter pylori*, themselves can be a trigger but also noninfectious inflammatory processes. This is well established for *Helicobacter pylori*-negative gastritis, and in my own experience, several patients recorded that the severity of urticaria symptoms correlates well with lifestyle factors which is having an impact on the severity of their gastritis as smoking or emotional distress.

While in chronic spontaneous urticaria, taking a history may reveal the triggering factor and allow a causal treatment, in inducible urticarias, in most instances the disease itself has to be regarded as idiopathic, and it is not helpful to go into an extensive diagnostic program. However also in these instances, a thorough history will help to better understand the situation of a patient and allow a better conception about the avoidance of triggering factors. Thus many patients, e.g., in pressure urticaria, have not really understood the correlation that pressure is defined by force per area and simple measurements like changing shoes and using cushioned soles or gloves may have a high impact. The same holds true for other subtypes of inducible urticarias, e.g., light urticaria, where consultation about the UV protection factor of clothes, the better understanding of their recreational habits, and the consultation about the proper use of sunscreens adapted to the wavelength which triggers the wheals is extremely helpful for patients. To offer a most perfect personalized treatment in the inducible physical urticaria subtypes, it is in general extremely important that the doctor pictures the daily life and also the working environment of the patients and knows the available items which can possibly give support, e.g., UV light protection screens for windows or specially worked tools causing less friction when being handled.

The guidelines propose a very clear and strict algorithm in treatment which is sufficient for the vast majority of patients, and a personalized approach is limited to those few patients needing other forms of treatment but should also take into account when using the standard algorithm which of the treatments supposed are fitting best for the individual requirements (Fig. 8.2). However, in this aspect, it also has to be noted that the treatment mentioned in the algorithm is not in all cases licensed, and certainly the alternative treatments are off-label. In fact until recently, only antihistamines had been licensed for all kinds for urticaria, and only in March 2014, omalizumab has been licensed by the EMA and FDA for chronic spontaneous urticaria.

Regarding the very strong recommendation against the use of first-generation sedating antihistamines in the guidelines as shown in Fig. 8.3, it must be noted that in a personalized approach, the guideline of course leaves room for the individual patient to be treated with these drugs. However, the reason why also some patients do like first-generation antihistamines at night is the obligatory sedating effect which helps patients to fall asleep despite of the itch and is sometimes also considered as slightly anxiolytic in the more anxious patient. Thus in a case where a patient already has been treated with sedating antihistamines and feels dependent on them, it may be warranted to continue this for a short period of a few days and at the same time treat them with a quadruple dose of nonsedating modern antihistamines and suggest a withdrawal of the sedating antihistamine after complete symptom control.

The next step in the algorithm is clearly to up-dose modern nonsedating antihistamines up to fourfold (see Fig. 8.1).

An individual choice here needs to be made about which of the currently available

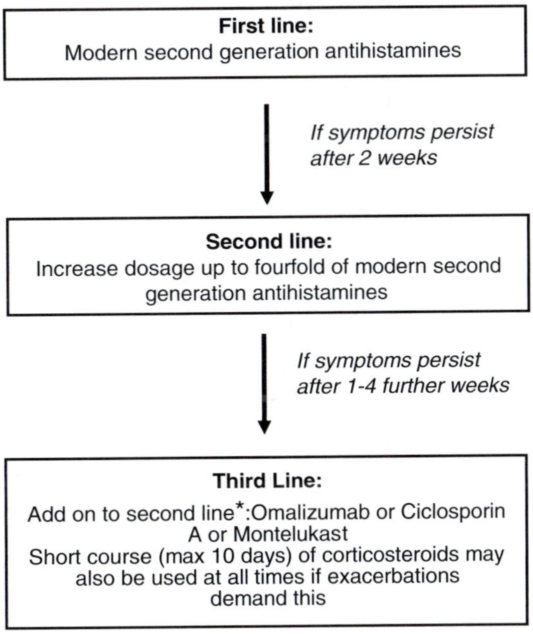

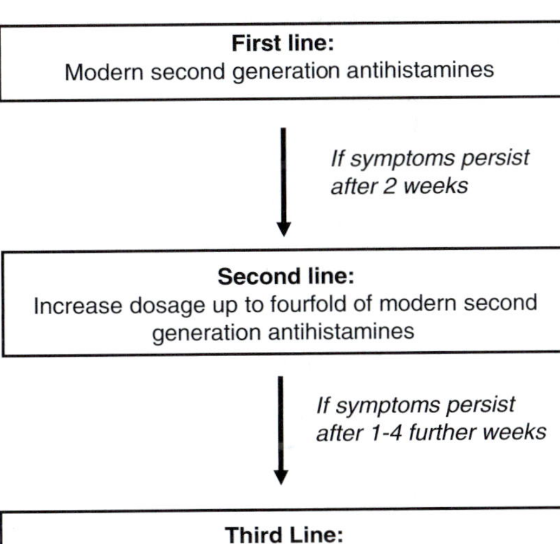

Fig. 8.2 Recommended treatment algorithm for urticaria [1]

Are modern second generation H1-antihistamines to be preferred over first generation H1-antihistamines in treatment of urticaria?

Summary:
We recommend that modern second generation H1-antihistamines are to be preferred over first generation H1-antihistamines in the treatment of urticaria (strong recommendation/high level of evidence)

Consented by voting
Voting result: 95 % of audience and the panel members agreed.

Fig. 8.3 Recommendation and voting results [5]

second-generation antihistamines should be used. As there are no head-to-head trials except in one case comparing desloratadine and levocetirizine in a higher dosage, the practical approach is to start with the antihistamine which has been used as single dose. If the up-dosing in this case does not show sufficient response, it can be discussed with the patient if, in conformity with the guidelines, the third step in the algorithm should be made or if a possible switch to another antihistamine may be useful. This latter approach had been recommended in the previous guidelines but due to the lack of evidence was omitted in the current version.

However there are some points which are in favor of this approach as scientifically the second-generation antihistamines differ from the first-generation antihistamines in the aspect that they also inhibit the release of pro-inflammatory mast cell mediators other than histamine. This property may be different comparing the different compounds available but has not been studied in extension. Some patients however clearly report that they have a better response to one or the other antihistamine without a clear tendency which one to prefer.

In addition, switching the antihistamine at a higher dosage has also the advantage of gaining more time to discuss the possibilities of third-line treatment with the patient and, in case of choosing one of the non-licensed medications, allows for the time to file an application with the insurance companies which are required in many countries of the world.

However very important is to mention to the patient that the high-dose antihistamine treatment in fact is also off-label although regarded by insurance companies and general medical practice as one of the most frequent treatment strategies which is also known from other areas of medicine like using painkillers, blood pressure tablets, or others. Thus the principle is easy to explain to the patient, and in the majority of countries, no filing for regulatory authorities is required in this case, especially as the treatment itself is comparatively cheap with the availability of generic second-generation drugs at costs as low as 0.10€ per tablet.

8.5 Further Therapeutic Possibilities for Antihistamine-Refractory Patients

With the licensing of omalizumab for chronic spontaneous urticaria, it is clear that this is the drug of choice to stay in label treatment in the first instance but also the level of evidence is clearly the best for this drug with a very low adverse event profile.

8.6 An Individualized Approach in Therapy-Refractory Patients

In those patients where neither up-dosing nor the combination treatment of high-dose antihistamines with omalizumab has been successful or sufficiently successful, clearly an alternative strategy is needed. In the guideline itself, some drugs are mentioned as a very short comment:

> For H_2-antagonists and dapsone, still recommended in the previous version of the guideline, the evidence is too low to maintain this as recommendable in the algorithm, but they may still have relevance as they are very affordable in some poorer health care systems. For sulfasalazine, methotrexate, interferon, plasmapheresis, phototherapy, and intravenous immunoglobulins (IVIG), only trials of low-quality or case series have been published [6] (Table 5).
>
> Antagonists of tumor necrosis factor a (TNF-alpha) [7] and IVIG [8–11], which have been successfully used in case reports, are recommended currently only to be used in specialized centers as a last option (i.e., anti-TNF-alpha for delayed pressure urticaria and IVIG for chronic spontaneous urticaria) [1].

Regarding these drugs mentioned above in the guideline, it is worthwhile mentioning that although not based on high-quality evidence, there are in my own practice still a considerable number of patients who do profit from the additional treatment of H2 antagonist or dapsone, although these are different types of patients.

H2 antagonists are clearly not evidence based, but in my own experience, they are worthwhile to try in those patients who mention any, even if slight, symptoms of gastritis. In this case they appear to be better than the use of proton inhibitors like omeprazole, possibly because they both act on the gastric inflammation and on the stimulation of H2 receptors in the stomach and intestine. However, this is purely a personal recommendation and surely needs further research. The same holds true for dapsone.

While in the guideline there is a statement that the current evidence does neither allow to vote for nor against dapsone as some trials do exist, but the quality of these trials is not sufficient although the outcome of these trials is convincing. In my own practice, I do use dapsone especially in those patients with long-standing wheals which are at the edge of turning over into urticaria vasculitis. On histopathology, often in these patients, an increased leukocytic infiltrate is observed in a perivascular pattern. Again based on old literature, I tend to combine dapsone in these patients with pentoxifylline which has a mild anti-TNFα activity and has been recommended in the past as a combination treatment for patients with an urticaria vasculitis.

Another avenue of possible alternative treatments becomes more and more interesting. Based on recent findings, apparently in some subgroups of patients with chronic spontaneous urticaria, elevated D-dimers have been found [12].

Already in the past, case reports on the effect of treatment with anticoagulants as heparin or warfarin had been published [13]. In my own experience, I have tried both heparin and warfarin and still use this as an alternative possibility in refractory patients due to the mode of handling as oral therapy. I prescribe warfarin at a level to achieve a reduction of the prothrombin time to 50 %.

8.7 Treatment of Children and Pregnant and Lactating Women

Clearly the treatment of children and especially pregnant and lactating women is always a challenge to the treating physician. Especially in pregnancy, there is no hard evidence based on trials, and circumstantial evidence on the safety of possible therapeutic approaches needs to be taken into consideration. This always involves a very open discussion with the pregnant woman and thorough information; many countries prefer a written informed consent. Similar aspects hold true in children and in the lactating women. However, in urticaria luckily the standard treatments are comparatively safe to be used, and at least during times of pregnancy, it is also important to inform the frequently anxious patient that not treating the disease may also have an impact as consistently high levels of histamine flood the bloodstream and it is unknown which effects this may have on the unborn child. Regarding the therapeutic approach in these special populations, it can clearly be recommended to follow strictly only the guideline-recommended procedures which are quoted here:

The same considerations in principle apply to pregnant and lactating women. On one hand, use of any systemic treatment should generally be avoided in pregnant women, especially in the first trimester. On the other hand, pregnant women have the right to best possible therapy. While the safety of treatment has not been systematically studied in pregnant women with urticaria, it should be pointed out that the possible negative effects of increased levels of histamine occurring in urticaria have also not been studied in pregnancy. Regarding treatment, no reports of birth defects in women having used modern second generation antihistamines during pregnancy have been reported to date. However, only small sample size studies are available for cetirizine [14] and one large meta-analysis for loratadine [15]. Furthermore, as several modern second generation antihistamines are now prescription free and used widely in both allergic rhinitis and urticaria, it must be assumed that many women have used these drugs especially in the beginning of pregnancy, at least before the pregnancy was confirmed. Nevertheless, since the highest safety is mandatory in pregnancy, the suggestion for the use of modern second generation antihistamines is to prefer loratadine with the possible extrapolation to desloratadine and cetirizine with a possible extrapolation to levocetirizine. All H1-antihistamines are excreted in breast milk in low concentrations. Use of second-generation H1-antihistamines is advised, as nursing infants occasionally develop sedation from the old first-generation H1-antihistamines transmitted in breast milk.

The increased dosage of modern second generation antihistamines can only be carefully suggested in pregnancy since safety studies have not been done, and with loratadine it must be remembered that this drug is metabolized in the liver. First generation agents may be cautiously employed when symptoms dictate in the face of nonresponse to modern second generation antihistamines. Use of first-generation H1-antihistamines immediately before parturition may cause respiratory depression and other adverse effects in the neonate (the first-generation H1-antihistamines with the best safety track record in pregnancy are chlorpheniramine and diphenhydramine). All further steps should be based on individual considerations, with a preference for medications that have a satisfactory risk-to-benefit ratio in pregnant women and neonates with regard to teratogenicity and embryo toxicity. For example, cyclosporine, although not teratogenic, is embryo-toxic in animal models and is associated with preterm delivery and low birth weight in human infants (the median gestation duration of infants born to mothers taking cyclosporine is 35.7 weeks, and the median birth weight of their infants is 2.2 kilograms). Whether the benefits of cyclosporine in chronic urticaria are worth the risks in pregnant women will have to be determined on a case-by-case basis. However, all decisions should be reevaluated according to the current recommendations published by regulatory authorities. [1]

8.8 What Else Can Be Offered (and at Low Cost): The Value of Diets

Especially in chronic spontaneous urticaria (as well as in acute urticaria), many patients suspect food items to be responsible or partly responsible for their symptoms. The guideline gives clear advice to dietary management but comments on who is eligible in a personalized approach are clearly required:

> Dietary management. IgE-mediated food allergy is rarely the underlying cause of chronic spontaneous urticaria [16, 17]. If identified, the specific food allergens need to be omitted as far as possible. In a subgroup of chronic spontaneous urticaria patients, pseudoallergic reactions (non-IgE-mediated hypersensitivity reactions) to naturally occurring food ingredients and in some cases to food additives have been observed [16–20]. Since the last version of the guidelines, the proposed pseudoallergen free diet has now also been successfully tested in different countries [21].
>
> Similar to drugs, pseudoallergens can both elicit and aggravate chronic spontaneous urticaria

[22]. In these cases, a diet containing only low levels of natural as well as artificial food pseudoallergens should be instituted and maintained for a prolonged period, at least 3–6 months. It should be underlined that avoidance of type I-allergens clears urticaria symptoms within 24–48 h if the relevant allergens are eliminated rapidly, whereas in pseudoallergy, a diet must often be maintained for a minimum of 3 weeks before beneficial effects are observed. Detailed information about dietary control can be found in the referenced manuscripts. However, it should be pointed out that success rates may vary considerably due to regional differences in food and dietary habits. More research is necessary on the effect of foodstuffs in causing urticaria, particularly in areas where the daily diet is greatly different from the one in Western Europe. [1]

Especially this passage of the guideline has been a matter of debate, and there are strong differences in opinion and in the frequency of dietary approaches used between Europe and the United States.

Much of the misunderstanding is based on the fact that previously especially in publications from the United States pseudoallergy was dismissed if provocation tests with frequent food additives were negative. However it is clear that not only food additives but much more frequently naturally occurring ingredients in food like aromatic compounds [23] can be eliciting factors. Pseudoallergic reactions are especially frequently observed in patients who also have a pseudoallergic reaction to aspirin in their history (more than 35 % of patients with chronic spontaneous urticaria). In addition, in my own experience, it is valuable to offer patients the possibility to use an exploratory diagnostic diet for 3 weeks. This gives the patient the feeling to be involved in the treatment, and independent of the outcome, it is helpful. In case the diet reduces the symptoms or leads to complete remission, the patient is clearly happy, and the next steps in expanding the diet can be quickly made. In case the diet does not reduce the severity of the disease again, the patient is happy as now for himself, it is clear that food is not responsible, and the dietary restrictions many patients with urticaria oppose on themselves (more than 60 % [2]) are not required.

The diet itself has now been used and tested in many different countries and appears to be

Table 8.1 Pseudoallergen-free diet [16]

	Allowed	Forbidden
Basic food	Preservative-free bread, potatoes, rice, unprocessed cereals, flour	All others (e.g., noodles, potato chips)
Fat	Butter, cold-pressed plant oils	All others (e.g., margarine)
Milk products	Fresh milk, cream, white cheese, young gouda	All others
Meat, fish, eggs	Fresh meat	All others, including seafood
Vegetables	All, except those listed as forbidden	Artichokes, peas, mushrooms, rhubarb, tomatoes, olives, sweet pepper
Fruits	None	All
Herbs, spices	Salt, sugar, chives	All others
Sweets	None except honey	All (including chewing gum)
Beverages	Milk, water, coffee, black tea	All others

Strictly forbidden: All foods containing preservatives, dyes, or antioxidants (all kinds of industrially processed food should be regarded with suspicion)

helpful to a similar extent all over the world. However it needs to be mentioned that the grade of success clearly depends on the selection of patients and the time the doctors spend on explaining the background of the diet.

Patients profiting the most from the diet are those with chronic spontaneous urticaria with daily occurrence of wheals. Explaining the diet without time-consuming appointments is most easily made by employing a validated list (Table 8.1).

But not only the list itself should be handed out it should be accompanied by explanatory material. It is important to point out that if the diet is employed, it needs to be employed strictly and that the effect of the diet is in most cases only noted after 10–14 days. This is similar to the effect of an aspirin tablet which keeps on making symptoms for up to 2 weeks after a single tablet. As many patients tend to make involuntary dietary mistakes, it is also recommended to ask the patients to keep a detailed diary of what has been eaten and match this with the symptom protocol using UAS. Still in our experience, it is also valuable, instead of just giving the patient the list of what to eat and what to avoid, to hand out clearly written recipes for breakfast, lunch, and dinner which ensures a sufficient supply with all nutrients and nutritional components and is simple enough for the patient to prepare himself or herself.

Conclusion

In summary, like in most areas of medicine, the real skill of a physician is to understand at what time the personalized approach and at what time a standardized approach is the best for the patient. To be able to fulfill this, it is required to train new observational skills and surely also to train the physicians' intuition, a skill which cannot be trained by reading books alone but will only come with practice. However, just listening with interest to the story a patient tells is already the first step to a personalized approach, as many patients especially with chronic diseases like urticaria are just missing this personal attention of a doctor.

References

1. Zuberbier T, Aberer W, Asero R, Bindslev-Jensen C, Brzoza Z, Canonica GW, et al. The EAACI/GA2LEN/EDF/WAO guideline for the definition, classification, diagnosis, and management of urticaria. The 2013 revision and update. Allergy. 2014;69(7):868–87.
2. Baiardini I, Pasquali M, Braido F, Fumagalli F, Guerra L, Compalati E, et al. A new tool to evaluate the impact of chronic urticaria on quality of life: chronic urticaria quality of life questionnaire (CU-QoL). Allergy. 2005;60(8):1073–8.
3. Magerl M, Borzova E, Gimenez-Arnau A, Grattan CE, Lawlor F, Mathelier-Fusade P, et al. The definition and diagnostic testing of physical and cholinergic urticarias–EAACI/GA2LEN/EDF/UNEV consensus panel recommendations. Allergy. 2009;64(12): 1715–21.

4. Kurbacheva O, Zuberbier T. A visit to the mother in law–a hidden cause for urticaria. Allergy. 2007;62(6): 711–2.

5. Zuberbier T, Aberer W, Asero R, Bindslev Jensen C, Brzoza Z, Canonica G, et al. Methods report on the development of the 2013 revision and update of the EAACI/GA²LEN/EDF/WAO guideline for the definition, classification, diagnosis, and management of urticaria. Allergy. 2014;69:868–87.

6. Zuberbier T, Asero R, Bindslev-Jensen C, Walter Canonica G, Church MK, Gimenez-Arnau AM, et al. EAACI/GA(2)LEN/EDF/WAO guideline: management of urticaria. Allergy. 2009;64(10):1427–43.

7. Magerl M, Philipp S, Manasterski M, Friedrich M, Maurer M. Successful treatment of delayed pressure urticaria with anti-TNF-alpha. J Allergy Clin Immunol. 2007;119(3):752–4.

8. O'Donnell BF, Barr RM, Black AK, Francis DM, Kermani F, Niimi N, et al. Intravenous immunoglobulin in autoimmune chronic urticaria. Br J Dermatol. 1998;138(1):101–6.

9. Dawn G, Urcelay M, Ah-Weng A, O'Neill SM, Douglas WS. Effect of high-dose intravenous immunoglobulin in delayed pressure urticaria. Br J Dermatol. 2003;149(4):836–40.

10. Pereira C, Tavares B, Carrapatoso I, Loureiro G, Faria E, Machado D, et al. Low-dose intravenous gammaglobulin in the treatment of severe autoimmune urticaria. Eur Ann Allergy Clin Immunol. 2007;39(7):237–42.

11. Mitzel-Kaoukhov H, Staubach P, Muller-Brenne T. Effect of high-dose intravenous immunoglobulin treatment in therapy-resistant chronic spontaneous urticaria. Ann Allergy Asthma Immunol. 2010;104(3):253–8.

12. Asero R, Tedeschi A, Cugno M. Heparin and tranexamic Acid therapy may be effective in treatment-resistant chronic urticaria with elevated d-dimer: a pilot study. Int Arch Allergy Immunol. 2010;152(4): 384–9.

13. Zuberbier T, Bindslev-Jensen C, Canonica W, Grattan CE, Greaves MW, Henz BM, et al. EAACI/GA2LEN /EDF guideline: management of urticaria. Allergy. 2006;61(3):321–31.

14. Weber-Schoendorfer C, Schaefer C. The safety of cetirizine during pregnancy. A prospective observational cohort study. Reprod Toxicol. 2008;26(1):19–23.

15. Schwarz EB, Moretti ME, Nayak S, Koren G. Risk of hypospadias in offspring of women using loratadine during pregnancy: a systematic review and meta-analysis. Drug Saf. 2008;31(9):775–88.

16. Zuberbier T, Chantraine-Hess S, Hartmann K, Czarnetzki BM. Pseudoallergen-free diet in the treatment of chronic urticaria. A prospective study. Acta Derm Venereol. 1995;75(6):484–7.

17. Juhlin L. Recurrent urticaria: clinical investigation of 330 patients. Br J Dermatol. 1981;104(4):369–81.

18. Pfrommer C, Bastl R, Vieths S, Ehlers I, Henz BM, Zuberbier T. Characterization of naturally occurring pseudoallergens causing chronic urticaria. J Allergy Clin Immunol. 1996;97(1), part 3, p.367.

19. Pigatto PD, Valsecchi RH. Chronic urticaria: a mystery. Allergy. 2000;55(3):306–8.

20. Bunselmeyer B, Laubach HJ, Schiller M, Stanke M, Luger TA, Brehler R. Incremental build-up food challenge–a new diagnostic approach to evaluate pseudoallergic reactions in chronic urticaria: a pilot study: stepwise food challenge in chronic urticaria. Clin Exp Allergy. 2009;39(1):116–26.

21. Akoglu G, Atakan N, Cakir B, Kalayci O, Hayran M. Effects of low pseudoallergen diet on urticarial activity and leukotriene levels in chronic urticaria. Arch Dermatol Res. 2012;304(4):257–62.

22. Nettis E, Colanardi MC, Ferrannini A, Tursi A. Sodium benzoate-induced repeated episodes of acute urticaria/angio-oedema: randomized controlled trial. Br J Dermatol. 2004;151(4):898–902.

23. Zuberbier T, Pfrommer C, Specht K, Vieths S, Bastl-Borrmann R, Worm M, et al. Aromatic components of food as novel eliciting factors of pseudoallergic reactions in chronic urticaria. J Allergy Clin Immunol. 2002;109(2):343–8.

Acknowledging the Clinical Heterogeneity of Lupus Erythematosus

Joerg Wenzel

Contents

J. Wenzel, MD
Department of Dermatology, University Clinic Bonn,
Bonn 53105, Germany
e-mail: joerg.wenzel@ukb.uni-bonn.de

9.1 Lupus Erythematosus: Definition and Classification

The diagnosis "lupus erythematosus" (LE) encompasses a group of mostly photosensitive autoimmune diseases. The central common attribute of these diseases is the detection of circulating autoantibodies, which are directed against specific nuclear structures such as nucleic acids or nucleoproteins. LE patients may present with a broad spectrum of clinical signs, ranging from localized skin lesions to severe systemic disease with affection of internal organ systems. Generally, systemic (= systemic LE/SLE) and cutaneous (= cutaneous LE/CLE) courses of LE are distinguished, but overlapping cases are common. Cutaneous lesions occur in about two thirds of patients with SLE. They can develop at any stage of the disease, irrespective of disease activity, and represent the first sign in about 25 % of SLE patients [1].

The SLE criteria of the American College of Rheumatology (ACR) have been the most widely used criteria to classify SLE in individual patients. The 11 ACR criteria ((1) malar rash, (2) discoid rash, (3) photosensitivity, (4) oral ulcers, (5) nonerosive arthritis, (6) pleuritis or pericarditis, (7) renal disorder, (8) neurologic disorder, (9) hematologic disorder, (10) immunologic disorder, and (11) positive antinuclear antibody) provide an insight into the clinical heterogeneity of LE and can be helpful in distinguishing SLE from rheumatoid arthritis and other connective tissue diseases [2]. However,

T. Bieber, F. Nestle (eds.), *Personalized Treatment Options in Dermatology*,
DOI 10.1007/978-3-662-45840-2_9, © Springer-Verlag Berlin Heidelberg 2015

Table 9.1 Classification of SLE: clinical and immunologic criteria used in the SLICC classification

Clinical criteria	1. Acute cutaneous lupus	Including lupus malar rash (do not count if malar discoid)
		Bullous lupus
		Toxic epidermal necrolysis variant of SLE
		Maculopapular lupus rash
		Photosensitive lupus rash in the absence of dermatomyositis
		Or subacute cutaneous lupus
		Nonindurated psoriasiform and/or annular polycyclic lesions that resolve without scarring, although occasionally with postinflammatory dyspigmentation or telangiectasias
	2. Chronic cutaneous lupus	Including classical discoid rash
		Localized (above the neck)
		Generalized (above and below the neck)
		Hypertrophic (verrucous) lupus
		Lupus panniculitis (profundus)
		Mucosal lupus
		Lupus erythematosus tumidus
		Chilblain lupus
		Discoid lupus/lichen planus overlap
	3. Oral ulcers	Palate, buccal, tongue, or nasal ulcers
		In the absence of other causes such as vasculitis, Behcet's disease, infection (herpes), inflammatory bowel disease, reactive arthritis, and acidic foods
	4. Nonscarring alopecia	(Diffused thinning or hair fragility with visible broken hairs)
		In the absence of other causes such as alopecia areata, drugs, iron deficiency, and androgenic alopecia
	5. Synovitis	Involving two or more joints, characterized by swelling or effusion or tenderness in two or more joints and 30 min or more of morning stiffness
	6. Serositis	Typical pleurisy for more than 1 day
		Or pleural effusions
		Or pleural rub
		Typical pericardial pain (pain with recumbency improved by sitting forward) for more than 1 day
		Or pericardial effusion
		Or pericardial rub
		Or pericarditis by EKG
		In the absence of other causes, such as infection, uremia, and Dressler's pericarditis
	7. Renal	Urine protein/creatinine (or 24 h urine protein) representing 500 mg of protein/24 h
		Or
		Red blood cell casts
	8. Neurologic	Seizures, psychosis mononeuritis multiplex
		In the absence of other known causes such as primary vasculitis
		Myelitis, peripheral or cranial neuropathy
		In the absence of other known causes such as primary vasculitis, infection, and diabetes mellitus
		Acute confusional state
		In the absence of other causes, including toxic-metabolic, uremia, drugs

Table 9.1 (continued)

	9. Hemolytic anemia	
	10. Leukopenia or lymphopenia	Leukopenia ($<$4,000/mm^3 at least once)
		In the absence of other known causes such as Felty's syndrome, drugs, and portal hypertension
		Or
		Lymphopenia ($<$1,000/mm^3 at least once) in the absence of other known causes such as corticosteroids, drugs, and infection
	11. Thrombocytopenia	($<$100,000/mm^3) at least once
		In the absence of other known causes such as drugs, portal hypertension, and TTP
Immunological criteria	1. ANA	Positive, above laboratory reference range
	2. Anti-dsDNA	Positive, above laboratory reference range, except ELISA: twice above laboratory
		Reference range
	3. Anti-Sm	Positive
	4. Antiphospholipid antibody	Any of the following lupus anticoagulant:
		False-positive RPR
		Medium- or high-titer anticardiolipin (IgA, IgG, or IgM)
		Anti-β2 glycoprotein I (IgA, IgG or IgM)
	5. Low complement	Low C3
		Low C4
		Low CH50
	6. Direct Coombs test	Positive, in the absence of hemolytic anemia

Modified from Petri et al. [4]

Classify a patient as having SLE if the patient satisfies four of the criteria listed in the table, including at least one clinical criterion and one immunologic criterion, or the patient has a biopsy-proven nephritis compatible with SLE and with ANA or anti-dsDNA antibodies

the relatively high number of dermatological criteria (malar rash, discoid lesions, photosensitivity, and oral ulcers) diminishes their potential to distinguish SLE from CLE. Parodi et al. who investigated classification systems of SLE in CLE patients concluded that the ACR (formerly: ARA) criteria "should not be used in CLE patients as they are too sensitive, poorly specific and altogether misleading" [3]. These problems stimulated the revision of the ACR criteria by the Systemic Lupus International Collaborating Clinics (SLICC) group. The revised classification includes 17 criteria and allows a more detailed assessment of the clinical and immunological aspects (Table 9.1), but it will need time to prove their specificity and sensitivity in different conditions [4].

The Revised Cutaneous Lupus Erythematosus Disease Area and Severity Index (RCLASI) has specifically been developed to assess disease activity and damage in CLE. This disease activity index focuses on LE skin parameters, including scaling, hypertrophy, dyspigmentation, edema, infiltration, and subcutaneous nodules [1].

9.2 The Spectrum of Cutaneous LE

As indicated above, the spectrum of skin lesions which may appear in the context of LE is wide. To make a complex topic even more complicated, these LE-associated skin lesions are distinguished in two major groups: "LE-specific" and "LE-nonspecific" lesions. The LE-specific lesions encompass all the specific dermatological subsets of LE and are clinically subdivided into four different subtypes (acute LE/ACLE, subacute cutaneous LE/SCLE, intermediate cutaneous LE/ICLE, and chronic cutaneous CLE). Typical clinical examples for these CLE subsets are depicted in Fig. 9.1. Skin lesions typically associated with autoimmune diseases albeit not

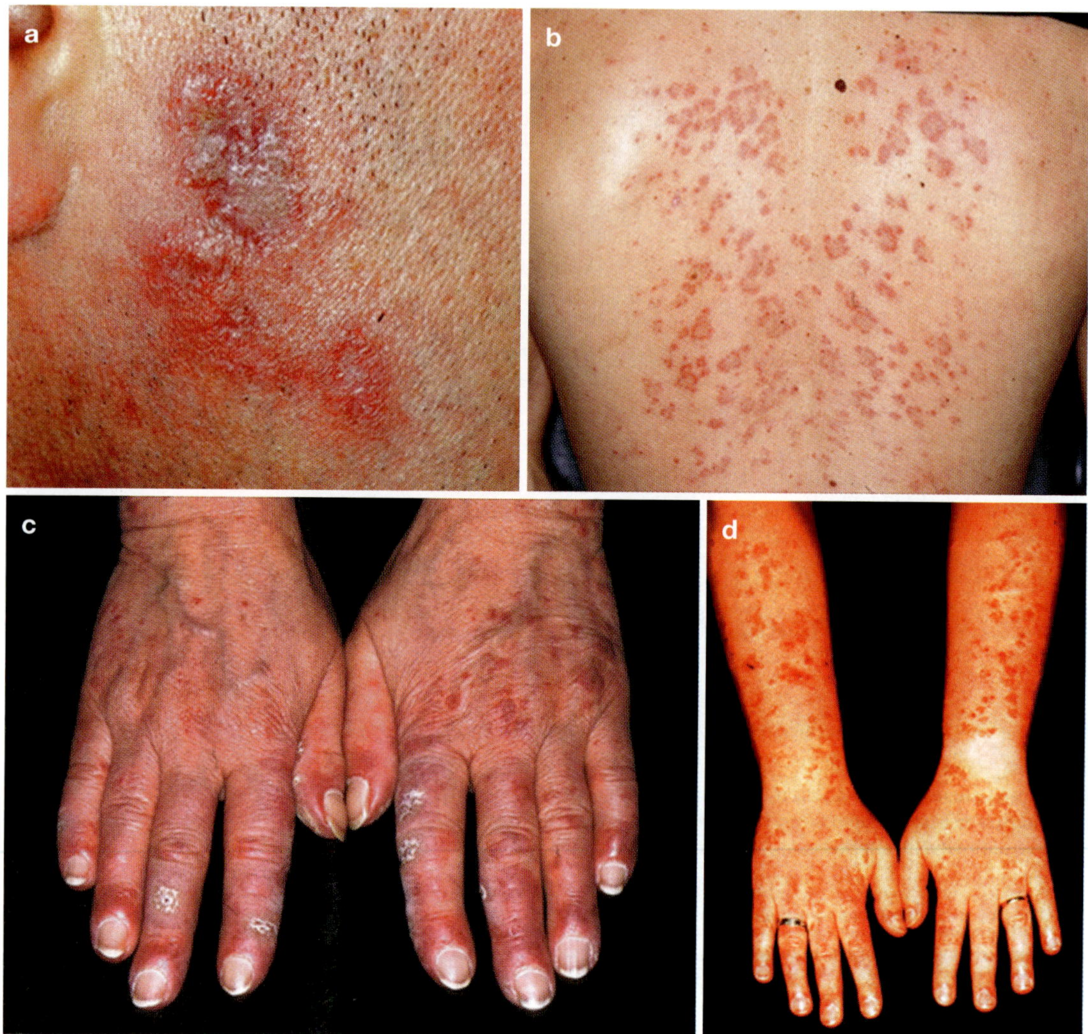

Fig. 9.1 The clinical heterogeneity of cutaneous lupus erythematosus skin lesions. Chronic discoid LE: (**a**) discoid erythrosquamous plaques in the face; (**b**) subacute cutaneous LE: annular maculae at the back; (**c**) chilblain LE: erythematous maculae and nodules of the hands; (**d**) bullous LE (vesicles and small bullae in sun-exposed skin)

LE-specific are, amongst others, vasculitis, livedo racemosa, calcinosis cutis, and skin ulcers [1].

As detailed in Table 9.2, two complementary strategies can be used to classify the different specific subsets of CLE: (1) a clinical classification, focusing on the different dynamics of the CLE subsets, and (2) a histological classification, which is based on the typical histological picture and the anatomical structures involved. The typical clinical and histological findings of the most common CLE subtypes are summarized in Table 9.3.

9.2.1 Acute CLE (ACLE)

Acute courses of CLE clinically present with plane redness in sun-exposed skin areas, particularly in the face, décolleté, and extensor sides of the arms. The most characteristic clinical sign is the butterfly rash, a symmetric, circumscribed, aliform erythema on both cheeks. This CLE subset shows a close association to SLE in younger female patients and may be accompanied by fever, myalgia, fatigue, and involvement of internal organ systems. In the peripheral blood,

Table 9.2 Clinical and histological classification of CLE

Clinical classification of CLE modified from Kuhn and Landmann [1]	
CLE	
Acute CLE (ACLE)	Localized form
	Generalized form
	Bullous LE
Subacute CLE (SCLE)	Annular form
	Papulosquamous form
Intermediate CLE (ICLE)	Lupus erythematosus tumidus (LET)
Chronic CLE (CCLE)	Discoid lupus erythematosus (DLE)
	Localized form
	Disseminated form
	Lupus erythematosus profundus (LEP; LE panniculitis)
	Chilblain lupus erythematosus (CHLE)
Histological classification of CLE:	
Histological pattern	**LE subtype**
Dermoepidermal LE	Acute LE
	Subacute LE
	Chronic discoid LE
	Bullous LE
	Chilblain LE
Dermal LE	LE tumidus
	Jessner's lymphocytic infiltration (JLI)
	Reticular erythematous mucinosis (REM)
	Papular mucinosis
Hypodermal LE	LE panniculitis (LE profundus)

often high-titer antinuclear antibodies with SLE-typical specificity (e.g., anti-dsDNA, anti-Sm) are detectable. In contrast to the impressive clinical picture, the histological changes may be discrete. The slides show a mild edema with only minor mucin deposits. However, some neutrophils may accompany the dermal and junctional inflammatory infiltrate. These are rarely found in other CLE subsets and may be indicative for ACLE [5].

9.2.2 Bullous CLE (BLE)

The BLE is a very rare subset of ACLE which presents clinically with confluating small vesicles on erythematous skin in sun-exposed skin areas. Circulating anti-collagen VII antibodies, which target structures in the basement membrane, are typically found in the peripheral blood of the patients affected. Histologically, skin lesions show a subepidermal blister (effect of the anti-collagen VII antibodies) and a neutrophil-rich inflammatory infiltrate (close association to ACLE/SLE).

9.2.3 Subacute Cutaneous LE (SCLE)

The SCLE presents clinically with widespread annular, gyrated, and/or plaque-like erythrosquamous lesions in sun-exposed skin areas including décolleté and extensor sides of the arms, while the face typically is not involved. The majority of SCLE patients are ANA-positive. Among the ANA, anti-SSA/Ro and anti-SSB/La antibodies are the most characteristic antibodies for this CLE subset. These antibodies not only are important diagnostic markers but also have a functional impact, since newborn babies of anti-SSA/Ro-positive mothers have an increased risk to develop SCLE-like skin lesions which diminish with the decline of the maternal postpartal immunoglobulin protection. From a histological point of view, SCLE shows a cell-poor interface dermatitis with vacuolar degeneration of the basal epidermal layer, colloid bodies, immigration of skin-homing lymphocytes, and dermal mucin deposits [6, 7].

9.2.4 LE Tumidus (LET)

LET clinically presents with infiltrated erythematous maculae and plaques without epidermal scaling which primarily appear in sun-exposed skin areas including the face. LET shows a dynamic which is between subacute CLE and chronic CLE and therefore was classified as "intermediate CLE type" in the Düsseldorf classification of CLE [1]. Histologically, the lesions are characterized by an extensive dermal spot-like perivascular and perifollicular inflammatory lymphoid infiltrate without any epidermal component. This inflammation is dominated by CD123-positive

Table 9.3 Clinical and histological findings of the most common CLE subtypes

	Clinical	Histological
Acute CLE (ACLE)	Butterfly rash	Edema and only mild lesional inflammation with a cell-poor interface dermatitis
	Erythema in sun-exposed skin	Neutrophils within the infiltrate
	Close association to SLE	
	ANA >90 % positive	
	Anti-dsDNA, anti-RNP, and anti-Sm often positive	
Subacute cutaneous LE (SCLE)	Annular, gyrated, or plaque-like erythrosquamous lesions in sun-exposed skin, but not the face	Cell-poor IFD with superficial lymphoid infiltrate
	ANA 60–80 % positive	Atrophic epidermal layer
	Anti-SSA/Ro and anti-SSB/La often positive	Mucin deposits in upper dermis
LE tumidus (LET)	Erythematous, pad-like, infiltrated lesions in sun-exposed skin (including the face)	Dense, patch-like, perivascular, and perifollicular lymphoid infiltrate (superficial and deep)
	No scaling	Large amounts of mucin within the dermal layer
	ANA 10–30 % positive	Clusters of CD123-positive pDCs
	Anti-SSA/Ro and anti-SSB/La negative	
Chronic discoid LE (CDLE)	Scarring, discoid, and erythrosquamous lesions	Dense, patch-like, perivascular, and perifollicular lymphoid infiltrate (superficial and deep)
	Predilection sites: capillitium and face	Cell-rich IFD, involvement of the follicular epithelium and follicular hyperkeratosis
	Positive tin-tack sign	Broadened basement membrane
	ANA 10–30 % positive	Lots of mucin within the dermis
LE profundus (LEP)	Early: subcutaneous nodules and indurations	Early: lobular panniculitis with numerous lymphocytes and pDCs
	Late: fat-tissue atrophy and skin retraction	Late: necrosis, fibrosis, and macrophages
	Predilection sites: gluteal region, thigh, upper arms, and face	Mucin deposits in the subcutis
	ANA ~75 % positive	Polyclonal TCR rearrangement (DD: cytotoxic T-cell lymphoma)
Chilblain LE (ChLE)	Livid and painful with erythemata and indurations and nodules of fingers and toes	Dense, perivascular lymphoid infiltrates within the dermis
	Special subset: familial ChLE with mutation on TREX1 gene	Fibrin deposits within small dermal vessels
		Sometimes additional typical findings of other CLE subsets (IFD, mucin)
Bullous LE	Small vesicles on erythematous skin in sun-exposed skin areas	Subepidermal blisters with neutrophils
	Close association to SLE	Direct immunofluorescence: linear deposits of IgG, IgM, IgA, and C3
	Anti-collagen VII positive	

plasmacytoid dendritic cells, which form clusters of more than ten cells together. This inflammation is accompanied by strong dermal mucin deposits. Most of the patients are ANA-negative, and SLE-typical organ manifestations are uncommon in LET. Particularly, anti-SSA/Ro and SSB/La, which are frequently found in other photosensitive CLE subsets, are almost completely lacking [8, 9].

9.2.5 Chronic Discoid LE (CDLE)

The most common CLE subset is the chronic discoid LE (CDLE). It presents clinically with chronic, discoid, scarring, erythrosquamous plaques particularly affecting the capillitium and face. Most manifestations remain localized to one body region, but extensive courses with widespread scarring lesions appear in up to 10 % of the cases. In contrast to the extensive lesional skin damage, CDLE patients have only a minor risk to develop SLE, and the ANA titers are usually low. The most typical clinical sign of CDLE is the so-called tintack sign: a painful hyperkeratosis with follicular plugging due to the follicular hyperkeratosis of CDLE. Histologically, the lesions show a dense periadnexal and perivascular lymphoid inflammation, accompanied by a cell-rich interface dermatitis with a broadened basement membrane. Older lesions are characterized by fibrosis, due to the scarring character of this CLE subset [5].

9.2.6 LE Profundus (LEP)

In early stages, patients suffering from LEP show subcutaneous nodules and pad-like indurations of the dermis and subcutis. During the course of the disease, the patients develop lipoatrophy with retractions of the skin. The gluteal region is the predilection site of the disease, but the thighs, upper arms, and the face may also be involved. Histologically, LEP (also called "lupus panniculitis") shows a lobular panniculitis with several CD8-positive cytotoxic T cells, accompanied by CD123-positive plasmacytoid dendritic cells and lesional expression of type I IFN-regulated cytokines. CLE-typical changes may also be seen in the dermis (e.g., mucin depositions) and at the dermoepidermal junction (interface dermatitis) in individual cases [10–12].

9.2.7 Chilblain LE (ChLE)

The classical chilblain LE (also called "lupus pernio") clinically presents with livid red, pad-like swellings, and nodules of the distal acra, which show tenderness to palpation. Particularly, fingers and toes are involved. Histologically, these lesions show a dermal inflammation with dense lymphoid perivascular infiltrates and fibrin deposits within the vessels. Some patients present CLE-typical changes like interface dermatitis and ANA positivity in the peripheral blood. These cases are easy to distinguish from real chilblains, but in other cases, the discrimination between these two entities may be impossible [13].

During the last years, a specific subset of very rare patients got into the focus of the lupus-research community. These patients suffer from the only known familial form of LE. The disease clinically presents with chilblain-like lesions and is therefore called "familial ChLE." The familial ChLE is due to a nonfunction mutation in the TREX1 gene and closely associated to the Aicardi-Goutières syndrome. If TREX1 (a DNase) is defective, cytosolic nucleic acids are able to activate the innate immune system via its cytoplasmatic receptors. This causes a continuous activation of the type I IFN-system with following activation of IFN-regulated proinflammatory pathways. The resulting skin lesions are similar to classical ChLE lesions, but the familial ChLE is a systemic disease with a high risk of progression into SLE. About 3 % of all SLE patients carry a TREX1 mutation. Histologically, the skin lesions may also resemble the classical ChLE. However, they carry a higher number of neutrophils, especially at the dermoepidermal junction. Within the CLE spectrum, neutrophils are exclusively found in ACLE/SLE lesions and may therefore be regarded as a warning signal for the potential SLE-like course of the disease [14].

9.3 Pathophysiology of LE

9.3.1 Lupus Erythematosus: An Autoimmune Disease with Inappropriate Activation of the Adaptive Immune System

The first functional approaches to understand the pathophysiology of LE focused on the autoimmune phenomena which became evident during the second half of the last century. The classification of LE as an autoimmune disorder was confirmed by immunofluorescence investigations, which revealed the presence of autoantibodies targeting human self-proteins, particularly nuclear antigens, in the peripheral blood of LE patients [15]. Additionally, histological investigations of CLE skin specimens identified the presence of autoaggressive lymphocytes within skin lesions which attack basal structures of the epidermal layer and force keratinocytes into apoptosis. These findings supported the assumption that LE is an autoimmune disease characterized by an inappropriate activation of the humoral (autoantibodies) and cellular (T lymphocytes) adaptive immune system. This was the rationale for the first targeted treatment strategies in LE, particularly for the use of immunosuppressive antilymphocytic drugs [16].

9.3.2 Hyperactivation of Innate Immune Pathways in LE

In the 1990s, Lars Rönnblom and others observed the iatrogenic induction of SLE in patients with malignant carcinoid tumors after treatment with interferon-α [17]. This observation confirmed the hypothesis that inadequate activation not only of adaptive but also of innate pathways of the immune system might have a functional impact on the pathogenesis of LE. This was further corroborated by subsequent gene expression analyses, which revealed a type I IFN signature in the peripheral blood of patients with severe SLE [18, 19]. The type I IFN serum levels in SLE mediate the typical flu-like clinical symptoms of LE patients like fever and fatigue and are directly associated with SLE disease activity as measured by SLEDAI [20].

Type I IFNs are also of pathophysiological relevance in CLE. CLE skin lesion are characterized by a strong expression of IFN-regulated proinflammatory chemokines and CLE patients with widespread skin lesions demonstrate high levels of the type I/III IFN-regulated protein MxA in the peripheral blood [21, 22]. Again, direct evidence for the functional impact of type I IFNs

resulted from clinical observations: subcutaneous administration of recombinant type I IFNs was reported to be able to induce CLE-like skin lesions at the injection site [23].

9.3.3 The Proinflammatory Vicious Circle of LE

The exact pathomechanisms of LE are still a matter of intensive research. But over the last years, it has become evident that the interconnection of misled adaptive and innate immune mechanisms most probably drives the lesional inflammation into a proinflammatory vicious circle, which is responsible for disease progression. The most important factor in LE is that mechanisms of the adaptive immune system, such as autoantibodies and cytotoxic lymphocytes, may activate the innate immune system which in turn restimulates the adaptive response [24]. In SLE, this phenomenon affects, for example, the "natural-IFN-producing" plasmacytoid dendritic cells (pDCs), which are able to produce large amounts of IFN upon adequate stimulation. Here, immune complexes composed of autoantibodies (part of the adaptive immune system) and cell debris are able to stimulate the pDCs to produce type I IFNs via CD32 and stimulation of the endosomal toll-like receptors (TLR) [25]. PDCs are also involved in CLE skin inflammation and are a major source of IFN within the lesions [10]. However, keratinocytes are also a robust source of type III IFNs, and the interconnection of these two cell populations in the skin as well as the potential role of lymphocytes has not yet been solved. Figure 9.2 depicts the current state of knowledge of the proinflammatory vicious circle in LE and details potential functional targets for therapeutic interventions.

9.4 Genomics and Transcriptomics of LE

Monozygotic twins have a high concordance of SLE (about 24 %). This indicates a profound role of genetic factors in the development of LE

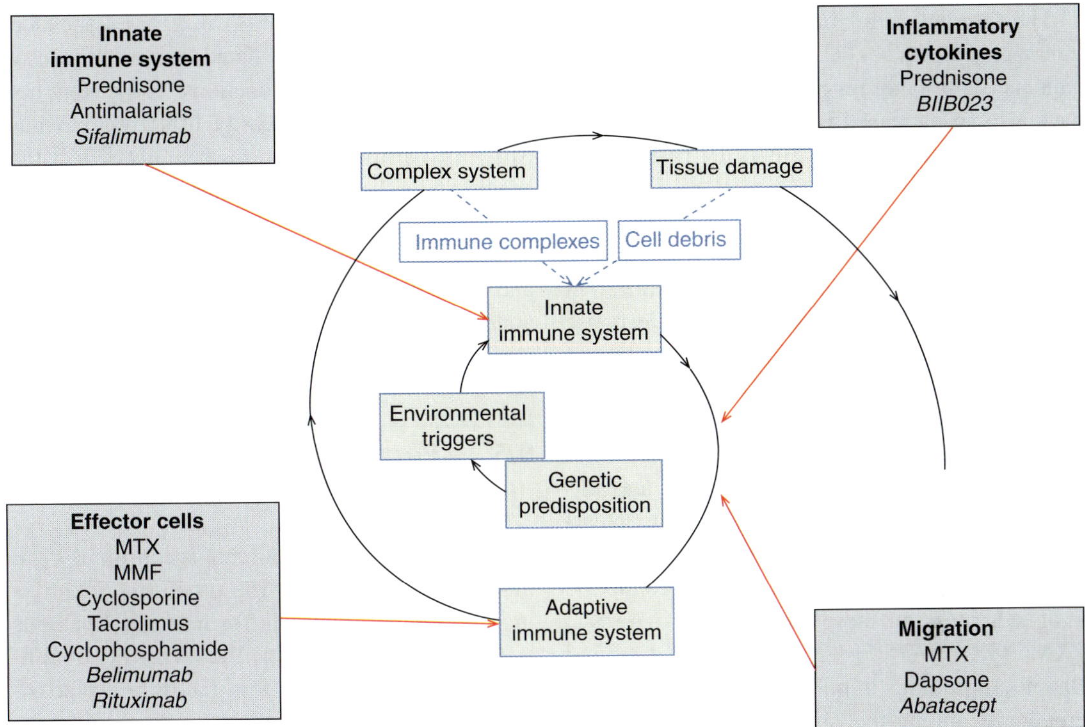

Fig. 9.2 Therapeutic targets in the proinflammatory vicious circle of LE. The figure illustrates the model of autoinflammatory immune responses in LE, which lead into a "spiral of disease progression and autoamplification" (Model adapted from Liu and Davidson [24]) and the resulting potential therapeutic targets. Environmental triggers activate the innate and subsequently the adaptive immune system and may initiate LE in genetically predisposed patients. Importantly, several factors induced by the adaptive immune response, including immune complexes as well as nuclear fragments within cell debris, in turn are able to activate the innate system and drive the proinflammatory vicious circle. This results in the identification of potential targets of the different drugs used in LE: Classic immunosuppressants target mainly the activity of different effector cell types or (like MTX) inhibit the migration of effector cells to their target organ. Prednisone has a broad effect on the innate immune system as well as on proinflammatory cytokines. Antimalarials have recently been shown to inhibit the innate immune system, thus opening up a promising new field for therapeutic strategies (see, e.g., studies using the anti-type-I-IFN antibody sifalimumab). *MTX* methotrexate, *MMF* mycophenolate mofetil, and *IFN* interferon. Drugs that are still in the status of clinical studies are given in italics

in individual patients. In the 1970s, the HLA locus was the first genetic factor which was proven to be associated with LE. The HLA class II alleles DR and DQ were shown to be associated with SLE, and HLA-DRB1*15, HLADRB1*16, and HLA-DRB1*03 alleles were noted to be present in two thirds of all SLE patients. The presence of the LE-characteristic autoantibodies anti-SSA/Ro and anti-SSB/La antibodies has been noted to be associated with HLA-B*08, HLA-DRB1*03, HLA-DQB1*02 (DQ2), and HLA-C4AQ0. The following investigations revealed associations with HLA class III, more specifically the complement system, including C2, C4, and C1q [26].

During the last years, several genome-wide association studies have focused on the genetic background of LE. These studies identified, next to confirming the associations with HLA and complement genes, multiple single nucleotide polymorphisms (SNPs) in more than 50 additional genes. Among these genes, HLA-DRB1*0301, HLA-DRB1*1501, PTPN22, IRF5, STAT4, BLK, ITGAM, and TNFAIP3 were confirmed to be associated with SLE in an extensive meta-analysis [26].

The familial chilblain LE is the only known monogenic form of CLE [27]. Interestingly, patients with heterozygous TREX1 mutations have also an increased risk to develop SLE, and about 2–3 % of the SLE patients are carriers of a TREX1 mutation [28].

Most of the LE-associated genes are involved in the activation and regulation of immune response mechanisms. They belong to different biological pathways: (1) innate immune response including TLR/interferon signaling pathways (IRF5, STAT4, TNFAIP3, and TREX1), (2) adaptive immune response pathways (HLA-DR, PTPN22, PDCD1, STAT4, LYN, BLK, and BANK1) including B and T cells and antigen-presenting cells, and (3) immune complex clearance mechanisms (FCGRs, CRP, and ITGAM). However, some of the genes identified cannot be assigned to one of these pathways (KIAA1542, PXK, XKR6, ATG5). As outlined by Lee and Bae, these findings implicate a wide genetic heterogeneity among the LE populations, thus providing new starting points to identify novel mechanisms and treatment strategies in LE [29].

In addition to the genetic investigations in LE, several gene expression analyses of cell and tissue samples have been performed during the last years. The most outstanding finding among those genes upregulated in LE patients (regardless of LE subtype or tissue subtype) was an enhanced expression of type I IFN-regulated genes, a so-called IFN signature comprising IFIT1, IFIT2, OAS1, OAS2, and Mx1. Other pathways which were found to be upregulated are associated with apoptosis, cell migration, cell differentiation, cell cycle progression, cytokines, chemokines, growth factors, and immunomodulatory genes [26].

A very recent study of the gene expression profile in the skin of CDLE patients demonstrated a distinct molecular signature that separated lesional from non-lesional skin including inflammatory pathways and processes, type I IFN mediated pathways, apoptotic/survival pathways, and dysregulated complement cascade elements. A large number of differentially expressed genes overlapped with those previously reported in SLE, and the authors found some transcriptional abnormalities in CLE that mirror those seen in SLE. However,

they also identified a number of genes associated with the T- and B-cell-mediated immune response, along with NK and DC functions. These were not included in the gene expression lists from previous SLE microarray studies, which might reflect the specificity of the lesional inflammation in the skin. Moreover, the downregulation of specific pathways including lipid and tryptophan metabolism and the ligand-independent activation of the androgen receptor might be important for the development of skin lesions [30].

9.5 Personalized Treatment of CLE Patients

As detailed above, the clinical spectrum of CLE manifestations is wide. The process of identifying the optimal treatment for individual patients is a complex one. Not only the variability of clinical manifestations, but also the different possibilities of systemic manifestations of the autoimmune disease, the individual background of the patients' history, and the personal preconditions (genetics, sex, age, pre-existing diseases) have to be taken into account.

This prompted the German Society of Dermatology to publish guidelines for the treatment of CLE (detailed in Table 9.4). However, guidelines mainly reflect evidence-based data and therefore depend considerably on the availability of clinical studies with larger sample sizes. This limits their potential to identify personalized treatment regimes in individual CLE patients. Therefore, we will discuss specific strategies for the use of selected drugs without claiming to be exhaustive.

9.5.1 Methotrexate (MTX): An Inhibitor of Lymphocyte Migration into the Skin

During the 1950s, MTX was developed as a folate analogue and antimetabolite chemotherapeutic drug for the treatment of leukemia.

Its anti-inflammatory properties became evident during the 1970s and led to its approval by

Table 9.4 Guidelines for the treatment of CLE

Recommendation	Drug	Indication	Dosage
1st choice	Topical corticosteroids	CLE	1–2×/day (occlusive application if necessary)
	Topical tacrolimus/pimecrolimus	CLE (face)	1–2×/day
	Hydroxychloroquine	CLE	6.0–6.5 mg/kg/day
	Chloroquine	CLE	3.5–4.0 mg/kg/day
	Mepacrine	Recalcitrant CLE (in combination with other antimalarials)	100 mg/day
	Prednisolone	Acute or severe CLE	0.5–1 mg/kg/day
2nd choice	Methotrexate	SCLE > CDLE	7.5–25 mg/week
	Acitretin/isotretinoin	Hypertrophic CDLE, SCLE, and LP overlap	0.2–1 mg/day / 0.5–1 mg/day
	Dapsone	BLE, LEP, SCLE, early CDLE, oral ulcers, and vasculitis	50–200 mg/day
	MMF	SCLE and ChLE	2 × 1,000 mg/day

The table details the 1st and 2nd choice treatment strategies of CLE as given by the guidelines of the German Dermatological Society (*LE* lupus erythematosus, *CLE* cutaneous lupus erythematosus, *CDLE* chronic discoid LE, *SCLE* subacute cutaneous LE, *LEP* LE profundus, *LP* lichen planus, *ChLE* chilblain LE, *MMF* mycophenolate mofetil; original publication accessible at www.awmf.de)

the US Food and Drug Administration for the treatment of rheumatoid arthritis in 1988. They are most probably independent of its chemotherapeutic properties but mediated by adenosine. Adenosine blocks the activity of antigen-presenting cells and inhibits the expression of cell adhesion molecules on endothelia and lymphocytes. The latter effect appears to be of specific interest in the treatment of CLE and related diseases like dermatomyositis. In CLE, MTX has been shown to be highly effective in treating patients with widespread skin lesions, especially those suffering from SCLE with a lesional lymphocytic inflammation. Interestingly, MTX is generally regarded as an immunosuppressive drug but shows a reciprocal effect on the number of circulating lymphocytes: patients with a diminished count of circulating lymphocytes in the peripheral blood showed an increase of these blood cells under treatment with MTX while the skin lesions cleared away at the same time. Since lymphocytes are the main effector cells seen in SCLE skin lesions, it is tempting to speculate that a main effect of MTX in this condition is the inhibition of the migration of these cells into their autoimmune target organ [16]. This hypothesis is supported by observations in patients suffering from dermatomyositis (DM), whose skin lesions are histologically very similar to SCLE lesions. In DM, MTX was found to be effective in the treatment of patients with cell-rich skin lesions, while the effect was clearly limited in patients with only a few lymphocytes in the skin biopsies taken prior to treatment [31].

In principle, these findings destine MTX as an ideal drug for the treatment of patients with lymphopenia and widespread SCLE lesions with a lymphocyte-rich inflammatory skin infiltrate. However, one distinct individual factor can limit the use of MTX in this condition dramatically: MTX should not be used in patients with reduced kidney function, and SCLE is one subset of CLE in which a mild systemic disease with involvement of the kidney is not uncommon.

9.5.2 Dapsone: Targeting Neutrophil Granulocytes

Dapsone (4,4′-diaminodiphenyl sulfone, DDS) is an old antibiotic drug which has been developed during the 1930s and has been used for the treatment of leprosy since 1949. Shortly after its first use as an antibiotic, the strong anti-inflammatory properties of the drug were discovered. Dapsone was observed to improve several inflammatory skin diseases, particularly those with a predominating neutrophilic inflammatory pattern, including dermatitis herpetiformis, subcorneal pustular dermatosis, and acne [32]. The drug inhibits the activation of neutrophilic granulocytes and their recruitment into the skin through a number of different pathways. It interferes with neutrophilic chemotactic migration by inhibiting IL8 and β2 integrin (CD11b/CD18)-mediated adherence of human neutrophils [32, 33].

Therefore, dapsone has its specific indication in CLE patients who show a neutrophil-rich inflammatory infiltrate in the lesional skin biopsy [34]. Generally, these cells are uncommon in CLE lesions, but they predominate in one LE subtype: the bullous LE. Importantly, dapsone has an impressive response rate of about 90 % in this subtype [34]. These findings underline the necessity of an individualized treatment of CLE patients. For CLE patients with a neutrophil-rich lesional infiltrate, dapsone provides a promising treatment option. However, the recommendation of dapsone in this condition is subject to one important restriction: prior to initiation of dapsone therapy, patients should be screened for glucose-6-phosphate dehydrogenase deficiency, as patients with decreased activity of this enzyme show a highly increased rate of adverse effects, particularly hemolytic anemia [34].

9.5.3 Antimalarials: Blocking the Proinflammatory Vicious Circle

Antimalarial drugs, particularly quinine and its synthetic successors chloroquine and hydroxychloroquine, are standard therapeutics in the treatment of several autoimmune diseases. They are also the first choice systemic treatment of CLE. Despite their extensive use in CLE for more than 100 years (the first documented use of quinacrine in CDLE dates back to 1894), their mode of action remained unknown for a long time.

Only recently, Kuznik et al. identified the DNA-binding capacity of antimalarials as an important anti-inflammatory factor [35]. They were able to demonstrate that antimalarials function by preventing immunostimulatory nucleic acids from activating the innate immune system. Specifically, the antimalarials have been shown to bind DNA-like structures in the endosome, thus inhibiting the activation of TLR9. As detailed above, this endosomal TLR9 activation through endogenous DNA is most probably an important step in the proinflammatory vicious circle of LE. These findings elucidate earlier observations of the clinical effects of antimalarials: They improve the course of the disease in most CLE patients over a longer time period of months, but they do not have direct immunosuppressive properties. Moreover, the understanding of this specific mode of action may help to identify specific groups of patients especially likely to benefit from this treatment. It may also help to exclude others: for example, in patients with familial ChLE, who suffer from a chronic overstimulation of the cytosolic (not the endosomal) innate immune receptor due to the defective TREX1-DNase, this drug should be used with care.

9.5.4 Outlook: Future Targeted Treatment Strategies in LE

The increasing knowledge of the pathomechanisms of LE and the growing insight into the interactions between innate and adaptive pathways of the immune system provide an opportunity for a number of potential new targets for future treatment strategies of the disease.

The shift from pure evidence-based to more functional approaches aiming to identify individual treatment strategies for specific diseases has only just begun. Table 9.5 details the ongoing clinical studies in the field of lupus as accessed at http://clinicaltrials.gov/ in July 2014. The table provides an overview of the therapeutic targets currently in the focus of the research companies. The main focus of the studies registered is still on the adaptive immune system: several drugs under clinical evaluation are directed against B and

Table 9.5 Outlook: targeted treatment strategies in LE

Drug	Indication	Mechanism
AMG 557	SLE	Anti-B7RP-1 (T-cell differentiation and cytokine production)
Omalizumab	SLE	Anti-IgE
Belimumab	SLE	Anti-B-cell activating factor (BAFF)
Blisibimod	SLE	Antagonist of B-cell activating factor (BAFF)
Atacicept	SLE	Anti-B-cell fusion protein (binds BlyS and blocks APRIL)
Nelfinavir	SLE	Protease inhibitors
Acthar	SLE	Preparation of adrenocorticotropic hormone
ABT-199	SLE	Anti-Bcl-2
Tabalumab	SLE	Anti-B-cell activating factor (BAFF)
Sirolimus	SLE	Prevents activation of T cells and B cells
Bortezomib	SLE	Proteasome inhibitor
Ala-Cpn10	SLE	Regulation of the innate immune system
Interleukin 2	SLE	Induction of regulatory T cells
Sifalimumab	SLE	Anti-IFNα antibody
MEDI-546	SLE	Anti-IFNa/b receptor antibody
Hydroxychloroquine	Neonatal lupus	DNA-binding molecule
Rituximab	Lupus nephritis	Anti-CD20 (B cell)
Leflunomide	Lupus nephritis	Pyrimidine synthesis inhibitor (antilymphocyte)
Voclosporin	Lupus nephritis	Calcineurin inhibitor (anti-T cells)
Abatacept	Lupus nephritis	IgG1/CTLA-4-fusion protein (inhibits T-cell migration and costimulation)
BIIB023	Lupus nephritis	Anti-TWEAK (block of proinflammatory mediators)
Ixazomib	Lupus nephritis	Proteasome inhibitor
R333	SLE, CLE	JAK/SYK inhibitor
Milatuzumab	SLE, CLE	Anti-CD74 antibody (B cells/monocytes)
CNTO 136	SLE, CLE	Anti-IL6
UVA1 radiation	CLE	Immunosuppression (via IL-10)

Overview of ongoing clinical trials in LE as registered by the US National Library of Medicine (NLM) and the National Institutes of Health (http://clinicaltrials.gov/) (accessed in April 2014) including the drugs' suggested mode of action (mechanism)

T cells and their cross talk. However, a rising number of studies concentrate on players of the innate immune system (e.g., anti-IFN-biologicals, DNA-binding molecules, kinase inhibitors, chaperonin 10-like drugs). It will be fascinating to observe the future developments in this field of research.

References

1. Kuhn A, Landmann A. The classification and diagnosis of cutaneous lupus erythematosus. J Autoimmun. 2014;48–49:14–9.
2. Tan EM, Cohen AS, Fries JF, Masi AT, McShane DJ, Rothfield NF, et al. The 1982 revised criteria for the classification of systemic lupus erythematosus. Arthritis Rheum. 1982;25(11):1271–7.
3. Parodi A, Rebora A. ARA and EADV criteria for classification of systemic lupus erythematosus in patients with cutaneous lupus erythematosus. Dermatology. 1997;194(3):217–20.
4. Petri M, Orbai AM, Alarcon GS, Gordon C, Merrill JT, Fortin PR, et al. Derivation and validation of the Systemic Lupus International Collaborating Clinics classification criteria for systemic lupus erythematosus. Arthritis Rheum. 2012;64(8):2677–86.
5. Baltaci M, Fritsch P. Histologic features of cutaneous lupus erythematosus. Autoimmun Rev. 2009;8(6):467–73.
6. Sontheimer RD. Subacute cutaneous lupus erythematosus: 25-year evolution of a prototypic subset (subphenotype) of lupus erythematosus defined by characteristic cutaneous, pathological, immunological, and genetic findings. Autoimmun Rev. 2005;4(5):253–63.
7. Sontheimer RD, Thomas JR, Gilliam JN. Subacute cutaneous lupus erythematosus: a cutaneous marker for a distinct lupus erythematosus subset. Arch Dermatol. 1979;115(12):1409–15.

8. Schmitt V, Meuth AM, Amler S, Kuehn E, Haust M, Messer G, et al. Lupus erythematosus tumidus is a separate subtype of cutaneous lupus erythematosus. Br J Dermatol. 2010;162(1):64–73.

9. Tomasini D, Mentzel T, Hantschke M, Cerri A, Paredes B, Rutten A, et al. Plasmacytoid dendritic cells: an overview of their presence and distribution in different inflammatory skin diseases, with special emphasis on Jessner's lymphocytic infiltrate of the skin and cutaneous lupus erythematosus. J Cutan Pathol. 2010;37(11):1132–9.

10. Wenzel J, Tuting T. Identification of type I interferon-associated inflammation in the pathogenesis of cutaneous lupus erythematosus opens up options for novel therapeutic approaches. Exp Dermatol. 2007;16(5):454–63.

11. Arai S, Katsuoka K. Clinical entity of Lupus erythematosus panniculitis/lupus erythematosus profundus. Autoimmun Rev. 2009;8(6):449–52.

12. Miyashita A, Fukushima S, Makino T, Yoshino Y, Yamashita J, Honda N, et al. Proportion of lymphocytic inflammation with CD123 positive cells in lupus erythematous profundus predict a clinical response to treatment. Acta Derm Venereol. 2014;94:563–7.

13. Millard LG, Rowell NR. Chilblain lupus erythematosus (Hutchinson). A clinical and laboratory study of 17 patients. Br J Dermatol. 1978;98(5):497–506.

14. Gunther C, Hillebrand M, Brunk J, Lee-Kirsch MA. Systemic involvement in TREX1-associated familial chilblain lupus. J Am Acad Dermatol. 2013;69(4):e179–81.

15. Wenzel J, Bauer R, Bieber T, Bohm I. Autoantibodies in patients with Lupus erythematosus: spectrum and frequencies. Dermatology. 2000;201(3):282–3.

16. Wenzel J, Brahler S, Bauer R, Bieber T, Tuting T. Efficacy and safety of methotrexate in recalcitrant cutaneous lupus erythematosus: results of a retrospective study in 43 patients. Br J Dermatol. 2005;153(1):157–62.

17. Ronnblom LE, Alm GV, Oberg KE. Possible induction of systemic lupus erythematosus by interferon-alpha treatment in a patient with a malignant carcinoid tumour. J Intern Med. 1990;227(3):207–10.

18. Baechler EC, Batliwalla FM, Karypis G, Gaffney PM, Ortmann WA, Espe KJ, et al. Interferon-inducible gene expression signature in peripheral blood cells of patients with severe lupus. Proc Natl Acad Sci U S A. 2003;100(5):2610–5.

19. Baechler EC, Batliwalla FM, Reed AM, Peterson EJ, Gaffney PM, Moser KL, et al. Gene expression profiling in human autoimmunity. Immunol Rev. 2006;210:120–37.

20. Dall'era MC, Cardarelli PM, Preston BT, Witte A, Davis Jr JC. Type I interferon correlates with serological and clinical manifestations of SLE. Ann Rheum Dis. 2005;64(12):1692–7.

21. Freutel S, Gaffal E, Zahn S, Bieber T, Tuting T, Wenzel J. Enhanced CCR5+/CCR3+ T helper cell ratio in patients with active cutaneous lupus erythematosus. Lupus. 2011;20(12):1300–4.

22. Wenzel J, Worenkamper E, Freutel S, Henze S, Haller O, Bieber T, et al. Enhanced type I interferon signalling promotes Th1-biased inflammation in cutaneous lupus erythematosus. J Pathol. 2005;205(4):435–42.

23. Arrue I, Saiz A, Ortiz-Romero PL, Rodriguez-Peralto JL. Lupus-like reaction to interferon at the injection site: report of five cases. J Cutan Pathol. 2007;34 Suppl 1:18–21.

24. Liu Z, Davidson A. Taming lupus-a new understanding of pathogenesis is leading to clinical advances. Nat Med. 2012;18(6):871–82.

25. Eloranta ML, Lovgren T, Finke D, Mathsson L, Ronnelid J, Kastner B, et al. Regulation of the interferon-alpha production induced by RNA-containing immune complexes in plasmacytoid dendritic cells. Arthritis Rheum. 2009;60(8):2418–27.

26. Arriens C, Mohan C. Systemic lupus erythematosus diagnostics in the 'omics' era. Int J Clin Rheumatol. 2013;8(6):671–87.

27. Gunther C, Meurer M, Stein A, Viehweg A, Lee-Kirsch MA. Familial chilblain lupus–a monogenic form of cutaneous lupus erythematosus due to a heterozygous mutation in TREX1. Dermatology. 2009;219(2):162–6.

28. Lee-Kirsch MA, Gong M, Chowdhury D, Senenko L, Engel K, Lee YA, et al. Mutations in the gene encoding the 3′-5′ DNA exonuclease TREX1 are associated with systemic lupus erythematosus. Nat Genet. 2007;39(9):1065–7.

29. Lee HS, Bae SC. What can we learn from genetic studies of systemic lupus erythematosus? Implications of genetic heterogeneity among populations in SLE. Lupus. 2010;19(12):1452–9.

30. Dey-Rao R, Smith JR, Chow S, Sinha AA. Differential gene expression analysis in CCLE lesions provides new insights regarding the genetics basis of skin vs. systemic disease. Genomics. 2014;104:144–55.

31. Hornung T, Ko A, Tuting T, Bieber T, Wenzel J. Efficacy of low-dose methotrexate in the treatment of dermatomyositis skin lesions. Clin Exp Dermatol. 2012;37(2):139–42.

32. Zhu YI, Stiller MJ. Dapsone and sulfones in dermatology: overview and update. J Am Acad Dermatol. 2001;45(3):420–34.

33. Kast RE, Scheuerle A, Wirtz CR, Karpel-Massler G, Halatsch ME. The rationale of targeting neutrophils with dapsone during glioblastoma treatment. Anticancer Agents Med Chem. 2011;11(8):756–61.

34. Piette EW, Werth VP. Dapsone in the management of autoimmune bullous diseases. Immunol Allergy Clin North Am. 2012;32(2):317–22, vii.

35. Kuznik A, Bencina M, Svajger U, Jeras M, Rozman B, Jerala R. Mechanism of endosomal TLR inhibition by antimalarial drugs and imidazoquinolines. J Immunol. 2011;186(8):4794–804.

Kyle T. Amber, Rüdiger Eming, and Michael Hertl

Contents

K.T. Amber, MD (✉)
Department of Dermatology and Cutaneous Surgery,
University of Miami Miller School of Medicine,
Miami, FL 33156, USA
e-mail: KAmber@med.miami.edu

R. Eming, MD • M. Hertl, MD
Department of Dermatology and Allergology,
Philipps-University, Marburg 35043, Germany
e-mail: hertl@med.uni-marburg.de

10.1   Introduction

The incidence of pemphigus, depending on the ethnic group, is low ranging from two to ten cases per one million inhabitants in central Europe [1]. Still, even though rare, this autoimmune bullous skin disorder is clinically relevant due to its high morbidity and mortality. The pathogenesis of pemphigus is linked to an intraepidermal loss of cell adhesion which is induced by IgG autoantibodies which target desmosomal adhesion proteins [2–4], specifically desmoglein 3 (Dsg3) and Dsg1. These adhesion proteins exert homophilic and heterophilic transinteraction mainly through their NH2 terminal extracellular subdomains [3, 5, 6]. In general, the serum concentrations of Dsg-reactive IgG autoantibodies correlate with the clinical disease activity of pemphigus [7, 8].

There is increasing evidence that the pathogenesis of PV is induced and regulated by autoaggressive T cells [9]. This contention is supported by the strong immunogenetic association of pemphigus vulgaris (PV) with HLA-DRß1*04:02 and HLA-DQß1*05:03. These HLA class II alleles play a critical role in the activation of CD4+ helper T cells which is presumably critical for the activation of autoaggressive B cells which differentiate into autoantibody-producing plasma cells. Moreover, the strong association of the clinically active phase of PV with serum autoantibodies of the IgG4 and IgE subclasses as well as the preferential detection of peripheral autoaggressive T helper 2 (Th2) cells

T. Bieber, F. Nestle (eds.), *Personalized Treatment Options in Dermatology*,
DOI 10.1007/978-3-662-45840-2_10, © Springer-Verlag Berlin Heidelberg 2015

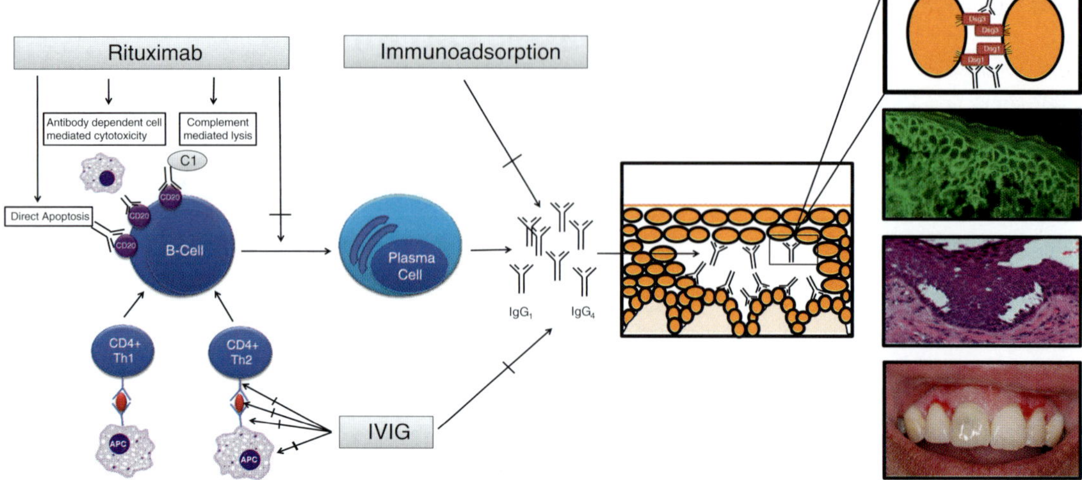

Fig. 10.1 Rituximab leads to B-cell depletion by a combination of antibody-dependent cell-mediated cytotoxicity, complement-mediated lysis, and direct apoptosis secondary to the binding of the monoclonal antibody to CD20. This decrease in the B-cell population leads to a subsequent decrease in the development of antibody-secreting plasma cells. IVIG targets pathogenic IgG autoantibodies in pemphigus by inducing an increased Ig catabolism via binding to the neonatal Fc receptor, as well as acting on numerous other immunologic sites. Immunoadsorption removes serum IgG with a very high specificity, reducing the circulation of pathogenic autoantibodies

strongly supports the concept that PV is a Th2-regulated autoimmune disorder [10, 11].

Despite the remarkable progress in our understanding of the immune pathogenesis of pemphigus, the currently practiced therapeutic regimens are based on high-dose systemic glucocorticoids and adjuvant immunosuppressants which are effective but bear the risk of considerable side effects. Recently, novel not yet fully validated, more specific therapies of pemphigus have been introduced which target critical effector cells and molecules in the pemphigus pathogenesis. These include therapeutic depletion of B cells with the monoclonal antibody, rituximab, and the removal or increased turnover of pathogenic IgG autoantibodies by the use of immunoadsorption and high-dose intravenous immunoglobulins [12, 13]. The mechanisms and major sites of action for each of these therapies are shown in Fig. 10.1.

10.2 Immunoadsorption (IA)

Immunoadsorption has recently gained major interest as a therapeutic option for pemphigus since it directly targets pathogenic IgG autoantibodies [14, 15]. In contrast to nonselective plasmapheresis, immunoadsorption removes serum IgG with a very high specificity. At present, the availability of immunoadsorption is limited since this therapeutic regimen is not available in many countries. A variety of immunoadsorption devices have been utilized including tryptophan adsorbers and regenerative adsorbers such as protein A or synthetic ligands (e.g., PGAM146, Globaffin) that have a high affinity to the Fc portion of human IgG. The efficacy of therapeutic immunoadsorption in pemphigus largely depends on the adsorber utilized and the treatment protocol. Depending on the absorption device, serum concentrations of IgG antibodies against desmogleins 1 and 3 are reduced by 30–80 % [16–19].

At present, the clinical efficacy of immunoadsorption in pemphigus is based on observations from uncontrolled single-case studies and case series. In most instances, immunoadsorption is performed in an adjuvant setting in combination with immunosuppressive drugs such as azathioprine, mycophenolate, methotrexate, or cyclosporin as 4-day cycles which can be repeated in monthly intervals [20]. There is generally agreement that removal of serum IgG autoantibodies by immunoadsorption is associated with improvement of mucocutaneous blistering. The long-term effects of immunoadsorption are not yet well characterized; long-term improvement after immunoadsorption has been reported in some studies. In patients with refractory pemphigus, immunoadsorption was successfully combined with treatment with rituximab and/or intravenous immunoglobulins [20, 21]. Most patients appear to tolerate immunoadsorption well. Among the reported adverse effects are hypotension, bradycardia, anaphylaxis, sepsis from the central catheter, and venous thrombosis [22]. Currently, a prospective multicenter trial in 24 German dermatology departments addresses the question of whether adjuvant treatment with immunoadsorption is superior to treatment with systemic glucocorticoids plus azathioprine or mycophenolate alone in patients with acute onset, chronic active, or relapsing pemphigus. The primary endpoint is time to clinical remission based on the initial observation that removal of pathogenic serum IgG autoantibodies by immunoadsorptions leads to faster clinical remissions.

10.3 High-Dose Intravenous Immunoglobulins (IVIG)

Similar to immunoadsorption, treatment with high-dose intravenous immunoglobulins (IVIG) has been introduced in pemphigus based on the contention that exogenous IgG blocks the action of pathogenic IgG autoantibodies [23, 24]. Current concepts suggest that IVIG targets pathogenic IgG autoantibodies in pemphigus by inducing an increased Ig catabolism via binding to the neonatal Fc receptor. Many single-case reports and case series suggest that IVIG, mostly applied in an adjuvant setting in combination with immunosuppressants such as azathioprine, mycophenolate, cyclophosphamide, and methotrexate, is efficacious [25]. In most instances, patients received IVIG at a dose of 2 g/kg/cycle over two to four consecutive days, and IVIG cycles were repeated in 4- to 6-week intervals. A glucocorticoid-sparing effect of adjuvant IVIG was suggested by a small retrospective study that found a significant reduction of systemic glucocorticoids upon IVIG treatment [26, 27]. IVIG therapy is well tolerated; side effects include headache and aseptic meningitis. Prior to initiating treatment, total IgA deficiency and reduced kidney function need to be excluded.

The best evidence for a beneficial therapeutic effect of IVIG in pemphigus is provided by a Japanese randomized multicenter trial in 61 adults with glucocorticoid-resistant pemphigus (defined as a failure to respond to ≥20 mg prednisolone/day) [28]. Patients either received 400 mg IVIG/kg/day over 5 consecutive days, 200 mg IVIG/kg/day over 5 days, or placebo infusions for 5 days. The primary endpoint of the trial was the time that the patients could be maintained on the previous treatment protocol (i.e., time to escape protocol). The study showed that the time to escape protocol was significantly longer in patients who had received 400 mg IVIG/kg/day compared to patients who had received the lower IVIG dose or placebo. However, the difference in the time to escape protocol for the 200 mg IVIG group and the placebo group was not statistically significant. Side effects are usually mild to moderate adverse events such as headache, back pain, increased blood pressure, and abdominal discomfort. Aseptic meningitis is a serious side effect of IVIG therapy that requires immediate termination of treatment. Anaphylaxis is a potential risk of IVIG treatment in patients with IgA deficiency.

10.4 Rituximab

10.4.1 B-Cell Depletion and Repopulation

Rituximab is a chimeric murine-human monoclonal IgG that targets CD20, approved by the Food and Drug Administration for the treatment of many B-cell lymphomas as well as rheumatoid arthritis and granulomatosis with polyangiitis. The off-label use of rituximab has been vast, including immunobullous disorders, systemic lupus erythematosus (SLE), and dermatomyositis. CD20 is a glycosylated phosphoprotein that is expressed on the surface of all B cells starting at the pro-B-cell phase which also corresponds with heavy chain variable, diversity, and joining region (VDJ) rearrangement. A case of a CD20-deficient patient suggests CD20 is also involved in T-cell-independent antibody response [29].

As B cells mature, CD20 expression increases. When mature B cells differentiate into plasma cells, expression of many common B-cell surface antigens, including CD20, is lost. Thus, rituximab destroys B-cell progenitor cells but not stem cells or antibody-secreting plasma cells. Peripheral B-cell depletion typically takes place between 2 and 4 weeks following infusion. B-cell repopulation takes place a mean 5–6 months following infusion, though in some cases B-cell depletion persists for up to 15 months [30–33]. As late pro-B cells are destroyed by rituximab, the new generation of immature B cells undergoes VDJ heavy chain arrangement and VJ light chain arrangement resulting in a novel antibody repertoire [30]. In PV, this likely results in the observed changes in IgG reactivity against particular subdomains within Dsg3, whereby patients may lose reactivity to certain subdomains following treatment, despite maintaining IgG antibodies against the ectodomain of Dsg3. Clinically, the recurrence of IgG autoantibodies targeting the patient's original pathogenic domain, most commonly Dsg3EC1, results in relapse [34]. Interestingly, anti-Dsg1 IgG titers also appear to be a more reliable indicator of clinical status of pemphigus than total anti-Dsg3 IgG [35].

Repopulation first occurs with the development of CD5$^+$/CD38^{high} naive B cells, followed by immature B cells (CD19$^-$/IgD$^-$/CD38^{high}/CD10^{low}/CD24^{high}). The return of CD27$^+$ memory B cells can remain reduced following treatment for up to 2 years [31, 36]. Repopulation with certain ratios of circulating B-cell subsets appears to have a predictive effect on disease relapse, with higher ratios of memory B cells at the time of repopulation related to relapse. Repopulation with certain subtypes additionally may predict treatment success. PV patients who achieved complete remission following treatment with rituximab had a greater number of transitional B cells and IL-10 secreting regulatory B cells as

well as a higher ratio of CD19$^+$/CD27$^-$ naïve B cells to CD19$^+$/CD27$^+$ memory B cells [37].

Short-lived plasma cells rather than long-lived plasma cells are more dependent on C20$^+$ memory B cells for replenishment. Thus, rituximab has a greater effect on the eventual depletion of short-lived plasma cells rather than long-lived plasma cells which can remain in circulation for an indefinite period of time. This may in part explain the more significant decrease in serum IgG autoantibodies relative to total immunoglobulin levels, as IgG autoantibodies appear to be produced more often by short-lived plasma cells [38–40]. In fact, following treatment with rituximab, IgG to common pathogens and recall antigens does not decrease [38, 41]. This can in part be explained by rituximab-mediated increases in B-cell-activating factor (BAFF) expression, which is associated with increased pathogen-specific IgG such as anti-Epstein-Barr-virus IgG and anti-varicella-zoster-virus IgG, but not autoantibodies in pemphigus [42]. Following repopulation with CD19$^+$ B cells, BAFF levels return to normal IgG. In a few reported cases of bullous pemphigoid patients treated with rituximab, early relapse was associated with lower peak serum levels of BAFF [43].

10.4.2 Mechanism of B-Cell Destruction

The mechanism by which rituximab-induced B-cell depletion occurs is complex and occurs by a combination of several mechanisms: antibody-dependent cell-mediated cytotoxicity (ADCC), complement-mediated lysis, and direct apoptosis. The degree to which each of these processes results in cell death is, however, somewhat disease specific, thus making comparison to lymphoma and other autoimmune disease more challenging.

Antibody-dependent cell-mediated cytotoxicity (ADCC) occurs when monocytes and macrophages are recruited via Fc and FcγR interaction [44, 45]. This interaction subsequently leads to the release of cytotoxic cytokines, proteases, and reactive oxygen species [46]. This process is primarily mediated by NK cells [47, 48]. NK cells function in a primarily IL-2-dependent manner and are enhanced following treatment with rituximab [49, 50]. FCγRIII (CD16) is the major Fc receptor involved in ADCC which leads to binding to the Fc portion of the antibody, subsequently resulting in the release of IFN-γ. FCγRIIB (CD32) is a potent regulator of ADCC, enhancing the internalization of rituximab. In follicular lymphoma, FCγRIIB predicts a poor response to rituximab [51]. Likewise, mice deficient in FCγRIIB demonstrated an increased ability to undergo ADCC [52]. Though less clear, pure blockage of the Fc receptor may additionally account for some of the short-term responses seen with rituximab [53].

Rituximab is able to bind to C1q inducing complement-mediated cell lysis [54] via the formation of reactive oxygen species [55]. In fact, in mice deficient in C1q, rituximab loses its efficacy against lymphoma cells [56]. Increases in C3b breakdown products additionally lead to increased rituximab-mediated cell death of CD20$^+$ cells [57]. Rituximab also causes redistribution of CD20 into Triton x-100-insoluble lipid rafts which cluster and enhance complement binding [58, 59]. In contrast, increased complement defense molecules such as CD55 and CD59 have been associated with resistance to treatment in lymphoma [60]. Likewise, in vivo studies of complement-deficient mice have demonstrated reduced anti-CD20 activity [61, 62]. In chronic lymphocytic leukemia, rituximab depletes complement, which in turn reduces its therapeutic function until fresh frozen plasma is given, restoring the complement pool [63]. As complement involvement plays a critical role in the acantholysis seen in pemphigus, it is unclear whether the effect of rituximab on this pathway plays a role in clinical response [64].

Rituximab can also influence apoptosis directly by causing cross-linking of CD20 and the monoclonal antibodies [65]. A caspase-independent mechanism of rituximab-induced cell death has also been described [66]. Rituximab's ability to directly induce apoptosis, however, appears to be marginal in comparison to other mechanisms [67].

10.4.3 Cellular Immunity

While immunobullous disorders may appear to be primarily a disorder of humoral immunity, T cells are in fact a critical component of the pathogenesis and maintenance of autoimmunity [9, 68–70]. Plasma cells appear to receive signaling from CD4$^+$ T cells and antigen-presenting cells, which may dictate their longevity [71, 72]. In patients with PV, treatment with rituximab led to a decrease in Dsg3-specific CD4$^+$ T cells, though the total quantity of CD4+ cells as well as the quantities of cytokines that they produce do not appear to change significantly [36, 73]. Interestingly, however, tetanus toxoid-reactive CD4+ T cells did not change following rituximab, thus demonstrating a role of B-cell-mediated regulation of autoreactive T-cell activation [33]. Likewise, rituximab was found to have an effect on regulatory T cells [74] and monocyte-derived macrophages [75] in SLE and rheumatoid arthritis, respectively. In idiopathic thrombocytopenic purpura, patients who received rituximab experienced a restoration in Th1/Th2 ratio with an increase in the number of Treg cells [76, 77]. Similar findings have been noted in SLE, yet not RA [74, 78, 79]. Rituximab also leads to a decrease in the expression of CD40 and CD80 on B cells which affects T-cell activation [80].

A small subset of T cells (1.6 %) expresses CD20 and exists in the normal population. These cells are split with 45 % expressing CD8 and 55 % expressing CD4. In RA, these cells constitutively express IL-1B and TNF-α and are depleted following treatment with rituximab. It is unclear whether these cells play a clinically meaningful role in other disease states such as in immunobullous disorders [81].

10.4.4 Mechanisms of Treatment Resistance

Multiple potential mechanisms for treatment resistance have been explored. Resistance can occur through the formation of anti-chimeric antibodies, as the murine sequences of the chimeric IgG_1 can contain immunogenic sequences. Interestingly, these anti-drug antibodies were more often observed in rituximab used for the treatment of autoimmune disease rather than lymphoma. The inhibitory effect of these anti-drug antibodies has been demonstrated to interfere with the ability of rituximab to bind to B cells in vitro [82] as well as decreased clinical response to treatment [83]. These anti-drug antibodies have also been associated with the development of serum-like sickness and infusion reactions.

Fc receptor polymorphisms additionally appear to provide a means for treatment resistance by decreasing the affinity of receptor binding to IgG. The FcγRIIIa polymorphism and FcγRIIa polymorphism correlated with a decreased response to rituximab treatment in lymphoma [84]. In SLE, the FcγRIIIa polymorphism was additionally found to be predictive of decreased treatment efficacy, with a tenfold increase in rituximab serum level necessary to achieve comparable B-cell depletion. This failure may be in part due to the observation that NK cells with the FcγRIIIa polymorphism require a significantly greater concentration of rituximab in order to induce the same level ADCC [85]. While these polymorphisms have known effects in other disease processes, it is unclear what effect they have in immunobullous disorders. For example, while a spliced mRNA transcript of CD20 (D393-CD20) has been associated with resistance to rituximab in lymphoma patients, this transcript was not found to be associated with failure to respond to rituximab therapy in patients with pemphigus [86].

Lastly, the inability of rituximab to effectively remove B cells occupying the bone marrow compartment may make rituximab ineffective in certain patients with central memory cells [87]. This is consistent with our finding that an increase in the duration of disease was associated with a decrease in the percentage of patients experiencing complete response versus partial response [88].

10.4.5 Clinical Studies

10.4.5.1 Pemphigus Vulgaris and Foliaceus

Large-scale clinical trials have been conducted demonstrating the clinical efficacy of rituximab in PF and PV [32, 89–93]. Approximately 60–80 % of PV and PF patients treated with rituximab experienced complete remissions [94, 95]. Most studies have used either the lymphoma protocol (375 mg/m²×4 weeks) or the rheumatology protocol (1,000 mg weekly × 2 weeks). In a review of 272 patients, Zakka et al. found a lower response rate with a higher mortality rate, yet a low rate of infection and relapse in patients treated with the lymphoma protocol in contrast to the rheumatology protocol [95]. Variations of these protocols have been described, with some groups halving the dosages in the original two protocols. In our analysis of patients responding to a single cycle of rituximab (those patients achieving either partial or complete remission following treatment), patients treated with the standard lymphoma protocol appeared to demonstrate an increase in the time until relapse. We additionally found the half rheumatology protocol (500 mg weekly × 2 weeks) to be the least efficacious, with a shorter time until relapse and fewer patients experiencing complete response [88]. Likewise, Kanwar et al. in a prospective blinded study comparing the full rheumatology protocol to the half rheumatology protocol demonstrated improved outcomes with the regular-dosed rheumatology protocol versus the half-dosed protocol [96]. Nevertheless, treatment preferences vary widely between physicians, and there remains significant controversy regarding protocol selection [97].

Despite its effectiveness, rituximab does not necessarily appear to alter the long-term relapse rate without maintenance therapy in comparison to conventional immunosuppressive therapy [35]. Nevertheless, certain therapeutic options exist to increase the length of time until relapse such as immunoadsorption [88] or the use of minimal maintenance therapy. In cases of relapse, however, Cianchini et al. demonstrated that repeated cycles of rituximab sufficiently mitigated clinical relapses without necessitating the use of concomitant immunosuppression [92].

10.4.5.2 Paraneoplastic Pemphigus

Paraneoplastic pemphigus carries a far worse prognosis than either PV or PF, as treatment must ultimately be directed against the underlying malignancy. In particular, patients presenting with erythema multiforme-like lesions with histologic keratinocyte necrosis carry an even worse prognosis [98]. Paraneoplastic pemphigus most commonly occurs secondary to lymphoproliferative disorders, particularly non-Hodgkin lymphoma [99]. Thus at times, rituximab may be indicated to treat the malignancy. Paraneoplastic pemphigus like PF and PV is, however, still an IgG-mediated disease with numerous autoantibodies present. Antibodies against envoplakin and periplakin are, however, the most sensitive and specific markers in a clinically suggestive setting [100]. The effect of the rituximab may thus be twofold by targeting the lymphoproliferative disease process while also leading to the destruction of B cells that may develop into IgG autoantibody-secreting plasma cells. Yet, clinical improvement in paraneoplastic pemphigus following treatment with rituximab has been mixed, with most case reports demonstrating only a marginal improvement [99]. A particularly interesting case is that presented by Schadlow et al. that described a patient with long-standing B-cell lymphoma who did not experience clinical improvement with rituximab [101]. This is both surprising and suggestive that perhaps the length of time with the primary malignancy may have an effect on the paraneoplastic pemphigus and its susceptibility to rituximab. Nevertheless, paraneoplastic pemphigus is a complex disease process that does not follow the similar pathogenic steps seen in other immunobullous disorders.

10.4.5.3 Other Autoimmune Blistering Diseases

Compared to PV, there have been far fewer studies and reported cases evaluating the efficacy of rituximab in bullous pemphigoid. In a 2013 review of 16 previously reported cases of BP patients treated with rituximab, Shetty et al. found that 69 % of patients experienced complete remission [102]. While this is comparable to the percentage of patients who experience complete remission in PV, this small sample size of reported cases prevents further analysis into factors associated with superior outcomes.

Several larger studies have examined the efficacy of rituximab in the treatment of mucous membrane pemphigoid. Le Roux-Villet et al. demonstrated complete response in all affected sites in 68 % (17/25) of patients while Heelan et al. reported 75 % (6/8) patients to have a complete remission following a single cycle of rituximab [103, 104]. Nevertheless, the significant relapse rate necessitating further cycles in a short period of time remains a concern [104, 105].

A handful of reports have described successful clinical outcomes in patients with epidermolysis bullosa acquisita treated with rituximab [106–114]. As the disease remains extremely rare with an estimated incidence of 0.2 per million per year [115], it is unlikely that larger studies will be possible. Nevertheless, despite the limited reports, treatment outcomes of epidermolysis bullosa acquisita appear comparable to that of other immunobullous disorders.

10.4.6 Safety

The relative risks associated with chronic steroid suppression and nonbiologic immunosuppressive medications must be weighed against the risks associated with rituximab. In a review of 153 pemphigus patients treated with rituximab, 7 % developed serious infections with 1.3 % fatalities [94]. In comparison, a large study in SLE demonstrated a 9.5 % risk of serious infection [116]. While this number may be of concern, patients treated with corticosteroids demonstrated an 8 % incidence of mild to severe infections, while 21 % those receiving corticosteroids plus mycophenolate mofetil developed an infection [117]. While the severity of the infections must be taken into account, rituximab does not lead to many of the chronic medical conditions to which corticosteroids lead. Interestingly, many of the rituximab patients who developed an infection also received high-dose corticosteroids and other forms of immunosuppression. Of the mucous membrane pemphigoid patients treated with rituximab, only those experiencing severe infectious complications were on concomitant immunosuppressants and high-dose corticosteroids [103]. It thus remains challenging to truly compare the risks of rituximab monotherapy or rituximab with concomitant low-dose corticosteroids with traditional immunosuppression.

The concomitant use of IVIG has not only demonstrated efficacy in treating immunobullous disorders but has also been suggested as a useful adjuvant to rituximab in decreasing the incidence of infections [93, 118]. While IVIG in theory repletes serum IgG during the time of B-cell depletion, it is unclear how the two medications interact with each other, complement and the Fc receptor. Additionally, the use of IVIG in itself comes with certain risks ranging from mild infusion reactions to severe reactions such as aseptic meningitis [119].

References

1. Langan SM, Smeeth L, Hubbard R, Fleming KM, Smith CJ, West J. Bullous pemphigoid and pemphigus vulgaris–incidence and mortality in the UK: population based cohort study. BMJ. 2008;337:a180.
2. Beutner EH, Jordon RE. Demonstration of skin antibodies in sera of pemphigus vulgaris patients by indirect immunofluorescent staining. Proc Soc Exp Biol Med. 1964;117:505–10.
3. Amagai M, Karpati S, Prussick R, Klaus-Kovtun V, Stanley JR. Autoantibodies against the amino-terminal cadherin-like binding domain of pemphigus vulgaris antigen are pathogenic. J Clin Invest. 1992;90: 919–26.
4. Amagai M, Nishikawa T, Nousari HC, Anhalt GJ, Hashimoto T. Antibodies against desmoglein 3 (pemphigus vulgaris antigen) are present in sera from patients with paraneoplastic pemphigus and cause acantholysis in vivo in neonatal mice. J Clin Invest. 1998;102:775–82.
5. Amagai M, Karpati S, Klaus-Kovtun V, Udey MC, Stanley JR. Extracellular domain of pemphigus vulgaris antigen (desmoglein 3) mediates weak homophilic adhesion. J Invest Dermatol. 1994;103:609–15.
6. Di Zenzo G, Di Lullo G, Corti D, et al. Pemphigus autoantibodies generated through somatic mutations target the desmoglein-3 cis-interface. J Clin Invest. 2012;122:3781–90.
7. Ishii K, Amagai M, Hall RP, et al. Characterization of autoantibodies in pemphigus using antigen-specific enzyme-linked immunosorbent assays with baculovirus-expressed recombinant desmogleins. J Immunol. 1997;159:2010–7.
8. Muller R, Svoboda V, Wenzel E, Muller HH, Hertl M. IgG against extracellular subdomains of desmoglein 3 relates to clinical phenotype of pemphigus vulgaris. Exp Dermatol. 2008;17:35–43.
9. Amber KT, Staropoli P, Shiman MI, Elgart GW, Hertl M. Autoreactive T cells in the immune pathogenesis of pemphigus vulgaris. Exp Dermatol. 2013; 22:699–704.
10. Hertl M, Eming R, Veldman C. T cell control in autoimmune bullous skin disorders. J Clin Invest. 2006;116:1159–66.
11. Nagel A, Lang A, Engel D, et al. Clinical activity of pemphigus vulgaris relates to IgE autoantibodies against desmoglein 3. Clin Immunol. 2010;134:320–30.
12. Kneisel A, Hertl M. Autoimmune bullous skin diseases. Part 2: diagnosis and therapy. J Dtsch Dermatol Ges. 2011;9:927–47.
13. Hertl M, Jedlickova H, Karpati S et al. Pemphigus. S2 Guideline for diagnosis and treatment - guided by the European Dermatology Forum (EDF) in cooperation with the European Academy of Dermatology and Venereology (EADV). J Eur Acad Dermatol Venereol. 2014. doi: 10.1111/jdv.12772. [Epub ahead of print].
14. Eming R, Hertl M. Immunoadsorption in pemphigus. Autoimmunity. 2006;39:609–16.
15. Schmidt E, Zillikens D. Immunoadsorption in dermatology. Arch Dermatol Res. 2010;302:241–53.
16. Schmidt E, Klinker E, Opitz A, et al. Protein A immunoadsorption: a novel and effective adjuvant treatment of severe pemphigus. Br J Dermatol. 2003;148:1222–9.
17. Luftl M, Stauber A, Mainka A, Klingel R, Schuler G, Hertl M. Successful removal of pathogenic autoantibodies in pemphigus by immunoadsorption with a tryptophan-linked polyvinylalcohol adsorber. Br J Dermatol. 2003;149:598–605.
18. Eming R, Rech J, Barth S, et al. Prolonged clinical remission of patients with severe pemphigus upon rapid removal of desmoglein-reactive autoantibodies by immunoadsorption. Dermatology. 2006;212: 177–87.
19. Gunther C, Laske J, Frind A, Julius U, Pfeiffer C. Successful therapy of pemphigus vulgaris with immunoadsorption using the TheraSorb adsorber. J Dtsch Dermatol Ges. 2008;6:661–3.

20. Kasperkiewicz M, Shimanovich I, Meier M, et al. Treatment of severe pemphigus with a combination of immunoadsorption, rituximab, pulsed dexamethasone and azathioprine/mycophenolate mofetil: a pilot study of 23 patients. Br J Dermatol. 2012;166: 154–60.

21. Behzad M, Mobs C, Kneisel A, et al. Combined treatment with immunoadsorption and rituximab leads to fast and prolonged clinical remission in difficult-to-treat pemphigus vulgaris. Br J Dermatol. 2012;166:844–52.

22. Kasperkiewicz M, Eming R, Behzad M, et al. Efficacy and safety of rituximab in pemphigus: experience of the German Registry of Autoimmune Diseases. J Dtsch Dermatol Ges. 2012;10:727–32.

23. Czernik A, Beutner EH, Bystryn JC. Intravenous immunoglobulin selectively decreases circulating autoantibodies in pemphigus. J Am Acad Dermatol. 2008;58:796–801.

24. Herzog S, Schmidt E, Goebeler M, Brocker EB, Zillikens D. Serum levels of autoantibodies to desmoglein 3 in patients with therapy-resistant pemphigus vulgaris successfully treated with adjuvant intravenous immunoglobulins. Acta Derm Venereol. 2004;84:48–52.

25. Seidling V, Hoffmann JH, Enk AH, Hadaschik EN. Analysis of high-dose intravenous immunoglobulin therapy in 16 patients with refractory autoimmune blistering skin disease: high efficacy and no serious adverse events. Acta Derm Venereol. 2013;93: 346–9.

26. Sami N, Qureshi A, Ruocco E, Ahmed AR. Corticosteroid-sparing effect of intravenous immunoglobulin therapy in patients with pemphigus vulgaris. Arch Dermatol. 2002;138:1158–62.

27. Green MG, Bystryn JC. Effect of intravenous immunoglobulin therapy on serum levels of IgG1 and IgG4 antidesmoglein 1 and antidesmoglein 3 antibodies in pemphigus vulgaris. Arch Dermatol. 2008;144:1621–4.

28. Amagai M, Ikeda S, Shimizu H, et al. A randomized double-blind trial of intravenous immunoglobulin for pemphigus. J Am Acad Dermatol. 2009;60:595–603.

29. Kuijpers TW, Bende RJ, Baars PA, et al. CD20 deficiency in humans results in impaired T cell-independent antibody responses. J Clin Invest. 2010;120:214–22.

30. Rouziere AS, Kneitz C, Palanichamy A, Dorner T, Tony HP. Regeneration of the immunoglobulin heavy-chain repertoire after transient B-cell depletion with an anti-CD20 antibody. Arthritis Res Ther. 2005;7:R714–24.

31. Leandro MJ, Cambridge G, Ehrenstein MR, Edwards JC. Reconstitution of peripheral blood B cells after depletion with rituximab in patients with rheumatoid arthritis. Arthritis Rheum. 2006;54:613–20.

32. Joly P, Mouquet H, Roujeau JC, et al. A single cycle of rituximab for the treatment of severe pemphigus. N Engl J Med. 2007;357:545–52.

33. Eming R, Nagel A, Wolff-Franke S, Podstawa E, Debus D, Hertl M. Rituximab exerts a dual effect in pemphigus vulgaris. J Invest Dermatol. 2008;128: 2850–8.

34. Muller R, Hunzelmann N, Baur V, et al. Targeted immunotherapy with rituximab leads to a transient alteration of the IgG autoantibody profile in pemphigus vulgaris. Dermatol Res Pract. 2010; 2010:321950.

35. Reguiai Z, Tabary T, Maizieres M, Bernard P. Rituximab treatment of severe pemphigus: long-term results including immunologic follow-up. J Am Acad Dermatol. 2012;67:623–9.

36. Mouquet H, Musette P, Gougeon ML, et al. B-cell depletion immunotherapy in pemphigus: effects on cellular and humoral immune responses. J Invest Dermatol. 2008;128:2859–69.

37. Colliou N, Picard D, Caillot F, et al. Long-term remissions of severe pemphigus after rituximab therapy are associated with prolonged failure of desmoglein B cell response. Sci Transl Med. 2013;5: 175ra130.

38. Cambridge G, Leandro MJ, Edwards JC, et al. Serologic changes following B lymphocyte depletion therapy for rheumatoid arthritis. Arthritis Rheum. 2003;48:2146–54.

39. Cambridge G, Isenberg DA, Edwards JC, et al. B cell depletion therapy in systemic lupus erythematosus: relationships among serum B lymphocyte stimulator levels, autoantibody profile and clinical response. Ann Rheum Dis. 2008;67:1011–6.

40. Teng YK, Wheater G, Hogan VE, et al. Induction of long-term B-cell depletion in refractory rheumatoid arthritis patients preferentially affects autoreactive more than protective humoral immunity. Arthritis Res Ther. 2012;14:R57.

41. Ferraro AJ, Drayson MT, Savage CO, MacLennan IC. Levels of autoantibodies, unlike antibodies to all extrinsic antigen groups, fall following B cell depletion with Rituximab. Eur J Immunol. 2008;38: 292–8.

42. Nagel A, Podstawa E, Eickmann M, Muller HH, Hertl M, Eming R. Rituximab mediates a strong elevation of B-cell-activating factor associated with increased pathogen-specific IgG but not autoantibodies in pemphigus vulgaris. J Invest Dermatol. 2009;129:2202–10.

43. Hall 3rd RP, Streilein RD, Hannah DL, et al. Association of serum B-cell activating factor level and proportion of memory and transitional B cells with clinical response after rituximab treatment of bullous pemphigoid patients. J Invest Dermatol. 2013;133:2786–8.

44. Hamaguchi Y, Xiu Y, Komura K, Nimmerjahn F, Tedder TF. Antibody isotype-specific engagement of Fcgamma receptors regulates B lymphocyte depletion during CD20 immunotherapy. J Exp Med. 2006;203:743–53.

45. Kaneko Y, Nimmerjahn F, Ravetch JV. Anti-inflammatory activity of immunoglobulin G resulting from Fc sialylation. Science. 2006;313: 670–3.

46. Glennie MJ, French RR, Cragg MS, Taylor RP. Mechanisms of killing by anti-CD20 monoclonal antibodies. Mol Immunol. 2007;44:3823–37.

47. Golay J, Manganini M, Facchinetti V, et al. Rituximab-mediated antibody-dependent cellular cytotoxicity against neoplastic B cells is stimulated strongly by interleukin-2. Haematologica. 2003;88: 1002–12.

48. Fischer L, Penack O, Gentilini C, et al. The anti-lymphoma effect of antibody-mediated immunotherapy is based on an increased degranulation of peripheral blood natural killer (NK) cells. Exp Hematol. 2006;34:753–9.

49. Bhat R, Watzl C. Serial killing of tumor cells by human natural killer cells–enhancement by therapeutic antibodies. PLoS One. 2007;2:e326.

50. Berdeja JG, Hess A, Lucas DM, et al. Systemic interleukin-2 and adoptive transfer of lymphokine-activated killer cells improves antibody-dependent cellular cytotoxicity in patients with relapsed B-cell lymphoma treated with rituximab. Clin Cancer Res. 2007;13:2392–9.

51. Lee CS, Ashton-Key M, Cogliatti S, et al. Expression of inhibitory Fc receptor (Fc?RIIB) is a marker of poor response to rituximab monotherapy in follicular lymphoma. Lancet. 2013;381:S63.

52. Clynes RA, Towers TL, Presta LG, Ravetch JV. Inhibitory Fc receptors modulate in vivo cytotoxicity against tumor targets. Nat Med. 2000;6:443–6.

53. Cooper N, Stasi R, Cunningham-Rundles S, et al. The efficacy and safety of B-cell depletion with anti-CD20 monoclonal antibody in adults with chronic immune thrombocytopenic purpura. Br J Haematol. 2004;125:232–9.

54. Reff ME, Carner K, Chambers KS, et al. Depletion of B cells in vivo by a chimeric mouse human monoclonal antibody to CD20. Blood. 1994;83:435–45.

55. Bellosillo B, Villamor N, Lopez-Guillermo A, et al. Complement-mediated cell death induced by rituximab in B-cell lymphoproliferative disorders is mediated in vitro by a caspase-independent mechanism involving the generation of reactive oxygen species. Blood. 2001;98:2771–7.

56. Di Gaetano N, Cittera E, Nota R, et al. Complement activation determines the therapeutic activity of rituximab in vivo. J Immunol. 2003;171:1581–7.

57. Kennedy AD, Solga MD, Schuman TA, et al. An anti-C3b(i) mAb enhances complement activation, C3b(i) deposition, and killing of CD20+ cells by rituximab. Blood. 2003;101:1071–9.

58. Cragg MS, Morgan SM, Chan HT, et al. Complement-mediated lysis by anti-CD20 mAb correlates with segregation into lipid rafts. Blood. 2003;101: 1045–52.

59. Cragg MS, Glennie MJ. Antibody specificity controls in vivo effector mechanisms of anti-CD20 reagents. Blood. 2004;103:2738–43.

60. Golay J, Zaffaroni L, Vaccari T, et al. Biologic response of B lymphoma cells to anti-CD20 monoclonal antibody rituximab in vitro: CD55 and CD59 regulate complement-mediated cell lysis. Blood. 2000;95:3900–8.

61. Treon SP, Mitsiades C, Mitsiades N, et al. Tumor cell expression of CD59 is associated with resistance to CD20 serotherapy in patients with B-cell malignancies. J Immunother. 2001;24:263–71.

62. Golay J, Cittera E, Di Gaetano N, et al. The role of complement in the therapeutic activity of rituximab in a murine B lymphoma model homing in lymph nodes. Haematologica. 2006;91:176–83.

63. Klepfish A, Rachmilewitz EA, Kotsianidis I, Patchenko P, Schattner A. Adding fresh frozen plasma to rituximab for the treatment of patients with refractory advanced CLL. QJM. 2008;101:737–40.

64. Lessey E, Li N, Diaz L, Liu Z. Complement and cutaneous autoimmune blistering diseases. Immunol Res. 2008;41:223–32.

65. Shan D, Ledbetter JA, Press OW. Apoptosis of malignant human B cells by ligation of CD20 with monoclonal antibodies. Blood. 1998;91:1644–52.

66. Chan HT, Hughes D, French RR, et al. CD20-induced lymphoma cell death is independent of both caspases and its redistribution into triton X-100 insoluble membrane rafts. Cancer Res. 2003;63:5480–9.

67. Taylor RP, Lindorfer MA. Immunotherapeutic mechanisms of anti-CD20 monoclonal antibodies. Curr Opin Immunol. 2008;20:444–9.

68. Tsunoda K, Ota T, Suzuki H, et al. Pathogenic auto-antibody production requires loss of tolerance against desmoglein 3 in both T and B cells in experimental pemphigus vulgaris. Eur J Immunol. 2002; 32:627–33.

69. Ujiie H, Shibaki A, Nishie W, et al. Noncollagenous 16A domain of type XVII collagen-reactive CD4+ T cells play a pivotal role in the development of active disease in experimental bullous pemphigoid model. Clin Immunol. 2012;142:167–75.

70. Sitaru AG, Sesarman A, Mihai S, et al. T cells are required for the production of blister-inducing auto-antibodies in experimental epidermolysis bullosa acquisita. J Immunol. 2010;184:1596–603.

71. Bortnick A, Allman D. What is and what should always have been: long-lived plasma cells induced by T cell-independent antigens. J Immunol. 2013;190: 5913–8.

72. Xu W, Banchereau J. The antigen presenting cells instruct plasma cell differentiation. Front Immunol. 2014;4:504.

73. Leshem Y A, David M, Hodak E, et al. A prospective study on clinical response and cell-mediated immunity of pemphigus patients treated with rituximab. Arch Dermatol Res. 2014;306(1):67–74.

74. Sfikakis PP, Souliotis VL, Fragiadaki KG, Moutsopoulos HM, Boletis JN, Theofilopoulos AN. Increased expression of the FoxP3 functional marker of regulatory T cells following B cell depletion with rituximab in patients with lupus nephritis. Clin Immunol. 2007;123:66–73.

75. Toubi E, Kessel A, Slobodin G, et al. Changes in macrophage function after rituximab treatment in patients with rheumatoid arthritis. Ann Rheum Dis. 2007;66:818–20.

76. Stasi R, Del Poeta G, Stipa E, et al. Response to B-cell depleting therapy with rituximab reverts the abnormalities of T-cell subsets in patients with idiopathic thrombocytopenic purpura. Blood. 2007;110: 2924–30.

77. Stasi R, Cooper N, Del Poeta G, et al. Analysis of regulatory T-cell changes in patients with idiopathic thrombocytopenic purpura receiving B cell-depleting therapy with rituximab. Blood. 2008;112:1147–50.

78. Vallerskog T, Gunnarsson I, Widhe M, et al. Treatment with rituximab affects both the cellular and the humoral arm of the immune system in patients with SLE. Clin Immunol. 2007;122:62–74.

79. Feuchtenberger M, Muller S, Roll P, et al. Frequency of regulatory T cells is not affected by transient B cell depletion using anti-CD20 antibodies in rheumatoid arthritis. Open Rheumatol J. 2008;2:81–8.

80. Sfikakis PP, Boletis JN, Lionaki S, et al. Remission of proliferative lupus nephritis following B cell depletion therapy is preceded by down-regulation of the T cell costimulatory molecule CD40 ligand: an open-label trial. Arthritis Rheum. 2005;52:501–13.

81. Wilk E, Witte T, Marquardt N, et al. Depletion of functionally active CD20+ T cells by rituximab treatment. Arthritis Rheum. 2009;60:3563–71.

82. Lunardon L, Payne AS. Inhibitory human antichimeric antibodies to rituximab in a patient with pemphigus. J Allergy Clin Immunol. 2012;130:800–3.

83. Schmidt E, Hennig K, Mengede C, Zillikens D, Kromminga A. Immunogenicity of rituximab in patients with severe pemphigus. Clin Immunol. 2009; 132:334–41.

84. Weng WK, Levy R. Two immunoglobulin G fragment C receptor polymorphisms independently predict response to rituximab in patients with follicular lymphoma. J Clin Oncol. 2003;21:3940–7.

85. Dall'Ozzo S, Tartas S, Paintaud G, et al. Rituximab-dependent cytotoxicity by natural killer cells: influence of FCGR3A polymorphism on the concentration-effect relationship. Cancer Res. 2004;64:4664–9.

86. Gamonet C, Ferrand C, Colliou N, et al. Lack of expression of an alternative CD20 transcript variant in circulating B cells from patients with pemphigus. Exp Dermatol. 2014;23:66–7.

87. Rehnberg M, Amu S, Tarkowski A, Bokarewa MI, Brisslert M. Short- and long-term effects of anti-CD20 treatment on B cell ontogeny in bone marrow of patients with rheumatoid arthritis. Arthritis Res Ther. 2009;11:R123.

88. Amber KT, Hertl M. An assessment of treatment history and its association with clinical outcomes and relapse in 155 pemphigus patients with response to a single cycle of rituximab. J Eur Acad Dermatol Venereol. 2014. doi: 10.1111/jdv.12678. [Epub ahead of print].

89. Leshem YA, Hodak E, David M, Anhalt GJ, Mimouni D. Successful treatment of pemphigus with biweekly 1-g infusions of rituximab: a retrospective study of 47 patients. J Am Acad Dermatol. 2013;68:404–11.

90. Balighi K, Daneshpazhooh M, Khezri S, Mahdavinia M, Hajiseyed-javadi M, Chams-Davatchi C. Adjuvant rituximab in the treatment of pemphigus vulgaris: a phase II clinical trial. Int J Dermatol. 2013;52:862–7.

91. Lunardon L, Tsai KJ, Propert KJ, et al. Adjuvant rituximab therapy of pemphigus: a single-center experience with 31 patients. Arch Dermatol. 2012;148:1031–6.

92. Cianchini G, Lupi F, Masini C, Corona R, Puddu P, De Pita O. Therapy with rituximab for autoimmune pemphigus: results from a single-center observational study on 42 cases with long-term follow-up. J Am Acad Dermatol. 2012;67:617–22.

93. Ahmed AR, Spigelman Z, Cavacini LA, Posner MR. Treatment of pemphigus vulgaris with rituximab and intravenous immune globulin. N Engl J Med. 2006;355:1772–9.

94. Feldman RJ, Ahmed AR. Relevance of rituximab therapy in pemphigus vulgaris: analysis of current data and the immunologic basis for its observed responses. Expert Rev Clin Immunol. 2011;7:529–41.

95. Zakka LR, Shetty SS, Ahmed AR. Rituximab in the treatment of pemphigus vulgaris. Dermatol Ther (Heidelb). 2012;2:17.

96. Kanwar AJ, Vinay K, Sawatkar GU, et al. Clinical and immunological outcomes of high and low dose rituximab treatments in pemphigus patients: a randomized comparative observer blinded study. Br J Dermatol. 2014;170(6):1341–9.

97. Mimouni D, Nousari CH, Cummins DL, Kouba DJ, David M, Anhalt GJ. Differences and similarities among expert opinions on the diagnosis and treatment of pemphigus vulgaris. J Am Acad Dermatol. 2003;49:1059–62.

98. Leger S, Picard D, Ingen-Housz-Oro S, et al. Prognostic factors of paraneoplastic pemphigus. Arch Dermatol. 2012;148:1165–72.

99. Vezzoli P, Berti E, Marzano AV. Rationale and efficacy for the use of rituximab in paraneoplastic pemphigus. Expert Rev Clin Immunol. 2008;4:351–63.

100. Joly P, Richard C, Gilbert D, et al. Sensitivity and specificity of clinical, histologic, and immunologic features in the diagnosis of paraneoplastic pemphigus. J Am Acad Dermatol. 2000;43:619–26.

101. Schadlow MB, Anhalt GJ, Sinha AA. Using rituximab (anti-CD20 antibody) in a patient with paraneoplastic pemphigus. J Drugs Dermatol. 2003;2:564–7.

102. Shetty S, Ahmed AR. Treatment of bullous pemphigoid with rituximab: critical analysis of the current literature. J Drugs Dermatol. 2013;12:672–7.

103. Le Roux-Villet C, Prost-Squarcioni C, Alexandre M, et al. Rituximab for patients with refractory mucous membrane pemphigoid. Arch Dermatol. 2011;147: 843–9.

104. Heelan K, Walsh S, Shear NH. Treatment of mucous membrane pemphigoid with rituximab. J Am Acad Dermatol. 2013;69:310–1.
105. Shetty S, Ahmed AR. Critical analysis of the use of rituximab in mucous membrane pemphigoid: a review of the literature. J Am Acad Dermatol. 2013; 68:499–506.
106. Niedermeier A, Eming R, Pfutze M, et al. Clinical response of severe mechanobullous epidermolysis bullosa acquisita to combined treatment with immunoadsorption and rituximab (anti-CD20 monoclonal antibodies). Arch Dermatol. 2007; 143:192–8.
107. McKinley SK, Huang JT, Tan J, Kroshinsky D, Gellis S. A case of recalcitrant epidermolysis bullosa acquisita responsive to rituximab therapy. Pediatr Dermatol. 2014;31(2):241–4.
108. Cavailhes A, Balme B, Gilbert D, Skowron F. Successful use of combined corticosteroids and rituximab in the treatment of recalcitrant epidermolysis bullosa acquisita. Ann Dermatol Venereol. 2009;136:795–9.
109. Schmidt E, Benoit S, Brocker EB, Zillikens D, Goebeler M. Successful adjuvant treatment of recalcitrant epidermolysis bullosa acquisita with anti-CD20 antibody rituximab. Arch Dermatol. 2006;142:147–50.
110. Kim JH, Lee SE, Kim SC. Successful treatment of epidermolysis bullosa acquisita with rituximab therapy. J Dermatol. 2012;39:477–9.
111. Kubisch I, Diessenbacher P, Schmidt E, Gollnick H, Leverkus M. Premonitory epidermolysis bullosa acquisita mimicking eyelid dermatitis: successful treatment with rituximab and protein A immunoapheresis. Am J Clin Dermatol. 2010; 11:289–93.
112. Saha M, Cutler T, Bhogal B, Black MM, Groves RW. Refractory epidermolysis bullosa acquisita: successful treatment with rituximab. Clin Exp Dermatol. 2009;34:e979–80.
113. Sadler E, Schafleitner B, Lanschuetzer C, et al. Treatment-resistant classical epidermolysis bullosa acquisita responding to rituximab. Br J Dermatol. 2007;157:417–9.
114. Crichlow SM, Mortimer NJ, Harman KE. A successful therapeutic trial of rituximab in the treatment of a patient with recalcitrant, high-titre epidermolysis bullosa acquisita. Br J Dermatol. 2007;156:194–6.
115. Ludwig RJ. Clinical presentation, pathogenesis, diagnosis, and treatment of epidermolysis bullosa acquisita. ISRN Dermatol. 2013;2013:812029.
116. Merrill JT, Neuwelt CM, Wallace DJ, et al. Efficacy and safety of rituximab in moderately-to-severely active systemic lupus erythematosus: the randomized, double-blind, phase II/III systemic lupus erythematosus evaluation of rituximab trial. Arthritis Rheum. 2010;62:222–33.
117. Beissert S, Mimouni D, Kanwar AJ, Solomons N, Kalia V, Anhalt GJ. Treating pemphigus vulgaris with prednisone and mycophenolate mofetil: a multicenter, randomized, placebo-controlled trial. J Invest Dermatol. 2010;130:2041–8.
118. Foster CS, Chang PY, Ahmed AR. Combination of rituximab and intravenous immunoglobulin for recalcitrant ocular cicatricial pemphigoid: a preliminary report. Ophthalmology. 2010;117:861–9.
119. Ventura F, Rocha J, Fernandes JC, Machado A, Brito C. Recalcitrant pemphigus vulgaris: aseptic meningitis associated with intravenous immunoglobulin therapy and successful treatment with rituximab. Int J Dermatol. 2013;52:501–2.